Vascular and Endovas
at a Glance

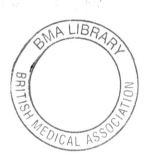

This title is also available as an e-book.
For more details, please see
www.wiley.com/buy/9781118496039
or scan this QR code:

Vascular and Endovascular Surgery at a Glance

Morgan McMonagle MB BCh BAO (Hons) MD FRCS (Gen Surg)

Consultant Vascular and Trauma Surgeon, HSE South Hospital Group and the Royal College of Surgeons in Ireland
Formerly Consultant Vascular and Lead Trauma Surgeon at St. Mary's Hospital and Imperial College
London, UK

Matthew Stephenson MB BS MSc FRCS (Gen Surg)

Consultant General Surgeon
Jersey General Hospital
Jersey

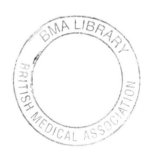

WILEY Blackwell

This edition first published 2014 © 2014 by John Wiley & Sons, Ltd.

Registered office: John Wiley & Sons, Ltd., The Atrium, Southern Gate, Chichester, West Sussex, PO19 8SQ, UK

Editorial offices: 9600 Garsington Road, Oxford, OX4 2DQ, UK
The Atrium, Southern Gate, Chichester, West Sussex, PO19 8SQ, UK
350 Main Street, Malden, MA 02148-5020, USA

For details of our global editorial offices, for customer services and for information about how to apply for permission to reuse the copyright material in this book please see our website at www.wiley.com/wiley-blackwell

The right of the authors to be identified as the authors of this work has been asserted in accordance with the UK Copyright, Designs and Patents Act 1988.

Library of Congress Cataloging-in-Publication Data

McMonagle, Morgan, author.
   Vascular and endovascular surgery at a glance / Morgan McMonagle, Matthew Stephenson.
      p. ; cm.
   Includes bibliographical references and index.
   ISBN 978-1-118-49603-9 (pbk. : alk. paper) – ISBN 978-1-118-49606-0 (epub) – ISBN 978-1-118-49610-7 (epdf) – ISBN 978-1-118-49614-5 – ISBN 978-1-118-78271-2 – ISBN 978-1-118-78281-1
   I. Stephenson, Matthew, author.   II. Title.
   [DNLM: 1. Vascular Diseases–surgery. 2. Blood Vessels–pathology. 3. Vascular Surgical Procedures. WG 170]
   RD598.5
   617.4′13–dc23
               2013026494

A catalogue record for this book is available from the British Library.

Wiley also publishes its books in a variety of electronic formats. Some content that appears in print may not be available in electronic books.

Cover image: Matthew Stephenson
Cover design by Meaden Creative

Set in 9/11.5 pt TimesLTStd-Roman by Toppan Best-set Premedia Limited
Printed and bound in Malaysia by Vivar Printing Sdn Bhd

1   2014

Contents

Preface

Although the *at a Glance* series originated as a unique visual, synopsis-style learning aid for undergraduate students, the conceptualisation underpinning *Vascular and Endovascular Surgery at a Glance* is to provide both breadth and depth to a completed vascular curriculum from undergraduate level through to postgraduate training and examinations. We have adhered to the powerfully simplistic, yet accurate approach of the *at a Glance* series with coloured illustrations, tables and clinical pictures supported by 'nuts and bolts' style didactics for rapid and effective learning. Great emphasis has been placed on the illustrations to simplify the understanding of disease processes, and, where possible, supported by clinical and intraoperative photographs. Although written with little reference to the evidence, for ease of readability, every effort has been made, where possible, to ensure that the facts presented, especially pertaining to the clinical management of vascular disease are both accurate and up-to-date. In addition, as vascular surgery is strongly driven by an evidence-based approach, we have included a chapter on the principal trials that students at all levels may be expected to know. In addition, we have emphasised the importance of the vascular surgeon's working knowledge and skill in vascular imaging, especially Duplex ultrasound, which forms a formal, in-depth part of training and examinations in the USA, Australia and Europe, and is now seen as an increasingly important skill armamentarium for the practising vascular specialist in Ireland and the UK.

Vascular surgery has often been considered by medical students and junior trainees to be poorly taught and perhaps 'too sub-specialised' for learning which often serves to generate learning barriers between the learner and subject matter. Yet vascular patients regularly appear on undergraduate examinations (both medical and surgical), MRCS-level postgraduate exams (written and clinical) and fellowship exams (including general surgery). Atherosclerosis is ubiquitous in the Western world, making vascular disease ubiquitous for all levels managing patients, including physicians, surgeons, emergency physicians, nurses, podiatrists, paramedics, physiotherapists and occupational therapists. *Vascular and Endovascular Surgery at a Glance* is a suitable and simplistic learning aid for all professionals dealing with vascular disease whilst remaining comprehensive. So whether a quick explanation is required or a more detailed overview of disease, *Vascular and Endovascular Surgery at a Glance* will serve as the perfect learning companion.

Vascular surgery has now become a stand-alone specialty within the UK (separate from general surgery), bringing it in line with Europe, North America and Australia. Evidence-based practice has driven improved expectations of care around the globe almost to international fellowship level, whereby outcomes from index vascular cases are now scrutinised and compared with best international practice. We feel *Vascular and Endovascular Surgery at a Glance* maintains this high standard and presents vascular disease and its management from basic science underpinning the pathology through to clinical examination, investigations and specific disease findings and its best treatments. Our book will serve as a learning tool for vascular disease (basic science and clinical) as well as a comprehensive curriculum for trainees and a last-minute study guide for examinees.

So whether you are looking for a simplified, easy-to-understand and readily accessible approach to vascular disease and its management at undergraduate level, or more complex knowledge for post-graduate MRCS examinations or even a quick but comprehensive knowledge and revision guide for vascular fellowship examinations, *Vascular and Endovascular Surgery at a Glance* will fulfill these requirements at all levels. We hope you will also agree.

Morgan McMonagle
Matthew Stephenson

List of abbreviations and symbols

List of abbreviations

AAA	abdominal aortic aneurysm
AAI	ankle-ankle index
ABG	arterial blood gas
ABPI	ankle Brachial Pressure Index
ACE	angiotensin-converting enzyme
ACEi	angiotensin-converting enzyme inhibitor
ACh	acetylcholine
ACT	activated clotting time
ADP	adenosine diphosphate
AI	angiotensin I
AII	angiotensin II
AK	above knee
AKA	above-knee amputation
AMI	acute mesenteric ischaemia
ANA	anti-nuclear antibody
APA	antiplatelet agent
APC	activated Protein C
APR	activated Protein C resistance
APS	antiphospholipid syndrome
APTT	activated partial thromboplastin time
ARBs	AII receptor blockers
ARDS	acute respiratory distress syndrome
AT	antithrombin
ATA	anterior tibial artery
ATLS	advanced trauma life support
A-TOS	arterial thoracic outlet syndrome
AVF	arteriovenous fistula
bFGF	basic fibroblast growth factor
BK	below knee
BKA	below-knee amputation
BMS	bare metal stent
BMT	best medical therapy
BP	blood pressure
bpm	beats per minute
Ca^{2+}	calcium
CABG	coronary artery bypass graft
cAMP	cyclic adenosine monophosphate
CBT	carotid body tumour
CCA	common carotid artery
CCF	congestive cardiac failure
CEA	carotid endarterectomy
CFA	common femoral artery
CFU	colony-forming unit
CFV	common femoral vein
cGMP	cyclic guanosine monophosphate
CIA	common iliac artery
CIN	contrast-induced nephropathy
CK	creatinine kinase
CKD	chronic kidney disease
CMI	chronic mesenteric ischaemia
COX	cyclooxygenase
CPEX	cardiopulmonary exercise testing
CS	compartment syndrome
CSVV	cutaneous small vessel vasculitis
CT	computed tomography
CTA	computed tomography angiography
CTD	connective tissue disease
CVM	congenital vascular malformation
CVP	central venous pressure
CVS	cardiovascular
CXR	chest X-ray
DES	drug-eluting stent
DIC	disseminated intravascular coagulopathy
DP	dorsalis pedis
DPA	dorsalis pedis artery
DVT	deep vein thrombosis
ECG	electrocardiogram
ECM	extracellular matrix
EDV	end-diastolic velocities
EEG	electroencephalogram
EEL	external elastic lamina
eGFR	estimated glomerular filtration rate
EIA	external iliac artery
ePTFE	expanded polytetrafluoroethylene (Teflon)
ET	endotracheal
EVAR	endovascular aneurysm repair
FBC	full blood count
FMD	fibromuscular dysplasia
FVII	factor VII
aFVII	activated factor VII
FX	factor X
aFX	activated Factor X
GA	general anaesthetic
GAGs	glycosaminoglycans
GFR	glomerular filtration rate
GI	gastrointestinal
GIT	gastrointestinal tract
GP	glycoprotein
GSW	gunshot wound
HbA1c	haemoglobin A1c
HDL	high-density lipoprotein
HIT	heparin-induced thrombocytopenia
HR	heart rate
HSPGs	heparan sulfate proteoglycans
HSV	herpes simplex virus
IC	intermittent claudication
ICA	internal carotid artery
IEL	internal elastic lamina
IHD	ischaemic heart disease
IMA	inferior mesenteric artery
IMH	intramural haematoma
INR	international normalized ratio
i.v.	intravenous
IVC	inferior vena cava
IVDU	intravenous drug user
JGA	juxta-glomerular apparatus
KTS	Klippel-Trenaunay syndrome
LA	local anaesthetic
LDL	low-density lipoprotein

LFT	liver function test		**SMA**	superior mesenteric artery
LMWH	low molecular weight heparin		**SMCs**	smooth muscle cells
LSV	long saphenous vein		**SNS**	sympathetic nervous system
MAL	median arcuate ligament		**SOB**	shortness of breath
MCA	middle cerebral artery		**SPJ**	saphenopopliteal junction
MI	myocardial infarction		**SSV**	short saphenous vein
MMP	metalloproteinase		**TAA**	thoracic aortic aneursym
MR	magnetic resonance		**TAAA**	thoracoabdominal aortic aneurysm
MRA	magnetic resonance angiography		**TAT**	thoracic aortic transection
MRI	magnetic resonance imaging		**TEVAR**	thoracic endovascular aneurysm repair
MTPJ	metatarso-phalyngeal joint		**TF**	tissue factor
MVI	minimal vascular injury		**TFPI**	tissue factor pathway inhibitor
MVT	mesenteric venous thrombosis		**TGF-β**	transforming growth factor beta
NO	nitric oxide		**TIA**	transient ischaemic attack
NSAIDs	non-steroidal anti-inflammatory drugs		**TOS**	thoracic outlet syndrome
NSF	nephrogenic systemic fibrosis		**tPA**	tissue plasminogen activator
N-TOS	neurogenic thoracic outlet syndrome		**TxA$_2$**	thromboxane A2
OTW	over the wire		**U&E**	urea and electrolytes
PA$_2$	phospholipase A2		**U/S**	ultrasound
PAD	phlegmasia alba dolens		**VA**	vertebral artery
PAN	polyarteritis nodosa		**Vd/Vs**	diastolic to systolic velocity ratio
PAR-1	protease activator receptor 1		**VHT**	venous hypertension
PAU	penetrating aortic ulcer		**VKA**	vitamin K antagonist
PCD	phlegmasia caerulea dolens		**VLDL**	very low-density lipoproteins
PDGF	platelet-derived growth factor		**V/Q**	ventilation/perfusion
PGs	prostaglandins		**VSMCs**	vascular smooth muscle cells
PAI-1	plasminogen activator inhibitor-1		**V-TOS**	venous thoracic outlet syndrome
PE	pulmonary embolism		**VV**	varicose vein
PICC	peripherally inserted central catheter		**vWF**	von Willebrand factor
PMNs	polymorphonuclear neutrophils		**VZV**	varicella zoster virus
PMT	percutaneous mechanical thrombectomy		**WCC**	white cell count
PPAM	pneumatic post amputation mobility			
PSV	pressure support ventilation			
PT	posterior tibialis			
PTA	posterior tibialis artery			
PUO	pyrexia of unknown origin			
PVD	peripheral vascular disease			
PVR	peripheral vascular resistance			
RAR	renal-aortic ratio			
RAS	renal artery stenosis			
REM	roentgen equivalent man			
RI	resistance index			
RP	retroperitoneal			
s.c.	subcutaneous			
SCA	subclavian artery			
SCDs	sequential compression devices			
SCV	subclavian vein			
SFA	superficial femoral artery			
SFJ	saphenofemoral junction			

List of symbols

+	and / plus
+/–	plus or minus
±	plus or minus
~	approximately
↑	increase / increases / increased
↓	decrease / decreases / decreased
×	multiplied by / times
=	equals
<	less than
>	greater than
≥	greater or equal to
°	degrees
μ	mu
α	alpha
β	beta
ρ	rho

About the companion website

Visit the companion website for this book at:

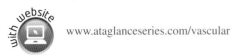 www.ataglanceseries.com/vascular

The website contains interactive MCQs for self-test.

The anytime, anywhere textbook

Wiley E-Text

Your book is also available to purchase as a **Wiley E-Text: Powered by VitalSource** version – a digital, interactive version of this book which you own as soon as you download it.

Your **Wiley E-Text** allows you to:

Search: Save time by finding terms and topics instantly in your book, your notes, even your whole library (once you've downloaded more textbooks)

Note and Highlight: Colour code, highlight and make digital notes right in the text so you can find them quickly and easily

Organize: Keep books, notes and class materials organized in folders inside the application

Share: Exchange notes and highlights with friends, classmates and study groups

Upgrade: Your textbook can be transferred when you need to change or upgrade computers

Link: Link directly from the page of your interactive textbook to all of the material contained on the companion website

The **Wiley E-Text** version will also allow you to copy and paste any photograph or illustration into assignments, presentations and your own notes.

CourseSmart

CourseSmart gives you instant access (via computer or mobile device) to this Wiley-Blackwell e-book and its extra electronic functionality, at 40% off the recommended retail print price. See all the benefits at: www.coursesmart.com/students

Instructors . . . receive your own digital desk copies!

CourseSmart also offers instructors an immediate, efficient, and environmentally-friendly way to review this book for your course.

For more information visit www.coursesmart.com/instructors.

With CourseSmart, you can create lecture notes quickly with copy and paste, and share pages and notes with your students. Access your **CourseSmart** digital book from your computer or mobile device instantly for evaluation, class preparation, and as a teaching tool in the classroom.

Simply sign in at http://instructors.coursesmart.com/bookshelf to download your Bookshelf and get started. To request your desk copy, hit 'Request Online Copy' on your search results or book product page.

We hope you enjoy using your new book. Good luck with your studies!

1 Overview of vascular disease

Figure 1.1 Prevalence of the multi-system nature of vascular disease. (Source: Prevalence of coexistence of coronary artery disease, peripheral arterial disease and atherosclerotic brain infarction in men and women > or = 62 years of age. Aronow WS, Ahn C. *Am J Cardiol* 1994;74:64–5. Reproduced with permission from Elsevier).

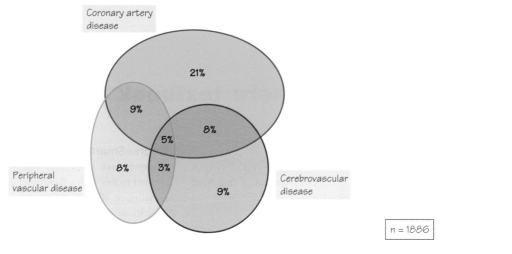

Figure 1.2 Diagrammatic representation of the age-related progression of atherosclerosis and its complications.

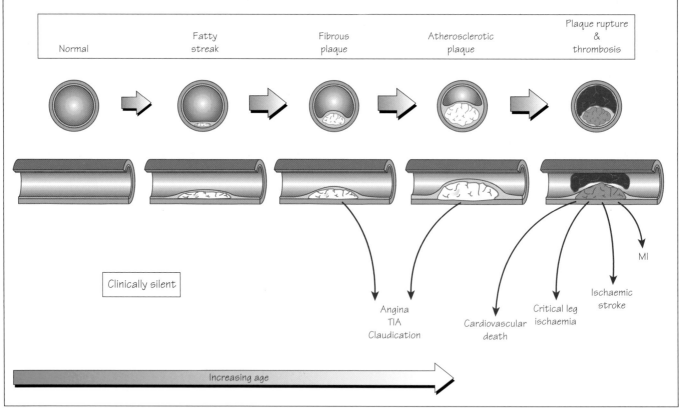

Abbreviations: MI, myocardial infarction: TIA, transient ischaemic attack

Vascular disease is a systemic disease typified by widespread atherosclerosis. The importance of this fact cannot be overemphasised both with regards to the multitude of medical conditions the vascular patient may present with in addition to the risks of intervention and surgical treatment in this patient group.

Being 'systemic', vascular disease affects a multitude of organs and tissues including the brain, heart, gut, kidneys and limbs. Therefore, the finding of atherosclerotic disease in one body region should prompt the examining physician to seek disease elsewhere in other high-risk vascular tissue (see Figure 1.1).

It is well documented that peripheral vascular disease is an independent marker for both coronary artery and cerebral vascular disease as well as an independent risk factor for an event in these tissues. In addition, vascular disease accounts for two out of the top five causes of death in the Western world (coronary artery disease and stroke). Furthermore, conditions afflicting the vascular patient account for an enormous number of lost disability-adjusted and quality-adjusted life years; including stroke, diabetes, obesity and chronic renal failure.

Because vascular disease is an age-related degenerative process developing over many years, by the time one tissue bed develops a complication often others do too, especially at times of great physiological stress such as illness or surgery. Certainly, the biggest complication among vascular patients, especially those undergoing intervention and surgery, is an acute myocardial infarction (MI). Figure 1.2 schematically demonstrates the age-related changes and advancement of atherosclerosis in the vascular patient, who will finally succumb to a 'plaque complication' with acute thrombosis and vessel occlusion.

However, there have been huge advancements in the care of the vascular patient over the past 25 years, not only in improved understanding and quality of medical management (especially antiplatelet agents and statins) but also in blood pressure control and long-term management of diabetes and chronic renal failure.

Endovascular treatment of vascular lesions including occlusions and aneurysms has also caused a shift in the demographics of patients being treated for disease who were once deemed too unwell or too risky for treatment. Many devices continue to be developed or improved at an alarming rate to the point that there is no absolute upper age limit for treatment. The vascular surgeon, in addition to the medical and surgical treatment of vascular disease, remains central to the multidisciplinary team that tends to our aging atherosclerotic population on a daily basis and includes staff from general surgery, cardiology, respiratory medicine, renal medicine, endocrinology and diabetology, ophthalmology, podiatry, stroke medicine, rheumatology, nutrition, physiotherapy, occupational therapy, speech and language, anaesthetics, intensive care, orthopaedics and prosthetics, rehabilitation and social work.

Furthermore, the vascular surgeon, not only being an endovascular specialist, is the only true 'open' surgeon who operates with any regularity in all body regions including abdomen–pelvis, thorax, neck, upper and lower limbs. This, combined with our expertise in dealing with massive haemorrhage and its consequences, has placed us at the fore of modern approaches to acute care surgery, and in particular trauma surgery, with numerous surgeons now practising in both fields.

Vascular surgery is held to a very high level of governance with more high-quality evidence-based practice than most other specialties (second only perhaps to cardiology). There are clear international best practice guidelines for best medical therapies, stroke risk management and aneurysm selection in addition to very strong and robust international trials contributing to the smorgasbord of evidence-based practice.

Vascular surgery is entering a new era in that it is now recognised as an independent specialty in the UK with its own recruitment and training system as well as fellowship exam. This brings it into line with other countries such as the USA, Canada, Australia and continental Europe for accreditation. This superspecialisation of the service, in addition to the endovascular requirements, will see the specialty concentrated into larger centres such as academic medical centres and major trauma centres, with the vascular specialist remaining central to any future developments for hospital network services.

2 Arterial anatomy

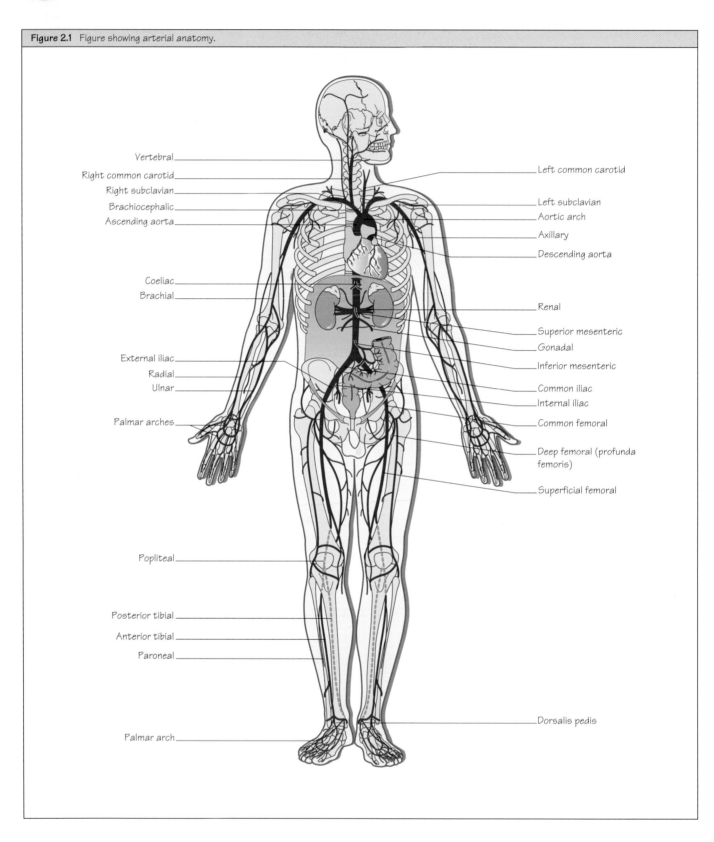

Figure 2.1 Figure showing arterial anatomy.

Vertebral
Right common carotid
Right subclavian
Brachiocephalic
Ascending aorta

Coeliac
Brachial

External iliac
Radial
Ulnar

Palmar arches

Popliteal

Posterior tibial
Anterior tibial
Paroneal

Palmar arch

Left common carotid
Left subclavian
Aortic arch
Axillary
Descending aorta

Renal
Superior mesenteric
Gonadal
Inferior mesenteric
Common iliac
Internal iliac
Common femoral
Deep femoral (profunda femoris)
Superficial femoral

Dorsalis pedis

Thoracic and neck

The **aorta** emerges from the left ventricle at the lower border of the third costal cartilage behind the sternum (slightly to the left). In the superior mediastinum it curves upwards, backwards and to the left, forming in turn the **ascending aorta**, **aortic arch** and then the **descending thoracic aorta**.

The ascending aorta gives branches to the heart – the right and left **coronary arteries**. The outer convexity of the aortic arch gives three branches:

1 **Brachiocephalic** (which is short and quickly divides into the right common carotid and right subclavian).

2 **Left common carotid**.

3 **Left subclavian**.

On each side then, the common carotid artery ascends in the neck almost and identically passing behind (although very deeply) the sternoclavicular joint to the upper border of the thyroid where it divides into the **external carotid** and **internal carotid**. The internal carotid has no branches and ascends into the skull via the carotid canal. The external carotid has several branches supplying the face and neck.

Meanwhile, the **descending thoracic aorta** passes through the thorax on the vertebral column, giving various branches in the mediastinum. It passes through the aortic hiatus in the diaphragm at T12 to become the **abdominal aorta**.

Upper limb

On each side (with the exception of the different origins), the path of the subclavian arteries (SCAs) is basically the same. It travels laterally over the first rib between the anterior and middle scalene muscles, which serve to 'divide' it into three different sections, with the second part lying behind the anterior scalene. The branches of the subclavian artery can be memorised by the mnemonic 'VIT C, D':

Part 1: Vertebral artery.

   Internal thoracic artery.

   Thyrocervical trunk.

Part 2: Costocervical trunk.

Part 3: Dorsal scapular artery.

At the outer border of the first rib the subclavian artery becomes the **axillary artery**, which passes through the axilla surrounded by the brachial plexus and is similarly divided into three parts by the pectoralis minor with branches that can be remembered using the mnemonic 'She Tastes Like Sweet Apple Pie'.

Part 1: Superior thoracic artery.

Part 2: Thoracoacromial artery.

   Lateral thoracic artery.

Part 3: Subscapular artery.

   Anterior circumflex humeral artery.

   Posterior circumflex humeral artery

The axillary artery becomes the **brachial artery** after passing the lower margin of teres major.

The brachial artery continues in the anterior compartment through the cubital fossa and becomes easily palpable medial to the tendon of biceps. It provides some deep branches in the upper arm but principally bifurcates into the **radial** and **ulnar arteries** in the cubital fossa.

The radial artery runs in the anterior compartment on the lateral side giving some branches; it winds laterally crossing the anatomical snuffbox over the trapezium, enters the dorsum of the hand and contributes to the palmar arch. The ulnar artery, which gives a large common interosseus branch early, also passes through the anterior compartment, but more on the medial side, and crosses the wrist, similarly providing supply to the palmar arches.

Abdomen

The abdominal aorta continues the journey on the vertebral column, slightly to the left, giving some pairs of small posterior lumbar arteries, and then bifurcates into the **right and left common iliac arteries** (and a small **median sacral artery**) at L4, approximately the level of the umbilicus. From its anterior surface it bears three visceral arteries:

1 **Coeliac trunk**.

2 **Superior mesenteric**.

3 **Inferior mesenteric**.

And laterally it gives off three paired arteries:

1 **Adrenal/suprarenal**.

2 **Renal**.

3 **Gonadal**.

Lower limbs

The common iliac arteries each bifurcate after about 4cm, anterior to the sacroiliac joint, into the **internal iliac**, supplying the pelvis, and the **external iliac**. The external iliac proceeds anteroinferiorly to enter the thigh by passing under the inguinal ligament, halfway from the pubic symphysis to the anterior superior iliac spine (midinguinal point). At this point it becomes the **common femoral artery**, which has several small branches but then divides into the **profunda femoris** and the **superficial femoral artery**. The profunda femoris passes deeply to supply the musculature of the thigh while the superficial femoral passes inferomedially through the femoral triangle (superior: inguinal ligament; lateral: medial border of sartorius; and medial: medial border of adductor longus) through the subsartorial canal and through the adductor hiatus to enter the popliteal fossa, where it becomes the **popliteal artery**.

The popliteal artery descends through the popliteal fossa as the deepest structure, passing then under the soleal arch, and immediately divides into the **anterior tibial** and the **tibioperoneal trunk**. The anterior tibial soon passes through the interosseus membrane to enter the anterior compartment, which it exits passing over the dorsum of the foot to become the **dorsalis pedis**. The tibioperoneal trunk bifurcates into the **posterior tibial** and **peroneal** arteries. (Note: anatomy books often call the tibioperoneal trunk simply the first part of the posterior tibial, from which the peroneal comes; however, vascular surgeons have this separate name.) The posterior tibial passes through the deep compartment and enters the sole of the foot by passing behind the medial malleolus where it can be easily palpated; it then divides into the **medial** and **lateral plantar arteries** in the sole. The peroneal artery meanwhile runs deep to the fibula; it doesn't itself cross the ankle but it may provide branches to the dorsalis pedis.

3 Venous anatomy

Figure 3.1 Figure showing venous anatomy.

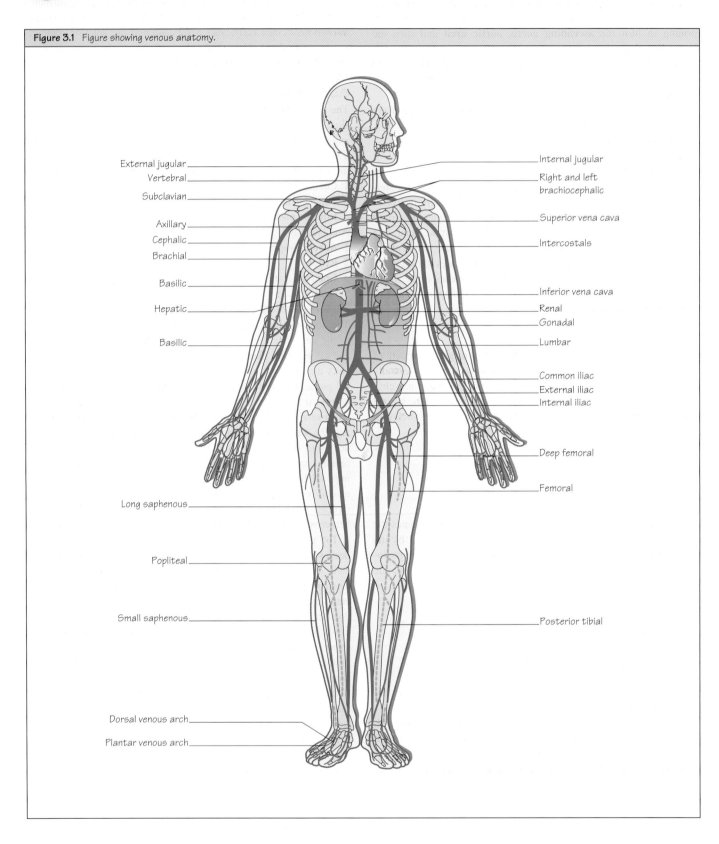

External jugular
Vertebral
Subclavian
Axillary
Cephalic
Brachial
Basilic
Hepatic
Basilic
Long saphenous
Popliteal
Small saphenous
Dorsal venous arch
Plantar venous arch

Internal jugular
Right and left brachiocephalic
Superior vena cava
Intercostals
Inferior vena cava
Renal
Gonadal
Lumbar
Common iliac
External iliac
Internal iliac
Deep femoral
Femoral
Posterior tibial

Vascular and Endovascular Surgery at a Glance, First Edition. Morgan McMonagle and Matthew Stephenson.

14 © 2014 John Wiley & Sons, Ltd. Published 2014 by John Wiley & Sons, Ltd. Companion website: www.ataglanceseries.com/vascular

You will need to remember the venous system in the leg because this is the most common site of venous problems (e.g. varicose veins and deep venous thrombosis). However, for vascular access the upper limb and central veins are very important.

Venous anatomy

The venous circulation is different from the arterial system in the following ways:

- There is **more interperson variability**.
- There is also **more functional reserve** – we can manage without many of our veins without any ill effect. Even some of the major veins like the **inferior vena cava (IVC)** can be ligated in an emergency without a devastating effect: blood will find its way back via other routes (i.e. collateral vessels).
- In keeping with this, there is often more than one vein serving the distribution of one artery, especially in the limbs. These are called **venae comitantes** and are seen usually as a pair of veins in close relation to an artery and often with many branches between them.
- In the limbs there is a clear distinction between **two sets of veins**: the superficial and deep, the former running enveloped by the superficial fascia and the latter running with the arteries.
- Veins do not have branches, they have **tributaries** – everything is in reverse order.

Lower limb

Blood drains from the foot into the **dorsal venous arch**, which is often visible on the dorsum of the foot. The lateral end of the dorsal venous arch continues as the **short saphenous vein** and passes posteriorly to the lateral malleolus, lying with the sural nerve. It passes up the posterolateral side of the calf in the subcutaneous fat towards the midline of the leg. It then turns deeply to pierce the deep fascia and continues on to join the **popliteal vein** at an oblique angle, the join being called the **saphenopopliteal junction**. The precise point at which the saphenopopliteal junction exists varies from person to person. It is most commonly at the skin crease but may be several centimetres above or below this.

The medial end of the dorsal venous arch continues as the **long saphenous vein**, passing anteriorly to the medial malleolus then up the medial side of the calf. It is its position just anterior to the medial malleolus that makes it an easily accessible vein for a 'saphenous cut down', when emergency intravenous access is required and nothing else is available. It passes up the medial calf swerving slightly posterior to run a handsbreadth behind the patella, and then swerving slightly anteriorly again as it ascends the thigh. It passes deeply through the cribriform fascia at an almost 90° angle to join the femoral vein, the **saphenofemoral junction**, 4 cm inferior and 4 cm lateral to the pubic tubercle. Along the way it has several connections, called **perforators**, with the deep veins. These perforators allow blood to pass from superficial to deep but not vice versa because of their unidirectional valves. There are usually also several other tributaries to the long saphenous vein and frequently a communication between the long and short saphenous vein called the **vein of Giacomini**.

The deep veins comprise the **posterior tibial**, **anterior tibial** and **peroneal veins** (which are in fact each usually duplicate) that converge to form the **popliteal vein**. The popliteal vein then ascends superficial to the popliteal artery, enters the thigh via the adductor canal and becomes the **femoral vein**. The femoral vein receives the **profunda femoris vein** and the long saphenous vein, as well as the various perforators described earlier.

The femoral vein passes medially to the common femoral artery in the groin and, as it ascends behind the inguinal ligament, it becomes the **external iliac vein**. It joins the **internal iliac vein**, which has drained the pelvis, to form the **common iliac vein**. The iliac veins lie just behind their artery counterparts.

Abdomen

The common iliac veins join at L5 to form the IVC, just to the right of the abdominal aorta. This ascends the retroperitoneum taking tributaries from the abdomen and passes through the caval opening in the diaphragm at T8 to almost immediately enter the **right atrium**. Along the way the IVC receives several tributaries:

- Lumbar veins.
- Gonadal veins.
- Renal veins.
- Adrenal veins.
- Hepatic veins.

It is the **hepatic veins** that drain the liver, which has received the portal circulation via the **portal vein**; this in turn is formed by the confluence of the **superior mesenteric vein** and **splenic vein**.

Upper limb

Venous blood from the hand drains into the **dorsal venous network**. Two principal veins drain this: on the lateral side, the **cephalic vein**; and on the medial side, the **basilic vein**. The cephalic vein runs superficially over the lateral wrist where it is easily cannulated (hence the nickname, the 'Houseman's friend'. It continues up to the cubital fossa where it communicates with the basilic vein via the **median cubital vein**. It continues up the lateral side of the arm and eventually turns deeply between deltoid and pectoralis major to empty into the **axillary vein**. The basilic vein continues on the medial side of the forearm and arm where it is latterly quite deep and joins the **deep brachial veins** to form the axillary vein.

Just like in the leg, there is also a deep venous system that begins with the **radial** and **ulnar veins**, which again are in fact venae comitantes around the artery. These join to form the brachial veins which, as described earlier, join the basilic to form the axillary vein. The axillary vein, which is usually singular, passes through the axilla in close relation to the artery and becomes the **subclavian vein** at the outer border of the first rib, running in front of the subclavian artery.

Thoracic and neck

On each side the subclavian vein joins the internal jugular vein to form the left and **right brachiocephalic (or innominate) veins**; these then join to form the **superior vena cava**, which passes directly into the right atrium. The left brachiocephalic has a longer course because it must cross the mediastinum. The head is drained superficially by the **external jugular vein** and deeply by the **internal jugular vein**. The former drains into the subclavian; the latter joins the subclavian to form the brachiocephalic veins.

Figure 4.1 Diagrammatic representation of arterial histology including cross-section of the wall with its divisional layers and contents.

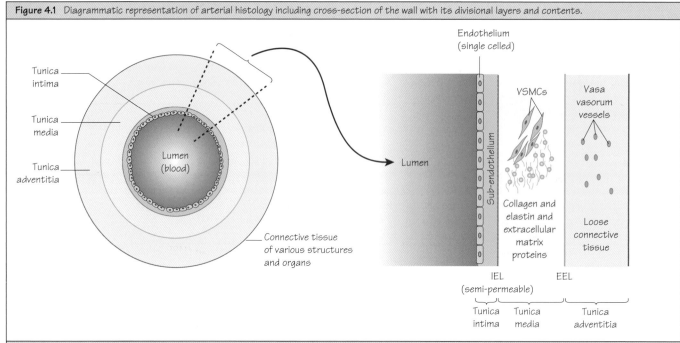

Figure 4.2 Diagram illustrating the histological divisional layers that make up arteries and veins.

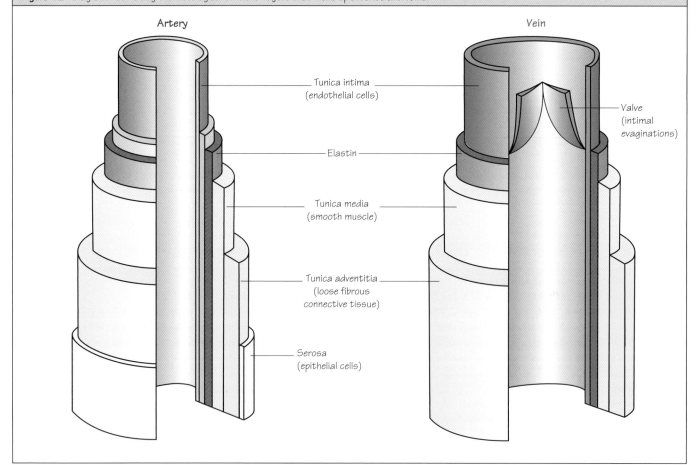

Abbreviations: EEL, external elastic lamina; IEL, internal elastic lamina; VSMCs, vascular smooth muscle cells

Vascular and Endovascular Surgery at a Glance, First Edition. Morgan McMonagle and Matthew Stephenson.

Structure of an artery

There are three basic histological layers ('tunics') in a vessel:
1 **Tunica intima (TI)** (innermost layer).
2 **Tunica media (TM)** (middle layer).
3 **Tunica adventitia (TA)** (outer layer).

Tunica intima

This is a thin layer consisting of the innermost, single-celled and physiologically active *endothelium* housed on a dense connective tissue basement membrane (*internal elastic lamina*).

Tunica media

This is the thickest layer of the wall and its content varies according to arterial subtype, anatomical location and exposure to fluid-mechanical stress. It is composed principally of vascular smooth muscle cells (VSMCs) within a connective tissue matrix.

Tunica adventitia

This is a poorly defined, heterogeneous, outermost layer of investing connective tissue consisting of a variable amount of smooth muscle cells (SMCs) and fibroblasts along with numerous autonomic nerve endings and *vasa vasora* (small, microscopic nutritional vessels traversing the layer). Its thickness varies according to location.

Blood vessel nutrition

In large and medium-sized arteries, cells in the innermost media acquire oxygen and nutrition from the blood in the lumen (direct diffusion) while the vasa vasora serve the outer half to two-thirds of the wall.

Arterial subtypes

There are two subtypes:
1 Elastic arteries.
2 Muscular arteries.
These are distinguished according to the histological contents of the tunica media.

Elastic arteries

These are larger vessels (e.g. the aorta and its major branches) and are rich in elastic tissue to allow compliant expansion followed by recoil during the cardiac cycle. This aids prograde blood flow by the conversion of potential energy into kinetic energy. These vessels appear to be more susceptible to atherosclerotic degeneration.

Muscular arteries

These are smaller (20–100 μm) vessels rich in SMCs (e.g. renal, coronary). They branch from the larger elastic arteries and serve to regulate capillary blood flow (end-organ and peripheries), thereby controlling peripheral vascular resistance.

Ancillary cells and structures
Endothelium

This is a single-celled (hexagonal-shaped) layer responsible for vessel tone and structure. It acts as selectively permeable membrane to control molecular transfer through the vessel wall (e.g. response to shock, vasoactive substances such as histamine), as well as co-ordinating platelet aggregation and coagulation after injury.

Endothelial regulation of coagulation

• Forms a non-thrombogenic blood-tissue interface for flowing blood by secreting the anticoagulant heparan sulfate (also limits thrombus formation after activation of coagulation).
• Secretes procoagulants plasminogen activator inhibitor (PAI-1) and von Willebrand factor (vWF).
• Synthesises various prostaglandins (PGs) including PGI2 (procoagulant, vasodilator and platelet inhibitor). PGI2 inhibits platelet aggregation by converting the platelet agonist adenosine diphosphate (ADP) to adenosine.
• Synthesises tissue plasminogen activator (tPA).
• Expresses the thrombin receptor thrombomodulin, which (after binding) activates protein C (integral to the coagulation cascade).

Internal elastic lamina (IEL)

This is a thin layer of condensed connective tissue (type IV collagen, laminin) and complex chemically active macromolecules (e.g. heparin sulfate proteoglycans [HSPGs]). It regulates and actively prohibits the movement of molecules and cells through its microscopic fenestrae.

Vascular smooth muscle cells

These SMCs are the predominant cell type in the tunica media. Under normal conditions, they exist in a predominantly non-proliferative, quiescent (but contractile) state responsible for vessel contraction and relaxation. Under certain conditions (e.g. endothelial injury), they become activated by growth factors (e.g. platelet-derived growth factor [PDGF]) and transform to a proliferative, more mobile phenotype capable of synthesising collagen, elastin and proteoglycans as well as migration to the intima.

Extracellular matrix

This is a connective tissue matrix giving vessel structure and composition and providing a medium for cell signalling and interaction within the vessel wall. It is composed mainly of collagen, elastin, proteoglycans, glycoproteins (e.g. fibronectin, laminin) and glycosaminoglycans (GAGs). GAGs are specialised, sulfated proteoglycans of which there are six primary types (keratin sulfate, hyaluronic acid, chondroitin sulfate, dermatan sulfate, heparan sulfate and heparin). They have a diverse role in regulating connective tissue structure and permeability, as well as cell growth, differentiation, adhesion, proliferation and morphogenesis, because of their inherent ability to bind to other ligands.

External elastic lamina (EEL)

This is less developed in comparison with the IEL, but it has a regulatory role for the passage of molecules and cells.

Other cells
Neutrophils (polymorphonuclear neutrophils [PMNs])

These mainly appear after injury to the vessel wall from the blood, and adhere to the subendothelial layers via the cell adhesion molecule P-selectin.

5 Vascular pathobiology

Figure 5.1 Illustration of the histopathological changes that occur with the two most prevalent and troublesome pathological conditions in vascular surgery: Atherosclerosis (left) and neointima hyperplasia (right).

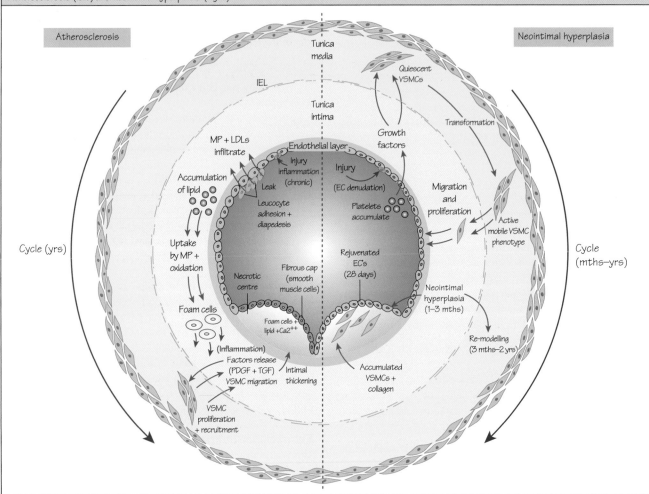

Figure 5.2 Gross spectrum of atherosclerotic plaque removed from carotid endarterectomy.

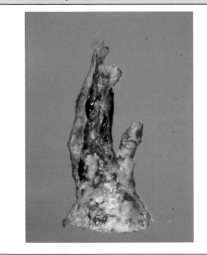

Figure 5.3 Neointimal hyperplasia as seen under high powered magnification in an artery six months post-angioplasty. Notice the severly narrowed lumen. This narrowing is secondary to the neointima (N), which is composed of hyperplastic cells and extracellular matrix proteins. There is also an abundance of SMCs in the media (M). A= adventitia.

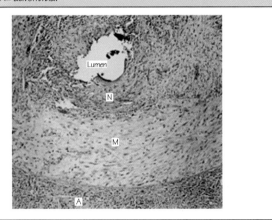

Abbreviations: Ca^{2+}, calcium; EC, endothelial cell; LDL, low density lipoprotein; MP, macrophage; PDGF, platelet-derived growth factor; TGF, transforming growth factor; VSMC, vascular smooth muscle cell

Vascular and Endovascular Surgery at a Glance, First Edition. Morgan McMonagle and Matthew Stephenson.

This is the study of the mechanisms behind vascular disease at a cellular level, which is dominated by atherosclerosis. Atherosclerosis is not only the most prolific vascular disease process, but it is the leading cause of death in Western society, contributing to two of the top five mortalities (cardiac and cerebrovascular disease).

Atherosclerosis

This principally affects large and medium-sized arteries (the aorta and its branches including coronaries, carotid, mesenteric and lower limb), but has a preponderance for occurring at branching sites (e.g. carotid bifurcation). Known risk factors for its development include male gender, advancing age, smoking, dyslipidaemia, diabetes mellitus and hypertension. Atherosclerotic lesions may occur in isolation, but, as a rule, atherosclerosis is a systemic disease affecting numerous arterial locations. Furthermore, an atherosclerotic lesion in one location (e.g. lower limbs) serves as a surrogate marker for disease elsewhere (e.g. coronary arteries).

Histology

The lesion forms primarily within the tunica intima consisting of a nodular accumulation of soft, yellowish material within a harder plaque. It is composed of modified macrophages (*foam cells*), cholesterol crystals and particulate calcification.

Pathophysiology

Probably multifactorial, of which vessel *injury* and *'vascular leak'* are the most accepted and popular theories.

Injury and vascular leak theory

• Atherosclerosis is a chronic inflammatory response over many decades in response to the biologic effects of various risk factors.
• There is a localised response to injury resulting in an increased permeability within the arterial wall ('vascular leak').
• Certain blood-borne cells (macrophages) and cholesterol-containing lipoproteins (LDL and VLDL [low-density lipoprotein and very low-density lipoprotein, respectively]) enter through the 'leaky' endothelium and deposit within the subendothelial space (i.e. the site of disease development).
• The lipoproteins are further oxidised by endothelial cells and later taken up by macrophages via 'scavenger' pathways, forming foam cells (pathognomonic of atherosclerosis).
• Over time there is a proliferation and accumulation of both endothelial cells and SMCs resulting in extracellular matrix (ECM) production and accumulation with a fibrous cap and eventual calcification of the plaque and arterial wall.
• Plaques may lead to blood flow limitation (stenosis) or may complicate by rupturing, leading to acute thrombosis due to the release of prothrombotic material from within the plaque core.

Neointimal (myointimal) hyperplasia

This is the vascular histological response to acute injury (e.g. surgery, angioplasty, stent insertion), initiated by endothelial injury or denudation (response is proportional to the severity [depth] of injury [i.e. if the media is also involved]).

Pathophysiology

After injury, growth factors are released, which in turn activate the normally quiescent VSMCs in the media. Activated VSMCs then change phenotype to their mobile and proliferative type (from quiescent and contractile type) and migrate to the intimal layer. Here they undergo proliferation and hyperplasia with synthesis and deposition of extracellular matrix proteins.

Histology

The lesion is firm, pale and homogenous lying between the endothelium and IEL (or media, depending on depth of injury). The lesion consists of VSMCs (about 20%) along with the newly synthesised ECM (about 80%), with smaller amounts of fibroblasts, macrophages and lymphocytes. The lesion may be typically localised and focal or occasionally diffuse throughout the vessel (or graft).

Clinical effects

Neointimal hyperplasia is the leading cause of vessel restenosis in both the medium and long term after vascular intervention, thereby complicating 30–50% of vascular treatments. Its peak effect occurs between 2 months (acute phase) and 2 years (chronic remodelling phase). After this time, there are chronic structural changes within the vessel (akin to atherosclerosis) with a similar risk of stenosis and plaque ulceration and rupture (leading to thrombosis).

Arteriosclerosis

This is a general term for sclerosis or 'hardening' of the arteries and is broadly subdivided into two types:

1 *Arteriosclerosis obliterans.* This is characterised by gradual fibrosis and calcification of the intima and media leading to stenosis and eventual obliteration, and it mostly affects the medium and large arteries of the lower extremities.

2 *Medial calcific sclerosis.* Also called *Monkeberg's arteriosclerosis*, this is characterised by dystrophic calcification of the media without intimal involvement or luminal narrowing, commonly affecting the extremities with advancing age.

Ischaemia-reperfusion injury

This phenomenon occurs after restoration of blood flow following a (variable) period of ischaemia resulting in further tissue damage (due to the reperfusion) with both systemic and local effects. It is caused by the uncontrolled release of oxygen-free radicals and superoxide moieties (especially the oxidation of hypoxanthine) that are generated in response to tissue ischaemia.

Local effects

Tissue *oedema* and *necrosis* leading to *compartment syndrome* (further potentiating the *ischaemia*).

Systemic effects

Acidosis and *hyperkalaemia* (release of accumulated acid moieties and intracellular potassium, respectively), *coagulopathy* (prothrombotic necrotic tissue) and *myoglobinuria* (*rhabdomyolysis* [↑ creatine kinase (CK)]) leading to *acute kidney injury*.

Aneurysmal degeneration

This is a degenerative condition of the vessel wall perhaps due to abnormal metalloproteinase (MMP) production and regulation. MMPs (especially MMP-2 and MMP-9) are thought to have enzymatic properties that degrade elastin, which in combination with years of increased wall stress leads to progressive vessel dilatation.

Chronic inflammatory infiltrates (especially in smokers) including T cells, B-cells, macrophages and plasma cells also occur, which in turn secrete cytokines that may activate MMPs. Although there appears to be an inflammatory aspect to aneurysm development, there is also a genetic and gender link that is poorly understood (note the higher familial incidence especially among first-degree male relatives).

6 Vascular physiology

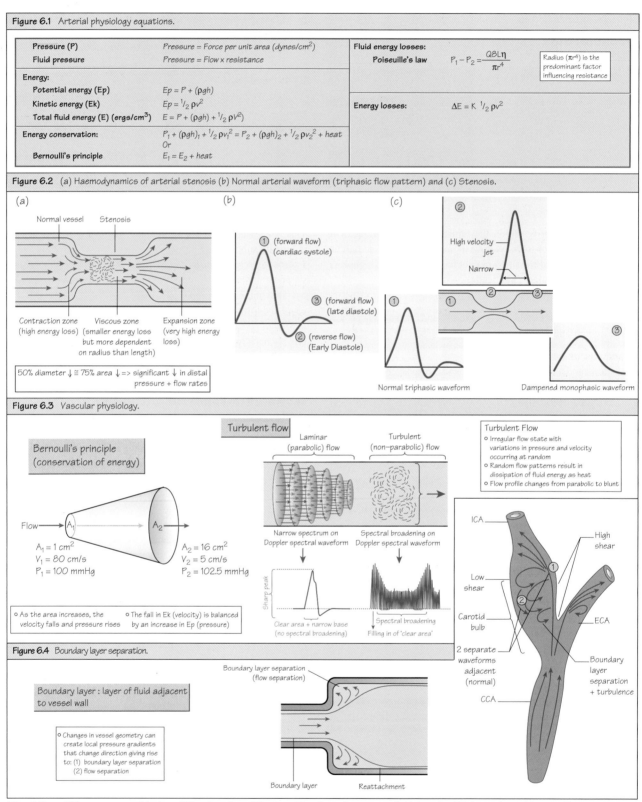

Figure 6.1 Arterial physiology equations.

| Pressure (P) | Pressure = Force per unit area (dynes/cm^2) |
| Fluid pressure | Pressure = Flow x resistance |

Energy:
Potential energy (Ep) — $Ep = P + (\rho gh)$
Kinetic energy (Ek) — $Ep = \frac{1}{2} \rho v^2$
Total fluid energy (E) (ergs/cm^3) — $E = P + (\rho gh) + \frac{1}{2} \rho v^2)$

Energy conservation:
$P_1 + (\rho gh)_1 + \frac{1}{2} \rho v_1^2 = P_2 + (\rho gh)_2 + \frac{1}{2} \rho v_2^2 + heat$
Or
Bernoulli's principle — $E_1 = E_2 + heat$

Fluid energy losses:
Poiseuille's law — $P_1 - P_2 = \dfrac{Q8L\eta}{\pi r^4}$

Radius (πr^4) is the predominant factor influencing resistance

Energy losses: — $\Delta E = K \frac{1}{2} \rho v^2$

Figure 6.2 (a) Haemodynamics of arterial stenosis (b) Normal arterial waveform (triphasic flow pattern) and (c) Stenosis.

(a)
Normal vessel   Stenosis
Contraction zone (high energy loss)   Viscous zone (smaller energy loss but more dependent on radius than length)   Expansion zone (very high energy loss)
50% diameter ↓ ≅ 75% area ↓ => significant ↓ in distal pressure + flow rates

(b)
① (forward flow) (cardiac systole)
③ (forward flow) (late diastole)
② (reverse flow) (Early Diastole)

(c)
② High velocity jet
Narrow
① ② ③
Normal triphasic waveform
③ Dampened monophasic waveform

Figure 6.3 Vascular physiology.

Bernoulli's principle (conservation of energy)
Flow → A_1 → A_2 →
$A_1 = 1$ cm^2
$V_1 = 80$ cm/s
$P_1 = 100$ mmHg
$A_2 = 16$ cm^2
$V_2 = 5$ cm/s
$P_2 = 102.5$ mmHg
○ As the area increases, the velocity falls and pressure rises   ○ The fall in Ek (velocity) is balanced by an increase in Ep (pressure)

Turbulent flow
Laminar (parabolic) flow   Turbulent (non–parabolic) flow
Narrow spectrum on Doppler spectral waveform   Spectral broadening on Doppler spectral waveform
Sharp peak
Clear area + narrow base (no spectral broadening)   Spectral broadening. Filling in of 'clear area'

Turbulent Flow
○ Irregular flow state with variations in pressure and velocity occurring at random
○ Random flow patterns result in dissipation of fluid energy as heat
○ Flow profile changes from parabolic to blunt

ICA
High shear
Low shear
Carotid bulb
2 separate waveforms adjacent (normal)
CCA
ECA
Boundary layer separation + turbulence

Figure 6.4 Boundary layer separation.

Boundary layer : layer of fluid adjacent to vessel wall
○ Changes in vessel geometry can create local pressure gradients that change direction giving rise to: (1) boundary layer separation (2) flow separation
Boundary layer separation (flow separation)
Boundary layer   Reattachment

Abbreviations: CCA, common carotid artery; ECA, external carotid artery; ΔE = change in energy; η, fluid viscosity; ICA, internal carotid artery; K = constant; L, length of tube; ρ (rho) = density of blood; ρgh; gravitational energy; P, intravascular pressure; P$_1$ – P$_2$, pressure gradient; Q, volume flow; r, tube radius; V = blood flow velocity

Vascular and Endovascular Surgery at a Glance, First Edition. Morgan McMonagle and Matthew Stephenson.

Arterial physiology

Fluid pressure and fluid energy

Fluid pressure is force that drives any fluid (blood) forward.
Fluid pressure is dependent on the available fluid energy.

Determinants of arterial pressure and flow

- *Dynamic pressure* (pulsatile cardiac contraction).
- *Hydrostatic pressure* (specific gravity of blood [$-\rho gh$]).
- *Static filling pressure* (pressure in an artery in the absence of cardiac contraction [i.e. tone]. It is low [5–10 mmHg] and relatively constant.

Fluid energy

- *Potential energy (Ep)* includes *intravascular pressure* (P) and *gravitational energy* ($+\rho gh$).
- *Kinetic energy (Ek)* is the ability of blood to do work based on its *velocity*.
- *Total fluid energy (E)* is the combination of Ep and Ek.

Energy conservation

Bernoulli's principle: *When fluid flows, the total energy (E) remains constant (in the absence of frictional losses).*

As fluid flows into an increased area, the velocity must fall so that the volume flow remains constant (i.e. falling kinetic energy). This is offset slightly by a small rise in the pressure (and a slight ↑ Ep).

Fluid energy losses in blood

- *Viscous losses.* Friction between adjacent layers of blood or between the blood and vessel wall.
- *Inertial losses.* Related to changes in velocity or direction of flow.

Poiseuille's law: *The volume flow rate (laminar flow) is given by the pressure difference divided by resistance to flow.*

This describes the viscous (frictional) energy losses occurring in an ideal fluid (Newtonian) and ideal system (non-pulsatile, straight cylindrical) and estimates the minimum pressure gradient for flow.

The inertial energy losses in arteries (acceleration–deceleration pulsations, changes in luminal diameter and turbulent flow patterns at branching vessels) will exceed the minimum pressure gradient. These effects are even greater in diseased vessels. *However, the energy losses are to the fourth power of the radius; therefore, the change in vessel radius will have an exponential effect on fluid flow.*

Peripheral vascular resistance (PVR)

This is the effect the pressure (energy) drop has on flow rates (akin to Poiseuille's law) and is dependent on *radius* of the vessel (r^4), *length* of vessel (L) and *viscosity* of fluid.

The radius is the predominant factor influencing resistance (πr^4) and the normal PVR occurs at the arterioles–capillaries (60–70%) and the medium-sized arteries (15–20%). In addition, the inertial effects of fluid (v^2) increase as velocity increases, thereby also increasing resistance (important with turbulence of disease).

Haemodynamics of disease

Any stenosis will also increase the PVR. Atherosclerosis commonly affects arteries that are *normally low resistance*. Therefore, the haemodynamic effects will have a significant impact on the normal flow physiology.

Arterial flow patterns are determined by *arterial geometry*, *vessel wall properties* and *flow velocities*, all of which are affected by atherosclerosis. In turbulent (non-laminar) flow, the random variations in pressure and velocity will cause significant energy losses (heat), which are reflected as '*spectral broadening*' on Duplex due to the non-parabolic flow (i.e. not flowing as a uniform column).

As flowing blood enters a stenosis, it undergoes a 'contraction zone' followed by an 'expansion zone' as it exits. Both zones are areas of large (kinetic) energy losses (especially the expansion zone) as the high velocity jet dissipates its energy (area of post-stenotic turbulence).

Thus, the radius of the stenosis will have a proportionately greater effect on energy losses than the length. In addition, an abrupt radius change will have a greater effect than a gradually tapering stenosis.

Critical arterial stenosis

This is the degree of narrowing required to produce a significant reduction in distal pressure and flow (*50% reduction in arterial diameter* or *75% reduction in area*). However, the exact narrowing also depends on the flow (i.e. it may be subcritical at rest, becoming significant during exercise when the flow velocities increase).

Venous physiology

Unlike arterial flow, venous flow is non-pulsatile. In addition, veins are thin-walled (little smooth muscle) displaying both elasticity and collapsibility. The combination of thin compliant walls with a larger lumen allows for accommodation of larger volumes of blood (65% of circulating volume is contained in the veins). In addition, venous flow must equal cardiac output!

Venous flow = cardiac output.

Venous capacitance

Large changes in volume will only produce small changes in venous transmural pressure (normally ~ 0 mmHg). Thus, veins tend to collapse at low pressures. Conversely, at very high distension volumes, the compliance is lost (important in bypass grafting).

Venous return

- *Venous tone and valves.* Muscular tone (albeit small) maintains an element of 'push' on the venous blood. In addition, the valves (intimal evaginations) maintain unidirectional flow as well as breaking the long column of blood (under gravitational influence) into multiple smaller volumes that are more easily forced antegrade (reducing venous pressure [otherwise >100 mmHg at the ankle]).
- *Vis-a-fronte* ('force from the front'). This is due to the cardiac 'suction' effect (right side diastole) and the low central venous pressure (CVP) (0 mmHg at atrial level) creating a pressure gradient from the periphery to the heart.
- *Vis-a-tergo* ('force from behind'). This is the pressure gradient between the capillary pressure (20–25 mmHg) and venous pressure (0 mmHg).
- *Muscle pump.* Lower limb muscle contractions will 'push' the segmentalised blood columns antegrade, thereby reducing the '*ambulatory venous pressure*' (close to 0 mmHg at the ankle).
- *Thoracic pump.* During expiration, abdominal pressure decreases, thereby increasing the pressure-flow gradient from the lower limbs.
- *Lymphatic drainage.* About 5% of capillary ultrafiltrate does not effectively return to the veins and instead is drained via the lymphatics to prevent swelling with venule compression and collapse.

7 Vascular pharmacology

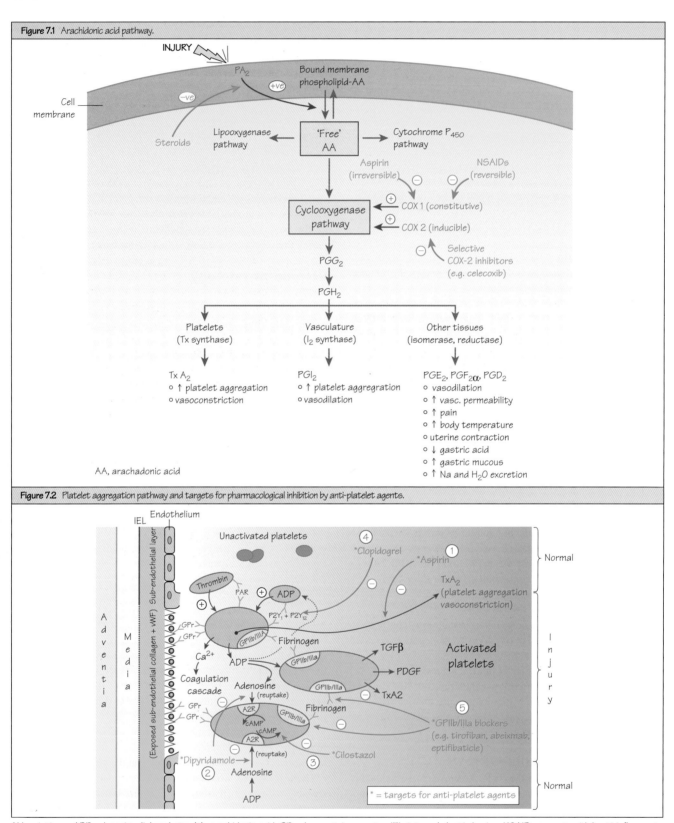

Figure 7.1 Arachidonic acid pathway.

Figure 7.2 Platelet aggregation pathway and targets for pharmacological inhibition by anti-platelet agents.

Abbreviations: ADP, adenosine diphosphate; AA, arachidonic acid; GPr, glycoprotein receptor; IEL, internal elastic lamina; NSAIDs, non-steroidal anti-inflammatory agents; PA₂, phospholipase; PDGF, platelet derived growth factor; TxA2, thromboxone; TGFβ, transforming growth factor β; vWF, von Willebrand factor; Tx, thromboxane

Vascular and Endovascular Surgery at a Glance, First Edition. Morgan McMonagle and Matthew Stephenson.

Arachidonic acid pathway

PGs are eicosanoid-compounds synthesised from arachadonic acid (normally found bound to cell membrane phospholipids). After injury, arachadonic acid (AA) is liberated from the cell membrane by the enzymatic action of phospholipase A_2 [PA_2]). Once liberated, free-AA may enter the cyclooxygenase (COX) pathway whereby COX enzymes transform AA into various PG's. There are two broad categories of active COX: COX-1 and COX-2. COX-1 is constitutively expressed in most tissues including gastrointestinal tract (GIT), platelets and kidney. COX-2 is mostly an inducible enzyme in response to injury (including endothelial injury) and inflammatory stimuli, and a major source of prostanoids. PGs have numerous effects, including acting as inflammatory mediators. Numerous PGs are also active in vascular tissue contributing to vasodilatation (PGI_2, PGE_2), vasoconstriction ($PGF_{2\alpha}$, thromboxane A_2 [TxA_2]), platelet aggregation (TxA_2) and platelet inhibition (PGI_2).

Targeting the arachadonic acid pathway

• **Corticosteroids** inhibit the phospholipase A_2 (PA_2)-mediated release of arachadonic acid from the cell membrane and down-regulate COX-2 expression (but not COX-1). However, steroids have not been shown to alter restenosis rates after treatment of vascular disease.
• **Non-steroidal anti-inflammatory agents** (NSAIDs) are reversible COX inhibitors (both COX-1 and COX-2), thus inhibiting PG synthesis. Induced COX-2 may be responsible for restenosis and platelet aggregation, and selective blockade of this isoform may inhibit this. However, inhibition of COX-2 is associated with increased rates of thrombosis (including coronary), thus prohibiting its use in vascular disease.

Platelet aggregation

• **Activation.** Platelets are activated by exposure to subendothelial collagen (P-selectin receptor), thrombin (PAR-1 [protease activator receptor 1] and ADP [adenosine diphosphate] receptors [$P2Y_1$ and $P2Y_{12}$]) expressed on platelet surfaces.
• **Binding.** Activated platelets bind to exposed collagen and (vWF) via glycoprotein receptors. Once bound, ADP (platelet aggregator) and calcium (Ca^{2+}) (involved in coagulation) are released.
• **Receptors.** The most abundant aggregating receptor is the calcium-dependent GP (glycoprotein) IIb/IIIa, which links various proteins (especially fibrinogen) to the platelets creating the platelet plug.
• **Modifying factors.** Released agents including TxA_2, PDGF (platelet derived growth factor) and TGF-B (transforming growth factor beta) are released, which further magnify the activation and aggregation (as well as activating endothelial smooth muscle cells).

Targeting platelet aggregation

• **Prostaglandin activity.** NSAIDs inactivate the COX-1 dependent synthesis of TxA_2 in platelets (**aspirin** is the most widely used and, unlike others, its action is irreversible). TxA_2 is both a potent vasoconstrictor and platelet aggregator (inactivation lasts for up to 10 days). Higher doses of aspirin will also inhibit endothelial PGI_2, which ironically is a vasodilator and platelet inhibitor (thus potentially having a reverse effect!). However, the endothelium quickly replenishes PGI_2 (thus negating this reverse effect) but platelets, being devoid of nuclei, cannot replenish TxA_2. Thus the net effect is inhibition of platelet aggregation lasting 7–10 days (when platelets are replenished).
• **Adenosine activity.** Dipyridamole (phosphodiesterase V inhibitor) inhibits adenosine re-uptake via the adenosine A2 receptor (which stimulates platelet adenylyl cyclase) resulting in increased intracellular cyclic adenosine monophosphate (cAMP). It is a vasodilator and antiplatelet agent (weak when used alone). **Cilostazol** (phosphodiesterase [type III] inhibitor) inhibits cAMP. It is a vasodilator and has an antiplatelet agent.
• **Adenosine diphosphate (ADP) receptor.** Selective inhibition of this will inhibit platelet aggregation. Agents such as **ticlopidine**, **clopidogrel** and **prasugrel** are thienopyridine compounds with both anti-inflammatory and antiplatelet properties. It selectively inhibits the $P2Y_{12}$ receptor, which in turn blocks activation of the GPIIb/IIIa pathway, thus inhibiting (ADP-dependent) platelet activity.
• **GPIIb/IIIa inhibitors.** The final common pathway in platelet aggregation–thrombosis involves the cross-linking of platelets by plasma proteins (especially fibrinogen) via GPIIb/IIIa receptors. GPIIb/IIIa receptor blockers (e.g. **tirofiban, abiximab**) are powerful antiplatelet agents (used primarily during coronary intervention).

Statins (HMG-CoA reductase inhibitors)

These are reversible, competitive inhibitors of HMG-CoA reductase (converting HMG-CoA to mevalonic acid), which is the rate-limiting step in cholesterol synthesis leading to decreased cholesterol synthesis and an up-regulation of LDL (low-density lipoprotein) receptors with increased plasma clearance. The net effect is a reduction in plasma levels of cholesterol, LDL and triglycerides with a corresponding increase in plasma high-density lipoproteins (HDL).

Statins also have other auxiliary pleotrophic properties independent of their lipid-lowering effects, probably *via* the inhibition of mevalonate-dependent vascular enzymes (including endothelial nitric oxide synthase). Effects include anti-inflammatory, improved endothelial function, ↓ platelet aggregation, atherosclerotic plaque stabilisation, anti-thrombosis and inhibition of cellular proliferation.

Renin-angiotensin system pathway

As well as a regulator of systemic blood pressure and homeostasis, this pathway also has effects on vascular biology. Angiotensin-converting enzyme (ACE) is membrane-bound and converts inactive angiotensin I (AI) to the active form AII (and inactivates bradykinin). AII binds to receptors AT_1 (VSMCs) and AT_2 (endothelium). After vessel injury, there is an increase in angiotensinogen gene expression and an up-regulation of AT_2, which induces PDGF, TGF-B and basic fibroblast growth factor (bFGF), and therefore may have a role in thrombosis, atherosclerosis and neointimal hyperplasia. ACE inhibition has cardiovascular health benefits independent of its blood pressure (BP)-lowering properties.

Ca^{2+} channel blockers

Calcium has a multifactorial role in vascular biology including platelet aggregation, PDGF release, coagulation and VSMC proliferation–migration. Blockage of voltage-dependent Ca^{2+} channels in VSMCs blocks atherosclerosis in animal studies.

Nitric oxide pathway

Nitric oxide (NO) is endothelium-derived (from arginine) and is responsible for vasodilatation (in response to vessel wall stress) and for the resting tone of vessels by its effects on VSMC (↑ cyclic guanosine monophosphate [cGMP]). It also inhibits leucocyte adhesion and platelet aggregation, and its impaired production has been implicated in hypertension, ischaemia–reperfusion, atherosclerosis and neointimal hyperplasia.

8 Coagulation and thrombosis

Figure 8.1 Major steps in coagulation.

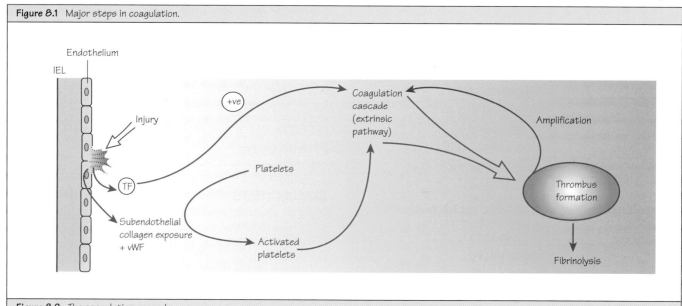

Figure 8.2 The coagulation cascade.

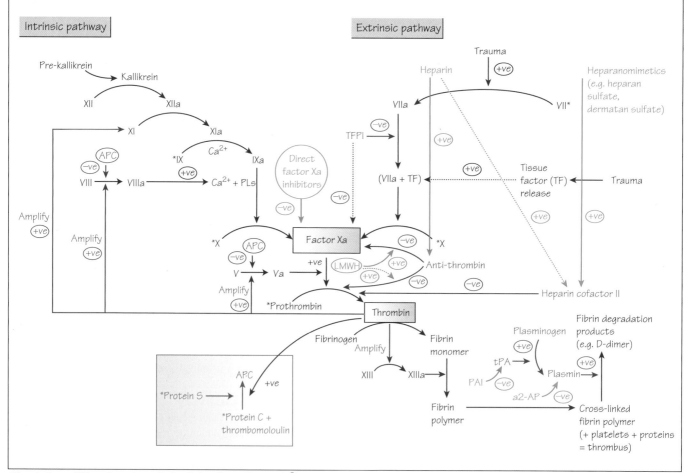

Abbreviations: APC, activated protein C; a2–Ap, a2 antiplasmin; Ca^{2+}, calcium; IEL, internal elastic lamina; LMWH, low molecular weight heparin; PL, phospholipid; PAI, plasminogen activator inhibitor; TF, tissue factor; TFPI, tissue factor pathway inhibitor; tPA, tissue plasminogen activator; *, vitamin K dependent factors; vWF, von Willebrand factor; Prothrombin, factor II

Vascular and Endovascular Surgery at a Glance, First Edition. Morgan McMonagle and Matthew Stephenson.

The coagulation cascade as described in manuscripts is an over simplification of a very complex phenomenon. Traditionally this cascade has been divided into intrinsic and extrinsic pathways. However, both these pathways are in fact intimately linked.

Steps in coagulation
- Vessel wall injury.
- Platelet aggregation.
- Tissue factor (TF) exposure.
- Coagulation cascade (intrinsic and extrinsic pathways).

The extrinsic pathway is the most important pathway *in vivo*!

Steps in the coagulation cascade
- The extrinsic pathway is initiated by subendothelial collagen exposure, which in turn stimulates platelet aggregation and TF (thromboplastin) release.
- Factor VII (FVII) is then activated (aFVII), which in turn combines with TF and is inhibited by tissue factor pathway inhibitor (TFPI).
- aFVII-TF converts factor X (FX) to activated factor X (aFX) and is the point of convergence of the intrinsic and extrinsic pathways.
- aFX converts prothrombin to thrombin, which magnifies the coagulation cascade by positive feedback on numerous factors.
- Thrombin converts soluble fibrinogen to insoluble fibrin, which forms the thrombus plug (combined with aggregated platelets).
- Thrombin also independently activates platelets (PAR-1 and ADP receptors) and releases calcium (necessary for coagulation).

Inhibitory pathways
Antithrombin (AT). This inhibits factor Xa and thrombin by acting as a suicide substrate. It also works in conjunction with *heparin cofactor II*, which also has a direct inhibitory effect on thrombin.

Proteins C and S. These are activated by thrombin and degrade cofactors Va and VIIIa, thereby diminishing the activation of prothrombin and FX.

Tissue factor pathway inhibitor (TFPI). This binds to and inhibits factor Xa and the factor VIIa-tissue factor complex.

Fibrinolysis pathway
tPA: This is released by endothelial cells and binds directly to fibrin as well as converting plasminogen to plasmin. This in turn binds to and cleaves fibrin to its soluble form. *Plasminogen activator inhibitor (PAI-1+2)* inactivates circulating tPA and *a2-antiplasmin* inactivates plasmin.

Pharmacological targets
Factor X and the prothrombin–thrombin complex compose the final common pathway in the coagulation cascade and are principal targets for its inhibition.

Thrombin inhibitors (direct and indirect)
Direct
These experimental agents bind directly to thrombin blocking its interaction with substrates. They inactivate both fibrin-bound thrombin as well as the fluid phase thrombin (unlike heparin). There are no specific antidotes.

Indirect
Heparanoids. These are polysaccharides (sugars) of variable size (e.g. pentasaccharides, hexasaccharides). **Unfractionated heparin** is a heterogenous admixture of oligosaccharides (wide variation in size) whereas **fractionated heparin** is a purified compound of chemically selected (fractionated) lighter chained oligosaccharides (hence also referred to as *low molecular weight heparin* [LMWH]). LMWH is therefore a purer, more potent compound with predictable pharmacodynamics and pharmacokinetics in comparison to its unfractionated counterpart.

The heparanoids are potent thrombin inhibitors by binding to and magnifying AT activity (×300), and they display a similar effect on heparin cofactor II (which also inhibits thrombin). LMWH has a direct inhibitory effect on anti-FXa activity too. Because the effects of LMWH are more predictable, it is associated with a superior safety profile (lower mortality, lower incidence of HITS). But the antidote protamine is less effective against LMWH and dosing needs to be adjusted in renal impairment.

Factor Xa inhibitors (direct and indirect)
Direct
These are pentasaccharides that bind directly to and inhibit factor Xa.

Ximelagatran. This is an enteral pro-drug of melagatran, with both being licensed for thromboprophylaxis in hip and knee surgery. It displays equal or superior efficacy to LMWH and warfarin (prophylaxis and deep vein thrombosis/pulmonary embolism [DVT/PE] therapy) with no significant increased bleeding risk. Side effects include abnormal liver function tests (LFTs).

Hirudin. This bivalent inhibitor has a $T_{1/2}$ of 60 minutes i.v. and 120 minutes s.c., and is renally cleared (caution in renal failure!). At low doses it is more effective than LMWH and heparin for thromboprophylaxis (hip surgery) without documented increase in bleeding. It is currently approved for use in patients with heparin-induced thrombocytopenia (HITS).

Bivalirudin. This is a synthetic analogue of hirudin ($T_{1/2}$ 25 minutes) with less renal clearance.

Indirect
These inhibitors form a pentasaccharide–antithrombin complex that in turn binds factor Xa with high affinity.

Fondaparinux. Synthetic pentasaccharide that binds antithrombin, thereby indirectly blocking thrombin generation (enhancing antithrombin-dependent inhibition of factors). It has almost 100% bioavailability after s.c. injection ($T_{1/2}$ 17 hours) with exclusive renal clearance (caution in renal failure). It has a predictable anticoagulant response (negating monitoring) and may be given as a once-daily dose with no risk of HITS and a low risk of osteoporosis. There is no known effective antidote.

Idraparinux. Hypermethylated derivative of fondaparinux that binds antithrombin with very high affinity. It has a $T_{1/2}$ of 80 hours and therefore can be administered once weekly!

Other inhibitory agents
Dextrans. Polymers of variable weight (e.g. dextran-70 and dextran-40) with a potent dose-dependent effect on platelet aggregation (inhibition), factors VIII and vWF (decreases levels) and fibrinolysis (enhancement). Side effects include bleeding, allergy, nephrotoxicity and an adverse effect on blood cross-matching.

Warfarin. Antagonist of vitamin K, thereby inhibiting the hepatic formation of factors II, VII, IX and X (vitamin K-dependent factors) as well as the anticoagulant proteins, Factors C and S. Warfarin inhibits the enzyme vitamin K epoxide reductase, thereby blocking the release of vitamin K in the liver (necessary for the carboxylation and activation of these factors). There is no direct effect on the coagulation cascade *per se* or on circulating coagulating factors. Other vitamin K antagonists include; acenocoumarol, dicourmarol and phenindione.

9 Cardiovascular risk factors

Figure 9.1 Known significant vascular risk factors.

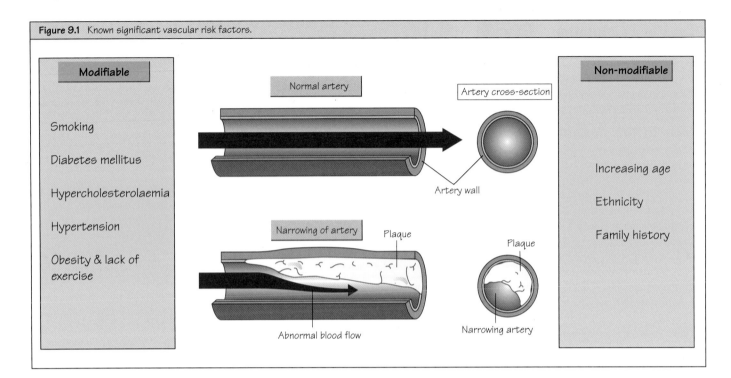

Vascular and Endovascular Surgery at a Glance, First Edition. Morgan McMonagle and Matthew Stephenson.

Atherosclerosis is a systemic disease. A patient is unlikely to have isolated cardiac, coronary or peripheral vascular disease (PVD). The risk factors are the same regardless of the vascular territory, although there is some evidence to suggest that diabetes and smoking particularly increase the risk in the lower limbs.

There are a number of well-known cardiovascular risk factors that are best divided into modifiable and non-modifiable:

Modifiable
- Smoking.
- Diabetes mellitus.
- Dyslipidaemia.
- Hypertension.
- Obesity and lack of exercise.
- Alcohol.

Non-modifiable
- Increasing age.
- Ethnicity.
- Family history.

The more that is learnt about these risk factors, the better the medical management of this problem can become. There are newer risk factors emerging such C-reactive protein, hyperhomocysteinaemia and elevated fibrinogen, although benefits of treating these have not been shown.

Modifiable
Smoking
Without doubt, the most significant modifiable risk factor for atherosclerotic disease is cigarette smoking, giving an odds ratio of about 4.5. Smokers are more likely to develop atherosclerotic disease, to develop complications of PVD and for it to deteriorate by continuing to smoke. The precise mechanism by which smoking causes atherosclerosis is still somewhat elusive despite the fact that the connection with claudication was recognised in 1911. There is a much smaller, but present, increased risk with passive smoking. Because of the high rates of smoking among vascular patients, it means that there are also higher rates of chronic obstructive airways disease and cancer in vascular patients.

Diabetes mellitus
This is the second most significant modifiable risk factor after smoking. Diabetics tend to develop more diffuse and distal disease, compounded by other diabetes-related complications such as neuropathy and increased susceptibility to infection. The lifetime risk of a major lower limb amputation is 10–16 times higher in a diabetic. The risk also rises the longer the patient has been diabetic and the more poorly the blood sugars are controlled. The UK Prospective Diabetes Study identified that, for every 1% increase in HbA1C, the risk of PVD increased by 28%. The effects of diabetes can be ameliorated by good glucose control but cannot be completely avoided.

The combination of diabetes with hypertension exacerbates the risk.

Dyslipidaemia
The Framingham Heart Study in Massachusetts, which commenced in 1948, is a very well-known ongoing longitudinal study that provided much of the basis for what we now know about risk factors for atherosclerotic disease. In this study, a fasting cholesterol >7 doubled the risk of claudication.

However, the story is slightly more complicated than this because the ratio of HDL:LDL cholesterol is also important. The higher this ratio, the lower the risk, because cholesterol, triglicerides and LDLs (the 'bad fats') are known to have a detrimental impact on plaque formation whereas HDLs are known to have a protective effect.

Hypertension
Again, the Framingham Heart Study was one of the first to show the epidemiological link between atherosclerotic disease and raised blood pressure. And again, the precise pathological link has not clearly been identified.

Obesity and lack of exercise
Obesity and lack of exercise increase the risk of atherosclerotic disease but this can be via the confounding factors of cholesterol profile, hypertension and diabetes mellitus.

Non-modifiable
Increasing age
There is clear evidence that atherosclerosis risk increases with age.

Ethnicity
People of South Asian descent are at higher risk of atherosclerotic disease, particularly with their higher risk of diabetes mellitus. People of Afro-Caribbean origin have higher rates of hypertension, which raises their risk.

Family history
This is almost certainly a complex polygenic issue. If you have a first-degree relative with atherosclerotic cardiovascular disease, this doubles your risk. Overall, another study from Framingham has indicated that family history is responsible for about 20% of a patient's total PVD risk.

Other
The effect of gender is variable on risk with some studies showing higher rates of disease in women, and others showing higher rates in men. Certainly the pre-menopausal state is protective against PVD such that pre-menopausal women have lower rates compared with age-matched controls.

Alcohol
Excessive alcohol raises LDL cholesterol and can increase BP resulting in raised risk.

However, the effects of alcohol on the development of PVD are contentious.

Figure 10.1 Nice guidence on hypertension treatment 2011. (Source: National Institute for Health and Care Excellence. Adapted from CG127 Hypertension: Clinical management of primary hypertension in adults, London: NICE 2011. Available from http://guidance. nice.org.uk/CG127. Reproduced with permission.)

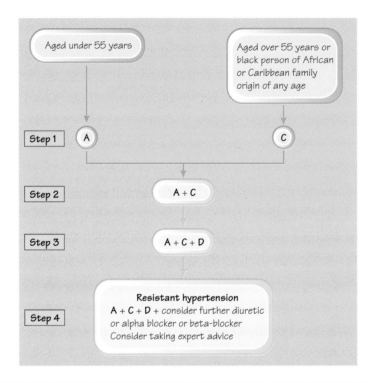

Abbreviations: **A**, ACE inhibitor or angiotensin II receptor blocker (ARB); **C**, calcium-channel blocker (CCB); **D**, thiazide-like diuretic

Vascular and Endovascular Surgery at a Glance, First Edition. Morgan McMonagle and Matthew Stephenson.

28 © 2014 John Wiley & Sons, Ltd. Published 2014 by John Wiley & Sons, Ltd. Companion website: www.ataglanceseries.com/vascular

Overview

Non-operative treatment does not necessarily mean 'conservative' treatment (i.e. doing nothing). Non-operative treatment should mean 'best medical therapy [BMT]', which is in fact an effective, proven treatment for atherosclerosis. If a patient comes with claudication and you successfully angioplasty their superficial femoral artery lesion, you may improve their walking distance, but you do nothing about the same disease process that is furring up their coronary vessels, or carotid vessels, etc. All patients should have BMT; sometimes they also need a specific intervention.

BMT partly centres around managing the risk factors described in Chapter 9; however, there are other interventions that do not quite relate to these.

Smoking cessation

Non-smokers should not underestimate how addictive smoking can be. Spontaneous cessation rates are very low (<15%). **Smoking cessation clinics** can be very beneficial and there are some important pharmacological adjuncts to consider that raise the chances of success:
- Nicotine replacement therapy.
- Bupropion (an antidepressant).
- Varenicline (a partial acetylcholine nicotinic receptor agonist).

A Cochrane database meta-analysis has shown these pharmacological agents to be superior to placebo.

Women can reduce their cardiovascular risk to age-matched controls within 2–3 years of smoking cessation, whereas men take longer.

Control of diabetes

Meticulous blood sugar control, as evidenced by acceptable sequential haemoglobin (Hb)A1C readings, are extremely important to cardiovascular risk, especially in the peripheral circulation. Patients should aim for a target HbA1C of <6.5% or 48 mmol/mol.

The UK Prospective Diabetes Study not only showed a strong association between HbA1C and peripheral artery disease but also that for every 10 mmHg reduction in systolic BP (in diabetics) the overall cardiovascular risk could be reduced by 12%.

Control of cholesterol

Cholesterol is principally endogenously produced by the liver. The remainder is absorbed from the diet. A meticulous diet strategy might hope to improve the cholesterol by about 10%, which is not sufficient for most patients. Most guidelines aim for an LDL cholesterol of <2.6 mmol/L, which is very difficult to attain without pharmacological agents.

Statins (e.g. simvastatin, atorvastatin, pravastatin) are HMG-CoA reductase inhibitors that affect the rate-limiting step in endogenous cholesterol synthesis. Even with standard doses, reaching this low cholesterol can be hard to achieve so some recommend high-dose statin agents. It is interesting to note that, regardless of a patient's baseline cholesterol, they still appear to benefit from statins. Statins have even been shown to improve claudication walking distance. In short, all patients with cardiovascular disease should be on a statin unless contraindicated.

Fibrates (bezafibrate, clofibrate, fenofibrate, etc.) are another class of drug that are usually only prescribed in combination with a statin for more aggressive lipid lowering, or as monotherapy in patients unable to take statins. The evidence for their use in monotherapy is poor.

There are a number of other agents occasionally used, such as niacin, bile acid sequestrants, exetimibe and orlistat.

BP control

The National Institute for Health and Care Excellence guideline advises that patients should have their BP diagnosed using 24-hour BP readings or home BP readings, rather than relying on high readings in clinic. Patients under 80 with BP readings >140/90, or 135/80 with other complicating issues, should be treated. As first line, patients aged <55 should be treated with ACE inhibitors whereas patients >55 or a black patient of any age should be treated with a calcium channel blocker. As second line, both drugs should be used together, and as third line a diuretic should be added (see Figure 10.1).

Antiplatelet agents

The evidence for aspirin in patients at increased cardiovascular risk is substantial. There is no significant evidence to suggest that it improves symptoms (i.e. claudication). The Clopidogrel versus Aspirin in Patients at Risk of Ischaemic Events (CAPRIE) trial identified that clopidogrel was more effective than aspirin in combined risk of stroke, MI and vascular death; however, cost considerations have made aspirin first line for most. There is evidence of benefit for both aspirin and clopidogrel in patients with unstable disease (e.g. acute coronary syndrome). However, the Clopidogrel for High Risk Atherothrombotic Risk and Ischaemic Stabilisation Management and Avoidance (CHARISMA) trial identified no benefit for patients with stable disease.

Dipyridamole inhibits phosphodiesterase enzymes and blocks thromboxane synthase. It is sometimes used in combination with aspirin.

Exercise

There is very good evidence that supervised exercise improves claudication distance. This is covered in more detail in Chapter 36, because this is not just risk factor modification but also specific treatment. Exercise can reduce obesity and subsequent insulin resistance too. The main drawback is compliance.

Dietary advice
- Reduce salt intake (to reduce hypertension).
- Avoid high-cholesterol foods.
- Eat fish regularly (providing two specific fatty acids, eicosapentaenoic acid and docosahexaenoic acid).
- Replace saturated fats with unsaturated fats.
- Regular fruit and vegetable consumption.

Figure 11.1 Typical outline of a vascular history. Use the **SOCRATES** approach for pain.

PC	What's been the problem?	Pain in my legs
HPC	Where do you get it? (**Site**)	In my left calf
	Where does it come on? (**Onset**)	Whenever I've been walking about 200 yards
	Can you describe it? (**Character**)	Aching, throbbing, tight
	Does it **radiate** anywhere?	No
	Do you get any other symptoms with it? (**Association**)	No
	How long does it last? (**Timing**)	A few minutes once I've stopped walking
	Are there any **exacerbating** or relieving factors? (And specifically) what about in bed at night when you're resting, do you get pain at all then?	Exercise makes it worse. Standing still makes it go away. I don't get any pain at night
	How **severe** is it?	Very severe
Risk factors	Are you diabetic? Do you smoke? Do you have high blood pressure? Do you have high cholesterol? Do you have any family history of.....	
PMH	Have you had any heart trouble? Have you ever had a stroke? Have you ever had any problems with your arteries before? Do you have any other medical problems? Have you ever had an operation?	
PSH	What medications are you on?	
DH	Are you allergic to anything?	
SH	What can you do for yourself at home? How do you get about? Do you have to use stairs?	

Abbreviations: DH, drug history; HPC, history of presenting complaint; PC, presenting complaint; PMH, past medical history; PSH, past surgical history; SH, social history

Vascular and Endovascular Surgery at a Glance, First Edition. Morgan McMonagle and Matthew Stephenson.

30 © 2014 John Wiley & Sons, Ltd. Published 2014 by John Wiley & Sons, Ltd. Companion website: www.ataglanceseries.com/vascular

Overview

Taking a vascular history tends to mean a focused history looking at arterial symptoms in the context of PVD.

The process should follow the usual history-taking sequence, with particular emphasis as described here.

Presenting complaint

Most commonly:
- Pain in the calf on walking.
- Pain in the foot at night.
- Noticed a toe has become discoloured.
- Ulceration.

History of presenting complaint

SOCRATES history of pain (see Figure 11.1). In **claudication**, the pain is typically:
- localised to the calf and sometimes the buttock
- aching/cramping/tight
- relieved with rest
- occurring after consistent distance
- relieved after consistent rest time
- inclined to pass without the patient needing to sit down (suggesting a load-bearing problem, e.g. hip pain).

In **rest pain**, the pain is:
- always distal (i.e. you can't have rest pain affecting the calf but not the foot)
- worse at night in bed (when cardiac output reduces)
- relieved by hanging the leg out of the bed (gravity helps circulation)
- severe, may only be relieved by opiates.

Past medical history

Divide this into these categories:
- Cardiovascular risk factors (see Figure 11.1):
  - Are they diabetic?
    - Type 1 or Type 2?
    - Are they on insulin?
    - For how long?
    - How well controlled (e.g. last HbA1C)?
  - Do they smoke?
    - How much do they smoke?
    - What do they smoke?
    - How long have they smoked for?
  - Do they know if they have high cholesterol?
    - What was the last reading?
    - Are they on a statin?
  - Do they have high blood pressure?
    - How well controlled?
  - Do they have a family history of specific conditions?
    - Heart disease?
    - Stroke?
    - Peripheral vascular disease?
    - Aneurysms (particularly men)?

- Cardiovascular history
  - Cardiac/cerebral:
    - Do they get chest pain?
    - Do they get shortness of breath (SOB)?
    - Ever had an MI?
    - Ever had a coronary angiogram?
    - Ever had a coronary artery bypass graft (CABG)?
    - Under a cardiologist?
    - Ever had a stroke or transient ischaemic attack (TIA)?
  - Vascular
    - Ever been seen by a vascular surgeon?
    - Ever had any investigations for PVD?
    - Ever had a peripheral angioplasty?
    - Ever had a bypass?
- General medical history – all the usual questions you would ask (i.e. chronic obstructive pulmonary disease [COPD], renal disease, arthritis) but pay particular attention to the chest.

Past surgical history

The vascular aspect of this should already have been covered in the past medical history but make sure that you know the full surgical history. An old appendicectomy scar might be mistaken for an iliac artery exposure, for instance.

Drug history

Specifically, and including doses:
- aspirin or clopidogrel
- statins
- warfarin
- antihypertensives
- oral hypoglycaemics and insulin
- naftidrofuryl or cilostazol (rarely used medications for claudication).

Family history

- Coronary artery disease?
- Aneurysmal disease?
- Hypertension?
- Diabetes?
- Renal failure?

Social history

Especially relevant in the elderly:
- Independence for activities of daily living:
  - Washing self.
  - Shopping.
  - Cleaning.
- Mobility:
  - Normal/1 stick/2 sticks/Zimmer frame/wheelchair.
  - Do they leave the home?
  - How many floors?
- Diet and alcohol intake.

Figure 12.1 Peripheral vascular examination.

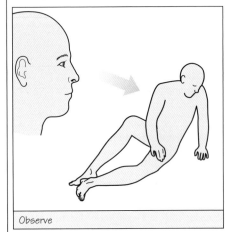

Observe

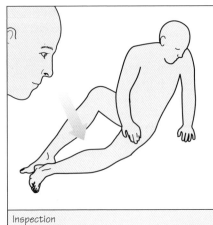

Inspection

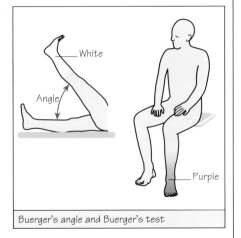

White

Angle

Purple

Buerger's angle and Buerger's test

Temperature

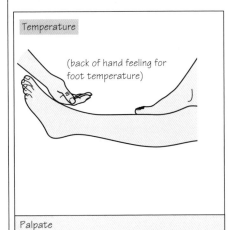

(back of hand feeling for foot temperature)

Palpate

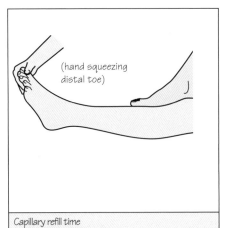

(hand squeezing distal toe)

Capillary refill time

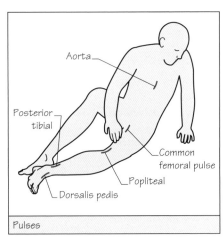

Aorta

Posterior tibial

Common femoral pulse

Popliteal

Dorsalis pedis

Pulses

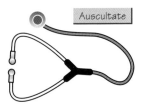

Auscultate

Problems finding the pulse?
o Your hand should be completely still – you're waiting for the artery to move, not your hand.
o Try pressing slightly firmer or slightly lighter.
o Line your fingers up in the line of the artery, not perpendicular to it (especially the femoral).
o Reconfirm the anatomical landmarks.
o If you're unsure whether the pulse you're feeling is the patient's or the one in your own fingers, use your other hand to time it with the patient's radial pulse.
o Learn to zone out everything else around you except what the mechanoreceptors in the skin of your fingertips are telling you.
o If unsure, always check with a Doppler probe.

Finally

I would examine the rest of the cardiovascular system

I would examine the venous system

I would check the sensation in the legs

I would check the ABPIs

Vascular and Endovascular Surgery at a Glance, First Edition. Morgan McMonagle and Matthew Stephenson.

Broadly there are three relevant vascular exams to learn:

1 Peripheral vascular examination – lower limb (Figure 12.1).

2 Varicose veins (Chapter 14).

3 Ulcers – essentially a matter of simply observing (Chapter 55).

Occasionally you may be asked to assess the upper limb arterial supply although this is unusual for undergraduates and even up to MRCS level. The principles are the same as for the lower limb arterial exam.

Peripheral vascular examination

The patient should be lying comfortably on the couch either supine or head slightly raised with the torso and legs exposed (can wear underwear for now).

Introduce and ask permission

Observe

Stand at the end of the bed and inspect:

• **around the bed** for paraphernalia of vascular or related diseases (e.g. prosthetic limb, nebuliser equipment)

• **the patient themselves** for obvious stigmata of vascular disease (e.g. median sternotomy wound, nicotine staining, SOB at rest).

Inspect

Legs for:

• colour

• scars from previous surgery (including in groins beneath any underwear)

• trophic changes (loss of tissue):
  • ulceration
  • gangrene
  • auto-amputation (count the toes; surprisingly it's not always immediately obvious if one is missing).

Note: be sure to check between the toes for interdigital ulcers.

Buerger's angle and test. Ask the patient to raise their leg off the bed (you can assist); inspect heel for ulceration. Keep raising slowly.

If leg **blanches**:

• note the angle – this is **Buerger's angle**; if it is less than 30°, this indicates severe ischaemia

• ask the patient to swing the leg out of bed to see if it becomes hyperaemic; if so – **Buerger's positive**.

If leg **doesn't blanche**:

• no Buerger's angle; no need for Buerger's test.

A secondary benefit of doing this now allows you to inspect the posterior aspect of the legs. Note: the leg needs to be quite ischaemic to blanche, so fairly unlikely in undergraduate exams.

Palpate

• **Temperature** (with back of your hand).

• **Capillary refill time** at a distal bony prominence (normal is <3 s in foot, <2 s in hand).

• **Pulses** (gradually move up leg):
  • **Dorsalis pedis** – located just lateral to the extensor hallucis longus tendon, which can be made prominent by asking the patient to extend the hallux.
  • **Posterior tibial** – 1/3 from medial malleolus to heel.
  • **Popliteal artery** – clasp both hands around upper calf with thumbs meeting on tibial tuberosity anteriorly and all the fingers creating a V-shape posteriorly in the popliteal fossa. Pull fingers anteriorly, pressing against the posterior aspect of the tibial plateau (usually lower than most people instinctively feel). Can be difficult to feel without practice.
  • **Femoral artery** – felt at the midpoint between the anterior superior iliac spine and the pubic symphysis.
  • **Abdominal aorta** – three steps:
    1 Press with both hands over the epigastrium. Remember the aorta is usually slightly to the left and can be compressed against the vertebral column.
    2 If pulsation present, place hands each side of epigastrium to see if pulsation pushes hands apart (expansile – aneurysmal) or pushes both out in same direction (transmitted – non-aneurysmal).
    3 Keep moving hands apart until can no longer feel pulsation – estimate size of aneurysm.
  • If any scars present in legs, palpate for any prosthetic grafts that may have been tunnelled subcutaneously.

Auscultate

Listen with a stethoscope for a bruit (indicates turbulent blood caused by a stenosed artery) over:

• the aorta (indicates aortic or renal stenosis)

• the common femoral (indicates iliac or common femoral stenosis)

• the adductor hiatus (indicates superficial femoral artery [SFA] stenosis).

Finally . . .

In an exam scenario, state that you would also:

• examine the rest of the cardiovascular system

• examine the venous system in the legs

• check the sensation in the legs

• check the Ankle Brachial Pressure Index (ABPI) measurements (Chapter 13).

Figure 13.1   The patient is supine and the probe is angled at 45–60 degrees over the brachial artery.

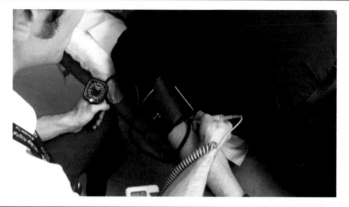

Figure 13.2   (a) The probe is angled over the DP artery and (b) over the PT artery.

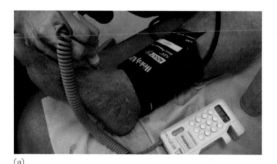

(a)

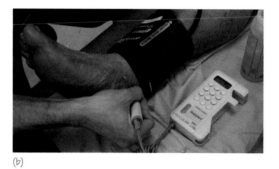

(b)

Resting	Disease severity
1.4 or greater	Calcification likely
0.9–1.3	Not suggestive of arterial disease
0.5–0.89	Suggests arterial minor disease (likely causing claudication)
0.40–0.3	Severe occlusive disease
Less than 0.3	Critical ischaemia with likely rest pain and tissue loss

Abbreviations: DP; dorsalis pedis, PT; posterior tibial

Vascular and Endovascular Surgery at a Glance, First Edition. Morgan McMonagle and Matthew Stephenson.
 Companion website: www.ataglanceseries.com/vascular

The ABPI is such a helpful and widely used test that it is worth devoting a whole chapter to it. It is:
• highly **sensitive** and **specific** for the presence of peripheral vascular disease
• **non-invasive**
• **quick**, **cheap** and **easy** to perform
• **reproducible**.

The premise of the ABPI lies in measuring a pressure difference between the arm, reflecting systemic pressure, and the foot. Because the arm is rarely affected by arterial occlusive disease, the arm pressure is used as the 'norm' (i.e. the denominator) and the foot pressure is the numerator. To be precise, it is the systolic pressure in one of the two foot pulses (whichever one is highest) divided by the brachial artery systolic pressure.

$$\frac{\text{Systolic dorsalis pedis (DP) or posterior tibialis (PT) pressure}}{\text{Systolic brachial pressure}} = \text{ABPI}$$

The pressure in the legs when you're supine should be about the same as the pressure in the foot; in fact, commonly the foot pressure might be a little higher, so the normal ratio is 0.9–1.2.

The lower the ratio, the more severe the arterial disease (see Figure 13.1). However, it is also possible for the ratio to be too high (i.e. above 1.2). This indicates that the arteries are heavily calcified and are therefore difficult for the cuff to compress. They may even be incompressible by the cuff, giving an ABPI value of infinity! Diabetics are particularly prone to this. The problem then comes with – what if you have arterial disease but you also have calcified arteries? This is the pitfall of the ABPI – it may appear reassuringly normal, or even high, despite severe arterial occlusive disease.

Fortunately however, there is a way of avoiding this confusion and it is explained by the Doppler waveform (i.e. the sound the Doppler machine makes).

Doppler waveforms

The sound created by the handheld Doppler machine is different depending on whether the artery is healthy and elastic or if it is diseased and calcified. These are the descriptions of the different sounds, from normal to most abnormal:
• **Triphasic:** You hear a loud whoosh and then two smaller whooshes per heartbeat. Listen to your own brachial artery to hear what this is like. This is the sound of a normal healthy artery.

• **Biphasic:** You hear a loud whoosh followed by only one more little whoosh per heartbeat. This may be normal but may also indicate some arterial disease.
• **Monophasic:** This indicates significant arterial disease. There is only one whoosh sound per heartbeat. Some divide this up further into monophasic pulsatile, in which there is a clear whoosh sound each heartbeat, and monophasic damped, in which there is an unimpressive but present sound of blood moving with each heartbeat.

So for those patients with normal or high ABPI in which you suspect calcification, you can put this together with the sound:

Normal ABPI + Triphasic foot signal = Normal arteries.

Normal/High ABPI + Monophasic signal = Arterial disease present, ABPI is unreliable.

High ABPI + Triphasic foot signal = Maybe normal, or consider upper arm arterial disease.

Procedure to perform ABPI

1 The patient must be lying supine and be rested.
2 The legs and arms should be fully exposed.
3 Apply a BP cuff snugly around the upper arm, elbow straight.
4 Palpate the brachial pulse to identify its position.
5 Apply ultrasound gel over the pulse.
6 Position tip of handheld Doppler machine over pulse and switch on – listen to the signal.
7 Inflate cuff until Doppler signal disappears.
8 Inflate another 20–30 mmHg.
9 Slowly deflate cuff until signal reappears.
10 Note this pressure: it is the brachial systolic pressure (the denominator).
11 Apply BP cuff around calf close to ankle.
12 Palpate DP, apply gel over it and position probe.
13 Inflate cuff until signal disappears.
14 Inflate another 20–30 mmHg.
15 Slowly deflate cuff until signal reappears.
16 Note this pressure.
17 Repeat with the PT and note this pressure.
18 Divide the higher of the two foot pulses by the brachial pulse.
19 Repeat with the other leg.

Note: if the patient has lower limb ulceration, the ulcers can be protected with cling film for the duration of the test; bandages will need to be removed. If this is not possible (for instance, because of pain) toe pressures can be checked in the vascular laboratory.

Figure 14.1   Examination (a) Observation (b) Inspection (c) Palpate and (d) Special tests.

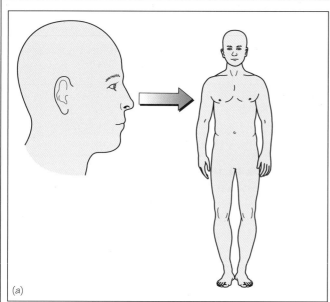

(a)

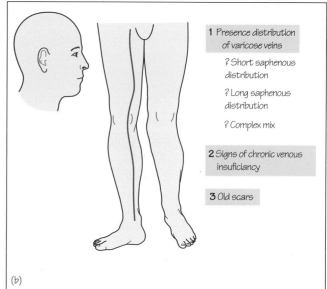

1 Presence distribution
   of varicose veins

   ? Short saphenous
   distribution

   ? Long saphenous
   distribution

   ? Complex mix

2 Signs of chronic venous
   insuficiancy

3 Old scars

(b)

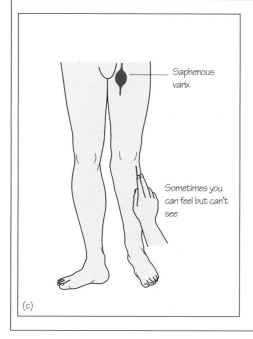

Saphenous
varix

Sometimes you
can feel but can't
see

(c)

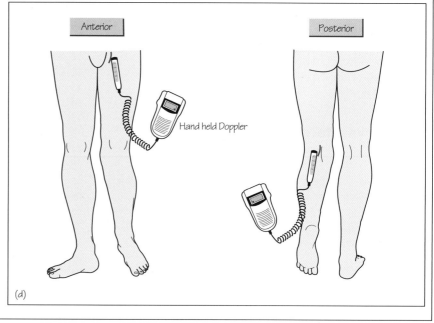

Anterior

Posterior

Hand held Doppler

(d)

Vascular and Endovascular Surgery at a Glance, First Edition. Morgan McMonagle and Matthew Stephenson.

36   © 2014 John Wiley & Sons, Ltd. Published 2014 by John Wiley & Sons, Ltd. Companion website: www.ataglanceseries.com/vascular

Varicose veins are extremely common, which means you will encounter them in real life and in exams, remarkably frequently. Fortunately examining the venous system is very easy and mainly requires observation and a simple handheld instrument – the Doppler probe. There are a myriad of other 'special' tests such as the tourniquet test, which are now considered obsolete because they are totally unreliable. It would be very unfair to ask you to perform them in an exam because they are never used now in clinical practice. The only people who would think it appropriate to include them would be ageing surgical dinosaurs who haven't practised vascular surgery in decades. Unfortunately, such people still exist in exam contexts, so the tests have been included here in basic format only, just for completeness.

Observation

The patient should be standing with the knee and hip slightly flexed. The whole leg must be exposed, with only underwear for cover; however, you will need even to look under this for the saphenofemoral junction. You should also be able to see the lower abdomen, as florid varices here suggest IVC obstruction. Inspect the leg looking for:

- the **presence of varicose veins**. Specifically look for dilated, tortuous, superficial veins. Also look in the saphenofemoral junction for a bluish swelling suggesting a saphena varix. Athletic and spider web veins are not varicose veins:
  - *Athletic veins*: dilated (>3 mm), superficial veins in the line of the long saphenous vein (LSV), but not tortuous. Usually in muscular legs. Simply physiological response.
  - *Spider web veins*: superficial, may be tortuous, but not dilated. These are just a cosmetic nuisance.
- signs of **chronic venous insufficiency**
  - Leg swelling (non-specific).
  - Pigmentation due to haemosiderin deposition.
  - Venous eczema.
  - Corona phlebectatica – a flare of intradermal veins around the medial malleolus.
  - Ulceration – usually above the medial malleolus. Shallow, sloping edges (very tender).
  - Atrophia blanche – whitish thin-looking skin that forms at the site of healed ulceration.
  - Note that lipodermatosclerosis is palpated, not seen, unless severe – in which case it forms a constricting band at the ankle causing the classic 'inverted champagne bottle'.
- the presence of **scars** from previous surgery
  - A very small (3–4 cm) scar in the groin crease suggests previous saphenofemoral junction ligation. Another small stab incision below the knee suggests the LSV has been stripped out between these two wounds. These can however be very difficult to see with time.
  - A transverse incision in the popliteal fossa may be from previous short saphenous vein ligation.

Palpation

- Palpate for varicose veins if you can't see them.
- Palpate the saphenofemoral junction for a saphena varix.
- Palpate for lipodermatosclerosis, which gives the skin and subcutaneous tissues a woody feel.

Handheld Doppler

This is a fundamental part of examining varicose veins and is very easy to do. Practise on a friend before your clinical exam – it would be very reasonable to ask you to perform it.

- Put some lubricating gel over the saphenofemoral junction which is 4 cm lateral and 4 cm inferior to the pubic tubercle.
- Place the tip of the Doppler probe over the same point and turn it on.
- If you can hear the sound of the femoral artery pulsating, you're too lateral; gently move medially until all you can hear is background buzzing.
- Gently squeeze the ipsilateral calf and listen for a whoosh sound.
- Release the calf – one of two things will happen:
  1 You hear no further sound, or just a very short fraction of a second whoosh (<0.5 s) – the saphenofemoral valve is functioning well.
  2 You hear a protracted whooshing sound (>0.5 s) – this is the blood refluxing back down the LSV through the defective saphenofemoral valve – you've found the site of venous reflux.
- Repeat for the short saphenous vein (SSV) in the middle of the popliteal fossa at the skin crease.

Other

- It may occasionally be appropriate to auscultate over large abnormal-looking venous clusters to detect a bruit suggesting an arteriovenous malformation.
- Examine the pulses: it is important to know that the arterial system is OK before embarking on venous surgery.
- To be complete, you would examine the abdomen including a rectal +/– pelvic examination.

Special (now obsolete) tests

- *Tap test:* Place one finger at the top of a varicose vein and the other at the bottom. Tap with the finger at the top and feel for a vibration with the lower finger. Feeling a vibration suggests there are defective valves within the varicose vein between your fingers.
- *Tourniquet test:* Lie the patient down and raise the legs to empty the superficial veins. Place a tourniquet as high on the thigh as you can, avoiding the pubic hair. Stand the patient up. If the veins still fill despite the tourniquet, it means the site of reflux must be below the tourniquet, so repeat but move the tourniquet ever lower on the thigh by a few centimetres each time. Once you reach a point where the veins no longer fill, you have found the level at which the valves are refluxing. Very unreliable.
- *Trendelenburg test:* Like the tourniquet test except it only involves using two fingers specifically on the saphenofemoral junction rather than a tourniquet (and therefore is only one stage). Very unreliable.
- *Perthes' test:* Raise the leg to empty the veins. Place a tourniquet around the leg. Stand the patient up. Ask the patient to walk or repeatedly stand on tiptoes, flexing and extending the ankle. If the superficial veins fill, it suggests deep venous obstruction. No longer recommended.

Figure 15.1 Interpreting vascular scars.

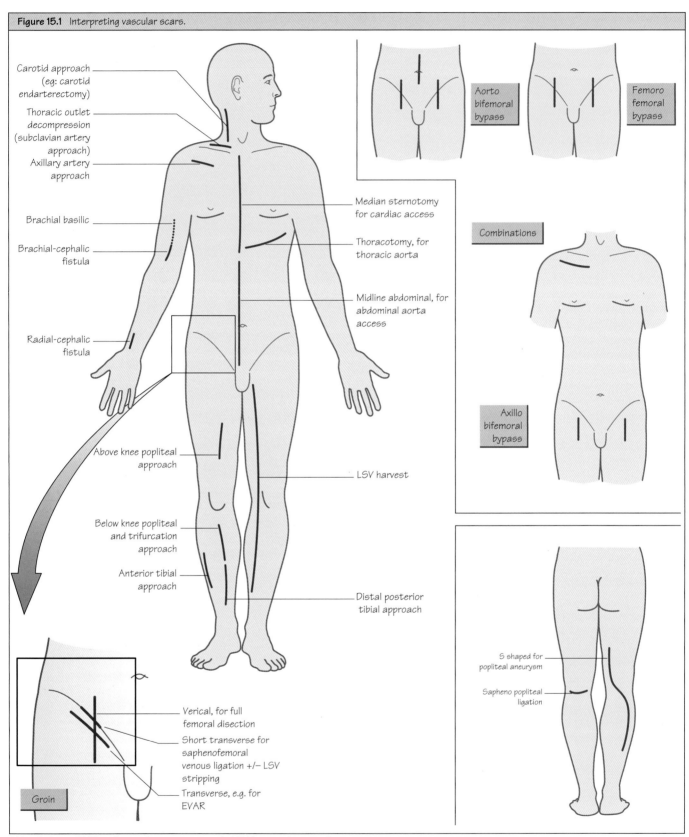

Carotid approach (eg: carotid endarterectomy)

Thoracic outlet decompression (subclavian artery approach)

Axillary artery approach

Brachial basilic

Brachial-cephalic fistula

Radial-cephalic fistula

Above knee popliteal approach

Below knee popliteal and trifurcation approach

Anterior tibial approach

Median sternotomy for cardiac access

Thoracotomy, for thoracic aorta

Midline abdominal, for abdominal aorta access

LSV harvest

Distal posterior tibial approach

Aorto bifemoral bypass

Femoro femoral bypass

Combinations

Axillo bifemoral bypass

S shaped for popliteal aneurysm

Sapheno popliteal ligation

Groin

Verical, for full femoral disection

Short transverse for saphenofemoral venous ligation +/– LSV stripping

Transverse, e.g. for EVAR

Abbreviations: EVAR, endovascular aneurysm repair; LSV, long saphenous vein

Vascular and Endovascular Surgery at a Glance, First Edition. Morgan McMonagle and Matthew Stephenson.

Overview

Vascular scars can be very confusing to the uninitiated. No scar is pathognomonic of a particular operation, and almost endless permutations of scars can exist together. Often two geographically quite distant scars can relate to the same operation because a bypass graft may be tunnelled between them (in these cases, always palpate between the scars because sometimes grafts are tunnelled subcutaneously). Gradually you will build up pattern recognition; however, it is not always possible to guess the exact operation from the scars, especially if the patient has had multiple trips to theatre.

Neck
Oblique incision in line with anterior border of sternocleidomastoid:
- *Carotid endarterectomy.*
- *Neck exploration for trauma.*
- *Excision of carotid body tumour.*
- *Carotid-subclavian bypass.*

Transverse incision above clavicle extending medially over sternocleidomastoid:
- *Thoracic outlet decompression.*
- *Subclavian access.*

Chest
Median sternotomy:
- Cardiac access, for example:
  - CABG.
  - Valvular replacements.

Infraclavicular transverse incision:
- to expose the *axillary artery.*

Small **stab incisions** in the third or fourth intercostal spaces:
- *Endoscopic thoracic sympathetcomy.*

Oblique incision in any of the left intercostal spaces:
- to expose the *descending thoracic aorta* (e.g. *thoracic aneurysm repair*).

Abdomen
Long midline:
- *Open repair of abdominal aortic aneurysm (AAA).*
- *Aortobi-iliac graft.*

Transverse/oblique lower quadrant:
- *Iliac artery exposure.*

Lower limb
Groin
Vertical/oblique/inverted hockey stick scar:
- to expose the *femoral artery*, for example:
  - *Femoral endarterectomy.*
  - *Femoral embolectomy.*

Transverse scar (long) (usually bilateral):
- to expose the *common femoral arteries*, for example:
  - *EVAR.*

Very short (3–4 cm) scar in groin crease:
- *Saphenofemoral junction ligation.*

Below the groin
Vertical scar above the knee on medial thigh:
- to expose the *above-knee (AK) popliteal artery.*

Vertical scar below the knee on the medial calf:
- to expose the *below-knee (BK) popliteal artery* or *proximal calf vessels.*

Vertical scar lateral to the tibial crest:
- to expose the anterior tibial artery.

Vertical scar posterior to the distal tibia:
- to expose the *distal posterior tibial artery* or *peroneal artery.*

Long scar along the line of the LSV:
- *Harvest of the LSV.* The patient may also have had ipsilateral arterial bypass through the same wound (femoropopliteal or femorodistal) or the vein harvested for CABG, for instance.

S-shaped scar over the popliteal fossa:
- *Popliteal artery aneurysm repair.*
- *Release of popliteal entrapment.*

Transverse scar over popliteal fossa:
- *Short saphenous vein ligation.*

Upper limb
Short vertical incision over distal radius:
- *Radial-cephalic fistula.*

Transverse or vertical antecubital fossa:
- *Brachial embolectomy.*
- *Brachial-cephalic fistula* (for renal access).

Long vertical incision up medial arm:
- *Brachial-basilic fistula* (for renal access).

Transverse incision in axilla:
- to expose the *axillary vein*, for example:
  - *Brachial-axillary graft* (for renal access).
  - *First rib resection for thoracic outlet syndrome.*

Combination
Midline abdominal + bilateral vertical femoral:
- *Aortobifemoral bypass.*

Bilateral vertical femoral:
- *Femorofemoral bypass graft.*

Infraclavicular transverse + unilateral vertical femoral:
- *Axillouniiliac bypass graft.*

Infraclavicular transverse + bilateral vertical femoral:
- *Axillobifemoral bypass graft.*

Bilateral transverse or vertical groin:
- *EVAR.*

Vertical groin + AK vertical:
- *Femoropopliteal (AK) bypass (with synthetic graft).*

Vertical groin + BK vertical:
- *Femoropopliteal (BK) bypass (with synthetic graft).*

Note: you know that synthetic graft has been used; otherwise there would also be an LSV harvest. To clarify, a long scar in the line of the LSV can only tell you the LSV was harvested – it cannot tell you whether the patient has also had an ipsilateral bypass; however, you may occasionally see:

Long LSV scar + vertical scar lateral to tibial crest:
- *Femorodistal (anterior tibial) bypass using LSV.*

Figure 16.1 Treadmill machine for measuring ABPIs before and after exercise.

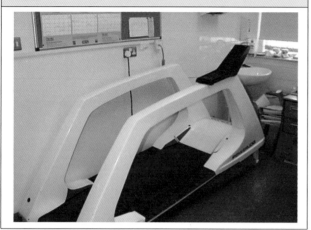

Figure 16.2 Equipment for measuring ABPI including hand-help Doppler device, BP cuff and manometer and ultrasound gel.

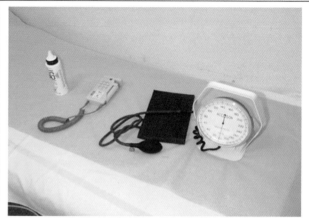

Figure 16.3 Measuring ABPI's at dorsalis pedis artery. Note BP cuff around calf.

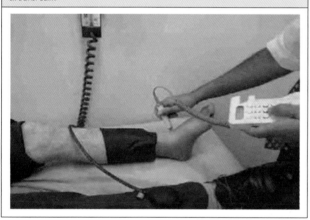

Figure 16.4 Typical state-of-the-art vascular ultrasound machine.

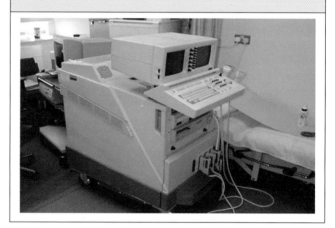

Figure 16.5 Outline of normal artery on colour flow Doppler (red).

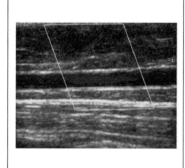

Figure 16.6 CT angiogram outlining left lower limb vessels including profunda femoris and SFA. Occlusion at level of adductor hiatus (AK popliteal artery).

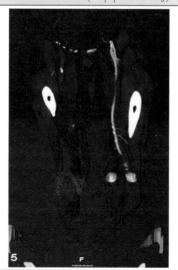

Figure 16.7 Catheter-directed angiogram showing occlusion at the AK popliteal artery with preserved collateral branches (geniculate vessel).

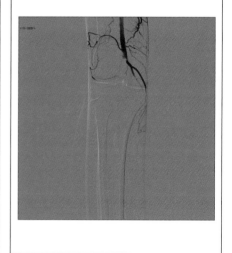

Abbreviations: AK, above knee; ABPI, ankle-brachial pressure index; BP, blood preaaure; CT, computed tomography; SFA, superficial femoral artery

Vascular and Endovascular Surgery at a Glance, First Edition. Morgan McMonagle and Matthew Stephenson.

General considerations

Vascular investigations are used in a hierarchical manner to give an objective assessment of disease and to determine if further intervention is necessary. Unfortunately, because of the widespread nature of atherosclerosis and the high incidence of recurrence of disease (and failure of invasive therapy), the vascular specialist must be satisfied that the disease process is serious enough to warrant the intervention. This will vary according to the presentation (e.g. symptomatic control in claudication, stroke prevention in carotid disease, aneurysm rupture risk in AAA). However, many vascular conditions do have internationally accepted, well-established evidence for best management, hence the need for objective investigations.

The general health of the patient is also important to consider before embarking on numerous and costly investigations, especially if the patient is deemed unfit for treatment regardless of the outcome of tests (less likely in modern practice because of the less invasive nature of angiointervention compared with historical open surgery).

Vascular investigations

For details on vascular U/S and catheter-based angiography, refer to Chapters 17–22.

Non-imaging

- Bedside investigations.
- Vascular laboratory:
  - Segmental pressure studies.
  - Toe pressure measurement.
  - Transcutaneous oximetry (for further details on these first three investigations, see Chapters 13, 34 and 35).
  - Digital waveform analysis.

Imaging

- Vascular ultrasound (vascular laboratory):
  - Grey-scale.
  - Doppler.
- Angiography (Radiology Department):
  - Non-invasive:
    - CT angiography.
    - MR angiography.
  - Invasive:
    - Catheter-directed angiography.

Bedside investigations
Hand-held Doppler and ABPI

- An 8 MHz probe is used to detect the presence and acoustic characteristic of the peripheral pulses (when they are impalpable), which may be classified as triphasic, biphasic or monophasic. However, this is of limited value unless ABPIs are also measured.
- The ABPI is the ratio of tibial (ankle) opening pressure to the brachial (systemic [normal] pressure), which can be measured at rest or before and after exercise (e.g. treadmill assessment).
- The brachial pressure is measured with a properly fitting BP cuff around the humerus, and the opening pressure is measured using the Doppler probe at the radial artery in the wrist. The ankle pressures are measured with the BP cuff around the calf and the Doppler probe held over the posterior tibialis artery (PTA) and dorsalis pedis artery (DPA). The cuff is inflated until the pulse wave disappears and then

slowly deflated. The moment the pulse wave returns is the 'opening pressure'.
- The highest brachial pressure is used and the ABPI for BOTH the DPA and PTA is recorded. *The highest ABPI is used.* An ABPI of <0.7 is associated with claudication and <0.3 with rest pain.
- An absolute ankle pressure of <50 mmHg is considered critical ischaemia (rest pain ± tissue loss), although higher pressures (>70 mmHg) are often needed for wound healing.
- The ABPI may be falsely elevated in calcified, poorly compliant, non-compressible vessels (e.g. diabetes, chronic renal failure) and toe pressures should be used instead (see Chapters 48 and 58).

Vascular U/S

Non-invasive, repeatable, sensitive and specific (see Chapter 17–19).

Computed tomography angiography (CTA)

This is now ubiquitous in modern hospital practice. Intravenous contrast with images taken during the *arterial phase* (± portal-venous phase) give very accurate contrast-enhanced images of vascular disease. It has the advantage over catheter-based angiography in that it is less invasive (save for contrast and radiation exposure) because the contrast is given intravenously rather than intra-arterial.

Modern computerised spiral (helical) CT scanners can 'reconstruct' images into 3D format with '*maximum intensity projection*' as well as subtraction of surrounding tissue to give an angiographic-like image.

CTA imaging detail includes vessel diameter and wall calcification, thrombus deposition, stenosis/occlusion, assessment of in-flow and run-off as well as surrounding tissue architecture (not seen on conventional angiography). Differentiating between contrast and calcium can be difficult in calcified, small-calibre vessels.

Magnetic resonance angiography (MRA)

MR imaging (MRI) uses a very strong pulsed magnetic field causing hydrogen ions to 'spin' from their normal axis and back again (as the magnet is deactivated) with the emission of a radiofrequency pulse (which gives very accurate images of tissues [including vessels] and blood flow).

The phase of the spin differs in flowing blood (white) compared with stationary images (tissue and vessels), which appear black (*phase-contrast angiography*). But, if there is a lot of turbulence, MRA may overestimate a stenosis (false-positive) or cause 'signal drop-out' reported as a false-positive total occlusion (black). Intravenous gadolinium contrast (para-magnetic element) is given as a bolus-chase to overcome this and a 'time-of-flight' acquisition (images taken before and after bolus for comparison) performed. The images undergo subtraction (T1 relaxation time) to increase the signal ratio between moving blood and stationary tissue to give sharper, more accurate images that can then be 3D reconstructed.

Disadvantages include difficulty interpreting disease in small vessels (due to contrast remaining in the small lumen), overestimation of a stenosis and poor visibility of in-stent stenosis (especially stainless steel). Contraindications to MRI include metal implants (e.g. pacemaker, cochlear, intracranial clip, ocular metallic foreign body) and severe claustrophobia (10%). The most serious side effect (albeit very rare) after gadolinium administration is *nephrogenic systemic fibrosis* (see Chapter 20).

Table 17.1 percentage (%) reduction in the vessel diameter and its corresponding percentage reduction in cross-sectional area of the same vessel (note it is not a direct linear relationship and assumes concentric narrowing).

% Stenosis (diameter)	% Cross-section area reduction
30	50
50	75
70	90

Percentage vessel diameter reduction calculation

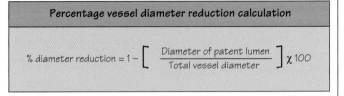

$$\% \text{ diameter reduction} = 1 - \left[\frac{\text{Diameter of patent lumen}}{\text{Total vessel diameter}} \right] \times 100$$

Figure 17.1 Illustrations of the normal arterial waveform (left) and the important features. This waveform will change shape and form as the stenosis progressively tightens (right).

Triphasic waveform (normal)

Peak systolic Velocity — 100%

Velocity

50%

End-diastolic velocity — 0

① Forward flow (cardiac systole)

Width at 50% amplitude

Time to peak

Base

(No spectral broadening)

③ Forward flow (late diastole)

② Reverse flow (early diastole)

Time (cardiac cycle) →

Features of an arterial waveform that the examiner should note:
a. Waveform shape
b. Peak systolic velocity
c. Is reverse component lost?
e. End-diastolic velocity
d. Presence of spectral broadening?
f. Is the waveform 'upstroke' delayed (tardus parvus)?
g. What are the waveforms like DISTAL to this one?

Spectral broadening: Represents the spread of frequencies present within a spectrum. There will be ↑ in 'time to peak' and ↑ 'width at 50% of peak amplitude'.

Biphasic
① 20–49% stenosis

Low acceleration monophasic
③ >75% stenosis

High acceleration monophasic
② >50% stenosis

Figure 17.2 Typical waveforms seen in the femoral artery and distal to iliac disease.

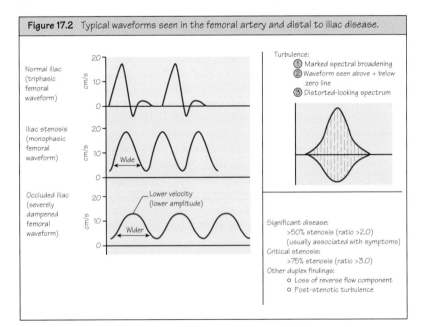

Normal iliac (triphasic femoral waveform)

Iliac stenosis (monophasic femoral waveform) — Wide

Occluded iliac (severely dampened femoral waveform) — Lower velocity (lower amplitude) — Wider

cm/s

Turbulence:
① Marked spectral broadening
② Waveform seen above + below zero line
③ Distorted-looking spectrum

Significant disease:
>50% stenosis (ratio >2.0)
(usually associated with symptoms)
Critical stenosis:
>75% stenosis (ratio >3.0)
Other duplex findings:
○ Loss of reverse flow component
○ Post-stenotic turbulence

Figure 17.3 Vascular wave patterns in carotid arteries.

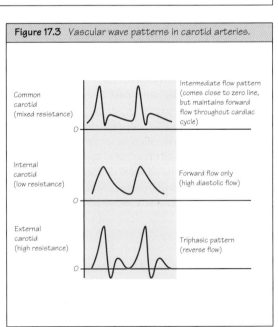

Common carotid (mixed resistance)

Internal carotid (low resistance)

External carotid (high resistance)

Intermediate flow pattern (comes close to zero line, but maintains forward flow throughout cardiac cycle)

Forward flow only (high diastolic flow)

Triphasic pattern (reverse flow)

Vascular and Endovascular Surgery at a Glance, First Edition. Morgan McMonagle and Matthew Stephenson.

Physics of Ultrasound

Ultrasound (*U/S*) *is a brief pulse of energy in the form of a high frequency sound wave that cannot be heard.*

An electric current is passed through quartz crystal (inside the handheld probe); this causes the crystal to oscillate rapidly, thereby generating ultrasonic waves (*piezoelectric effect*). The speed of the U/S wave is dependent on the density and compressibility of the medium it is travelling through, and the reflected waves (detected by the transducer) are generated into pictures for diagnostic assessment. These reflected waves are dependent on the *acoustic impedance* of the tissue. In addition, the angle of the beam will also affect the amplitude of the signal detected by the transducer.

Units of measurement

The unit of frequency is the hertz (Hz).
- 1 Hz = 1 cycle/second.
- 20–20,000 Hz = normal human audibility.
- >2 KHz = U/S.

The Doppler effect

This is the change in observed U/S frequency (as detected by the stationary probe) due to the relative motion of the source (in comparison to the transducer) and is useful for measuring blood flow velocity and flow direction. This alteration in observed frequency is known as the *Doppler shift*. In vascular U/S, the moving medium is blood, which may be 'moving away' or 'moving towards' the probe (stationary observer).

Risks of U/S

Theoretical risks relate to thermal tissue effects and cavitation (oscillation and collapse of gas-filled cavities in the U/S beam). However, U/S is considered safe, although, when imaging the pregnant patient and foetus, it is still considered good practice to keep exposure '*as low as reasonably achievable*' (ALARA).

U/S in vascular assessment

- The typical probe transmitting frequency is 5–10 MHz.
- U/S investigation is non-invasive, non-toxic, reproducible, accurate, sensitive and specific (but very user-dependent).
- It displays arterial disease along the vessel wall including degree of stenosis, intima thickness, plaque characteristics, anatomical shape and location as well as in-flow and run-off.
- Venous U/S is useful in assessing the size of veins, suitability for bypass or renal access, presence of thrombus and its compressibility (e.g. DVT), venous reflux, targeting for cannulation and instrumentation, and visualising endovenous ablation.
- It is used in graft surveillance (e.g. bypass, renal access) to identify critical restenosis for intervention before total occlusion occurs.

Vascular U/S modes

- Grey-scale U/S (also called B-mode or 2D Mode)
- Doppler U/S:
  - Colour Doppler.
  - Spectral Doppler.
- *Duplex* combines and displays both grey-scale and Doppler U/S.

Grey-scale (B-mode) U/S

- This visualises anatomic structural detail and is the most common format used in medical U/S (using simple pulse-echo imaging).

- It can visualise plaque morphology and identify thrombus as well as estimating luminal diameter, but is not useful in estimating the haemodynamic significance of a stenosis (Doppler required).

Doppler U/S

- This visualises the flow or movement of fluid (i.e. blood) through a structure (e.g. artery).
- The Doppler signal is analysed and displayed using either *colour flow* (colour-coded blood flowing in vessels) or *spectral analysis* (waveforms from moving blood) to provide a 'functional map' of vascular flow characteristics.

Colour flow Doppler

- Blood flow direction is colour coded corresponding to flow towards or away from the probe (***BART***: *Blue = Away, Red = Towards*).
- The actual colour or wavelength (*hue* [violet through to red as per displayed scale]) and its brightness (luminosity) will vary according to the velocity (i.e. brighter and more intense colour reflecting higher velocities).
- A whole mosaic of colours (*saturation*) is seen in very turbulent flow (reflects the magnitude of small eddy currents (turbulence) created at an irregular lesion).

Spectral Doppler analysis and vascular assessment

- This graphically displays blood flow as *velocity and direction over time*, producing a characteristic waveform and measurable *peak velocity*.
- As a stenosis tightens, the velocity across it also increases (to compensate for the same volume of blood flow continuously reaching the afferent side [up to the point of total occlusion]).
- In vascular assessment, the peak flow systolic velocities are most important in the assessment of a stenosis (critical [i.e. haemodynamically significant] versus non-critical) and may be compared with the velocities proximal to this.
- The velocity will also be affected by the resistance of the vascular bed into which it is flowing (e.g. the internal carotid artery [ICA] empties into a low-resistance bed [i.e. the brain] and its waveform will vary compared with the lower limbs [high resistance]).
- The *shape* of the spectral analysis waveform will change with the degree of stenosis: *triphasic* (normal), *biphasic* (moderate stenosis or stiffness), *monophasic* (dampened waveform).
- The waveform distal to a stenosis will demonstrate a monophasic, dampened waveform with reduced velocities.

The normal waveform explained

The normal waveform is *triphasic* and consists of brisk upstroke (forward flow) during systole (the *peak systolic velocity*). This is followed immediately by a short, reverse-flow component in early diastole, which represents the reflected waves from the (compliant) peripheries. This is followed by a short forward-flow component in late diastole (not always present and depends on the vascular bed).

The waveform shape may be affected by ambient and patient temperature, peripheral resistance (brain, renal and mesenteric tissues have 'low resistance' while the muscles and skin are 'high resistance'), and ability of the tissues to compensate and collateralise.

18 Vascular ultrasound II

Table 18.1 Table of the normal arterial diameter and its corresponding normal mean velocities in the lower limb vessels.

Artery	Mean diameter (cm)	Mean velocity (cm/s)*
Abdominal aorta	2	50–70
Common iliac	1.5–1.8	70–90
External iliac	0.8–1.0	100–140
Common femoral	0.8–1.0	90–130
SFA (proximal)	0.6–0.8	75–105
SFA (distal)	0.5–0.6	80–110
Popliteal	0.5–0.6	55–85
Tibial vessels	0.3–0.4	45–65

Figure 18.1 Illustration of the waveform analysis at the measured points across an arterial stenosis (corresponding to Table 18.2).

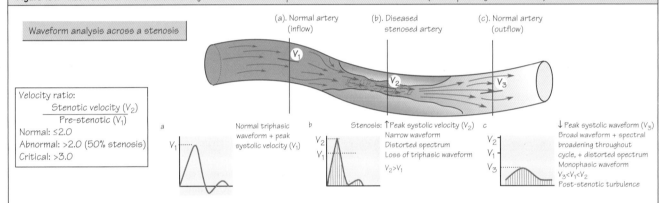

Waveform analysis across a stenosis

Velocity ratio:

$$\frac{\text{Stenotic velocity } (V_2)}{\text{Pre-stenotic } (V_1)}$$

Normal: ≤2.0
Abnormal: >2.0 (50% stenosis)
Critical: >3.0

(a). Normal artery (inflow)
Normal triphasic waveform + peak systolic velocity (V_1)

(b). Diseased stenosed artery
Stenosis: ↑Peak systolic velocity (V_2)
Narrow waveform
Distorted spectrum
Loss of triphasic waveform
$V_2 > V_1$

(c). Normal artery (outflow)
↓ Peak systolic waveform (V_3)
Broad waveform + spectral broadening throughout cycle, + distorted spectrum
Monophasic waveform
$V_3 < V_1 < V_2$
Post-stenotic turbulence

Table 18.2 Typical changes seen on ultrasound as stenotic disease progresses from normal to total occlusion (lower limb).

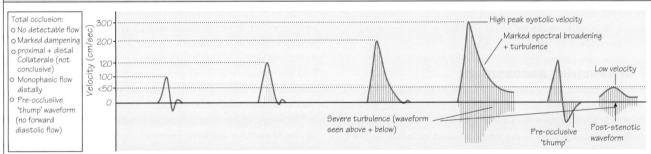

Total occlusion:
o No detectable flow
o Marked dampening
o proximal + distal Collaterals (not conclusive)
o Monophasic flow distally
o Pre-occlusiive 'thump' waveform (no forward diastolic flow)

High peak systolic velocity
Marked spectral broadening + turbulence
Low velocity
Severe turbulence (waveform seen above + below)
Pre-occlusive 'thump'
Post-stenotic waveform

Analysis	Normal parameters	<20% stenosis	20–49% stenosis	50–99% stenosis	Total occlusion
Waveform contour	Normal triphasic	Normal triphasic	Triphasic	Reverse flow pattern lost	Pre-occlusive 'thump' waveform (no forward diastolic flow)
Velocity	100cm/sec (±30%)	Focal velocity increase of <30%	Focal velocity increase of 30–100%	Focal velocity increase >100% or PSV >200cm/sec	No detectable flow
Spectral broadening	No	Yes (slight)	Yes (marked)	Yes (significant)	No detectable flow
Proximal-distal flow patterns	Normal flow	Normal flow	Normal flow	Post-stenotic turbulence	Marked dampening proximal and distal
Arterial wall (B-mode)	Normal	Minimal wall irregularity	Visible plaque	Plaque and acoustic shadowing	Occlusion ± visible collaterals

Abbreviations: PSV, peak systolic velocity
*Table 18.1, rule of thumb: 100cm/s +/– 30–50%

Vascular and Endovascular Surgery at a Glance, First Edition. Morgan McMonagle and Matthew Stephenson.

Duplex assessment of an arterial stenosis

The *raison d'etre* in the Duplex assessment of a vascular stenosis is to decide if it is *critical* or not. A critical stenosis is one that meets parameters that are considered haemodynamically significant (and hence intervention should be strongly considered). Duplex findings will help assess the need for intervention and its planning in addition to complementing other angiographic studies.

In addition, the lesion should be assessed in combination with the simultaneous assessment of proximal velocities (calculate the velocity ratio), distal waveform (effects on distal flow velocities), the number of lesions and their lengths.

Objectives of Duplex assessment
- Identify pathology (stenosis, occlusion, aneurysm).
- Localise (the lesion(s)).
- Grade (the severity of the lesion(s)).

Grading and assessment
1 *Peak systolic velocities**.
2 *Velocity ratio* across the lesion*.
3 *Waveform shape* (flow pattern)*.
4 *In-flow* and *run-off* (and their velocities).
5 *Flow direction.*
6 Vessel *size.*
7 Estimated *narrowing* (on grey-scale).
8 *Diastolic velocities* (more relevant low-resistance tissues).
9 *Plaque morphology and intimal thickness.*
10 *Flow quality* (disturbance).

Waveform analysis
- Measure the *peak systolic velocity* and *velocity ratios.*
- Analyse the *shape*:
  - Triphasic (normal waveform).
  - Biphasic (moderate stenosis).
  - Monophasic (dampened waveform ± critical stenosis).
- Establish presence or absence of *spectral broadening.*

Peak systolic velocity. As a vessel becomes narrowed (i.e. stenosis), the flow velocity will also increase (up to the point of occlusion). *This is akin to squeezing the tip of a running hosepipe. The tighter the grip, the faster the water will flow until complete occlusion.*
- Velocities >125 cm/s (>1.25 M/s) are abnormally high.
- >250 cm/s (>2.5 M/s) is haemodynamically significant (critical).

Velocity ratio. Ratio of the peak velocity across a stenosis to the peak velocity just proximal to it (i.e. its in-flow velocity).
- A doubling (×2) of the peak systolic velocity represents a 50% (i.e. halved) narrowing of the lumen.
- A × 2.5 increase represents >50% narrowing.
- ≥3 is critical (haemodynamically significant).

Waveform shape. Normal waveform is multiphasic (triphasic) with a 'forward-reverse-forward flow pattern'. A stenosis will alter this.

Spectral broadening. This is *widening of the base* of the waveform and represents the numerous velocities within the wave spectra sec-

*Most useful in vascular assessment.

ondary to turbulence. It reflects a dampened waveform (tight stenosis or the haemodynamic effects distal to a stenosis).

Duplex findings in stenosis progression
- The earliest sign is often a loss of the normal 'reverse-flow' component of the waveform.
- As narrowing progresses, 'spectral broadening' (early diastole) will develop as the flow decelerates eventually becoming *monophasic* (systolic up-stroke followed by deceleration to baseline).
- As narrowing progresses, the blood flow velocities will increase across the stenosis (increase in peak flow velocities), which is also reflected in an increase in the velocity ratio across the lesion.
- Flow velocities distal to a stenosis will become reduced ('dampened') with wide spectral broadening (there may be little discernable difference between systolic and diastolic velocities or between venous and arterial flow with very tight proximal lesions).

Venous Duplex
Duplex diagnosis of venous reflux
Venous duplex can define the sites of insufficiency (deep or superficial veins and perforators) as well as sites of venous obstruction (e.g. limb, abdomen, pelvis). Venous flow is low resistance and normal findings on Duplex include:
- spontaneous flow
- phasic flow (respiriophasic)
- flow ceases with valsalva
- flow is augmented by distal compression (e.g. squeeze the calf)
- unidirectional flow (due to valves)
- compressibility
- anechoic (black) lumen.

Respiriophasic describes the slight variations representing cardiac contraction and the respiratory cycle. Normally there is little or no flow in either the deep or superficial veins on standing or sitting. However, flow augmentation (e.g. calf squeeze) will produce venous flows of 20–30 cm/s, with rapid flow towards the heart followed by rapid valve closure and abrupt cessation of flow (although there may be slight normal retrograde flow). *Absence of flow augmentation represents obstruction to flow.*
- Reflux is diagnosed by sustained retrograde flow:
  - Normal: reflux <0.5 s.
  - Moderate: moderate reflux lasting 0.5–<1 s.
  - Significant: large volume reflux lasting ≥1 s.

Duplex diagnosis of DVT
- Loss of compressibility with the U/S probe (most important criterion). Partial collapse may indicate partial occlusion or very fresh thrombus. However, *thrombus may be excluded if on compression the vein lumen is seen to disappear completely!*
- A mobile, free-floating thrombus may be seen on B-mode imaging.
- Loss of the spontaneous phasic flow on colour flow Doppler.
- Loss of the spectral Doppler pattern on augmentation if the vein is occluded. An occluded iliac vein will have a low-volume continuous flow in the femoral vein with a loss of the normal augmentation to valsalva.

19 Vascular ultrasound III: Specific parameters

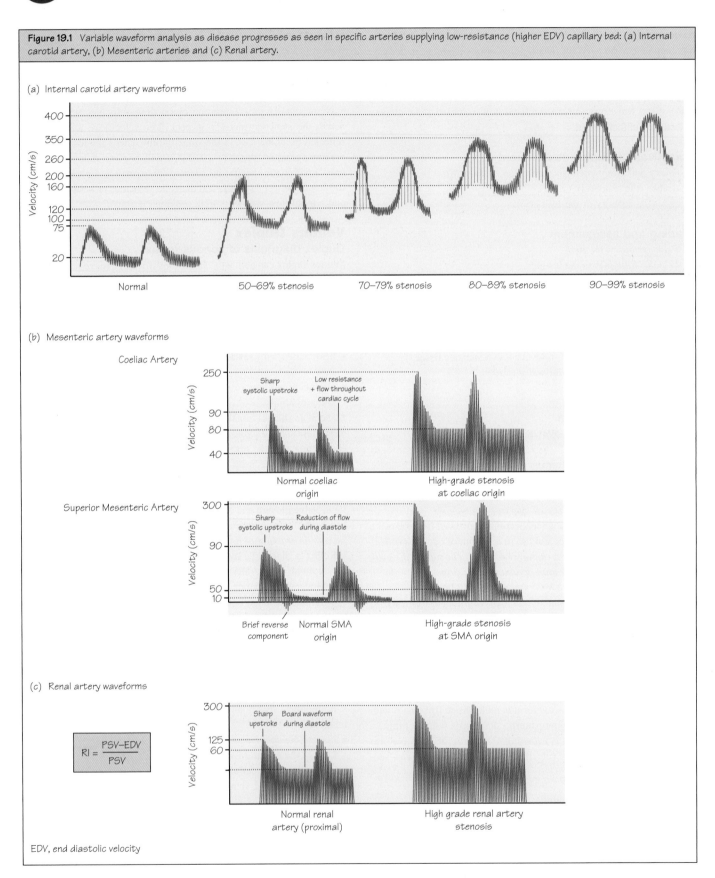

Figure 19.1 Variable waveform analysis as disease progresses as seen in specific arteries supplying low-resistance (higher EDV) capillary bed: (a) Internal carotid artery, (b) Mesenteric arteries and (c) Renal artery.

(a) Internal carotid artery waveforms

Normal   50–69% stenosis   70–79% stenosis   80–89% stenosis   90–99% stenosis

(b) Mesenteric artery waveforms

Coeliac Artery

Sharp systolic upstroke   Low resistance + flow throughout cardiac cycle

Normal coeliac origin   High-grade stenosis at coeliac origin

Superior Mesenteric Artery

Sharp systolic upstroke   Reduction of flow during diastole

Brief reverse component   Normal SMA origin   High-grade stenosis at SMA origin

(c) Renal artery waveforms

$$RI = \frac{PSV-EDV}{PSV}$$

Sharp upstroke   Board waveform during diastole

Normal renal artery (proximal)   High grade renal artery stenosis

EDV, end diastolic velocity

Vascular and Endovascular Surgery at a Glance, First Edition. Morgan McMonagle and Matthew Stephenson.

Lower limb assessment

As a 'rule of thumb' the mean velocity is 100 cm/s (±30–50%) including the aorta (peak systolic velocity [PSV] 100–150 cm/s) with triphasic morphology. There is a gradual decrease in velocities on moving distally down the arterial tree (loss of energy and increasing number of branches). The normal ratio is <2.0 and critical stenosis is defined as >2.5–3.0 (≥50% stenosis). Distal to a stenosis, there is loss of the reverse-flow component of the waveform with post-stenotic turbulence (spectral broadening). In addition, tandem lesions may have a greater magnitude effect than an isolated critical lesion (i.e. critical limb ischaemia due to multiple sub-critical lesions).

Upper limb arterial assessment

Duplex examination includes simultaneous provocative testing (positional changes in the arm and head) if thoracic outlet syndrome is suspected. Lesions in the SCA are more difficult to visualise because of the presence of the clavicle. The flow in the ipsilateral vertebral artery should also be assessed for evidence of reversed flow (i.e. steal syndrome).

The waveform is normally triphasic at rest, but with high diastolic flow rates on vasodilatation (e.g. post-exercise). The normal PSV is 80–120 cm/s for the SCA and axillary artery, 50–100 cm/s for the brachial and PSV 40–90 cm/s for the radial and ulnar arteries.

The criteria for grading critical stenosis in the upper limb is not well established because of its resistance to ischaemia (profunda brachii) with patients often remaining asymptomatic. However, a doubling of the PSV corresponds to a 50% lumen reduction and may be considered haemodynamically significant (i.e. PSV > 180 cm/s).

Carotid artery assessment

The carotid has high flow into a low resistance bed and therefore there is a significant amount of flow in diastole. Therefore, end-diastolic velocities (EDV) are also important along with PSV in assessments. The normal PSV and EDV in the ICA is <125 cm/s and <40 cm/s respectively with an ICA/common carotid artery (CCA) PSV ratio <2.0. A 50–69% stenosis corresponds to PSV 125–230 cm/s, EDV 40–100 cm/s and a ratio of 2.0–4.0. Surgery (+BMT) has superior long-term stroke prevention rates for critical stenosis (>70%):

- 70–79%: PSV > 230 cm/s, EDV > 100 cm/s and a ratio >4.0.
- 80–89%: PSV > 330 cm/s, EDV > 140 cm/s, ratio 4.0–5.0.
- 90–99%: PSV > 400 cm/s and EDV > 180 cm/s, ratio >5.

Mesenteric vessel assessment

High flow into low resistance capillary bed and therefore there is higher diastolic flow and EDVs are also relevant. Flow varies enormously from fasting to post-prandial (especially SMA).

Coeliac axis. Sharp systolic upstroke (narrow systolic window) with a very low resistance pattern (antegrade flow through the cardiac cycle). Typical PSV <125 cm/s. A significant stenosis (>70%): PSV > 200 cm/s, EDV ≥ 55 cm/s, mesenteric/aortic ratio >3.0. In addition, reversed flow in the common hepatic artery is always indicative of severe coeliac stenosis or occlusion.

SMA (fasting). Sharp upstroke (narrow systolic window) with triphasic morphology. There is a brief reverse-flow phase and little or no flow at end of arterial cycle. Typical PSV <125 cm/s. A significant stenosis (≥70%): PSV >275 cm/s; mesenteric/aortic ratio >3.0 and EDV ≥ 45 cm/s.

Renal artery assessment

High flow into a low resistance capillary bed and therefore there is significant blood flow during diastole (waveforms more pulsatile proximally and dampen distally). *The normal renal systolic velocity is 100–150 cm/s. A significant stenosis is PSV > 180–200 cm/s or renal-aortic ratio (RAR) ≥ 3.5.* PSV > 400 cm/s corresponds to a 90% stenosis.

In addition, the resistance index (RI) measured in an interlobar artery reflects diastolic flow and is calculated as:

$$RI = \frac{PSV - EDV}{PSV}$$

(Normal RI: 0.55–0.7)

Diastolic flow reduction is reflected by an increased RI (may predict response to revascularisation).

Renal access assessment

Pre-operative evaluation. Vein assessment includes compressibility, continuity (with the deep system, free from stenosis/occlusion and including the central veins) and minimal accepted venous diameter (>2.5–3 mm) for success. Arterial assessment includes patency, calcification, waveform, patent palmar arch, and absence of pressure differential between arms (>20 mmHg) and diameter (≥2 mm).

Post-operative surveillance. The proximal native artery above a surgically created arteriovenous fistula (AVF) is assessed as well as the AVF anastomosis. Important measurements include mid-graft and anastomotic PSV as well as the outflow vein and central veins. A normal graft should have pulsatile flow with low resistance and high diastolic forward flow. There should be a high amplitude (systolic and diastolic) with spectral broadening (similar to a stenotic ICA). Because of the high diastolic flow rates, the diastolic to systolic velocity ratio (Vd/Vs) is normally >0.4. A significant stenosis is present if it is <0.3. Volume flows in a fistula should be >500 ml/min. <450 ml/min is considered significantly stenosed. PSV (arteriovenous) >400 cm/s or ratio >3.0 also signify a stenosis.

Post-operative lower limb graft surveillance

Up to 20–30% of lower limb bypass grafts will develop a graft stenosis within one year of surgery and there is a high acute thrombosis rate with critical stenosis (>70%). The normal mean graft flow velocity is 60–70 cm/s, and this will be reduced if there is a significant stenosis (note: large [>6 mm] veins may have low, but normal, velocities). Salvage rates are much higher if the stenosis is revised before complete occlusion occurs.

The recommended Duplex velocity criteria for revision: PSV > 300 cm/s, Ratio >3.5 (pre-stenosis to stenosis) and Mean graft velocity <50 cm/s.

Figure 20.1 Layout of a typical hybrid angiography suite.

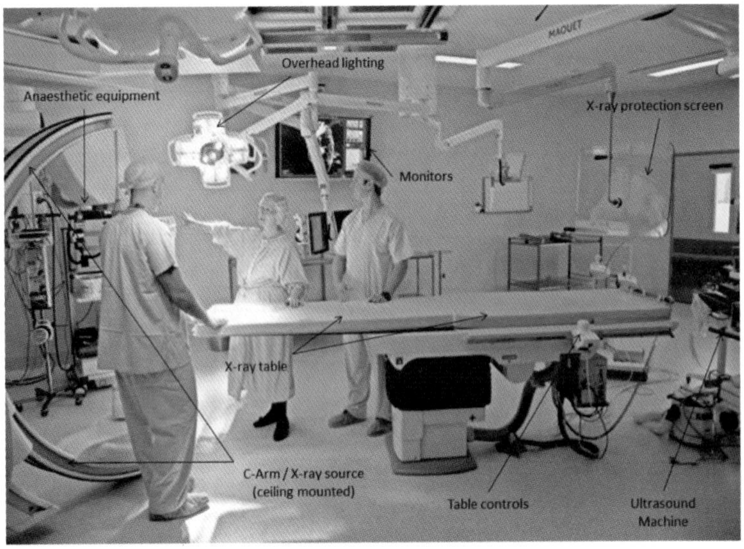

Figure 20.3 Potential side effects of intravenous iodinated contrast agents.

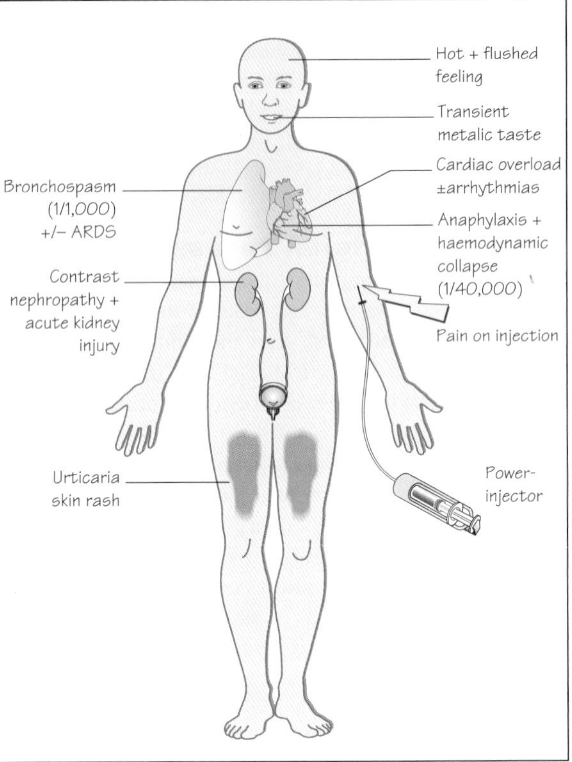

Figure 20.2 Layout of angiography suite.

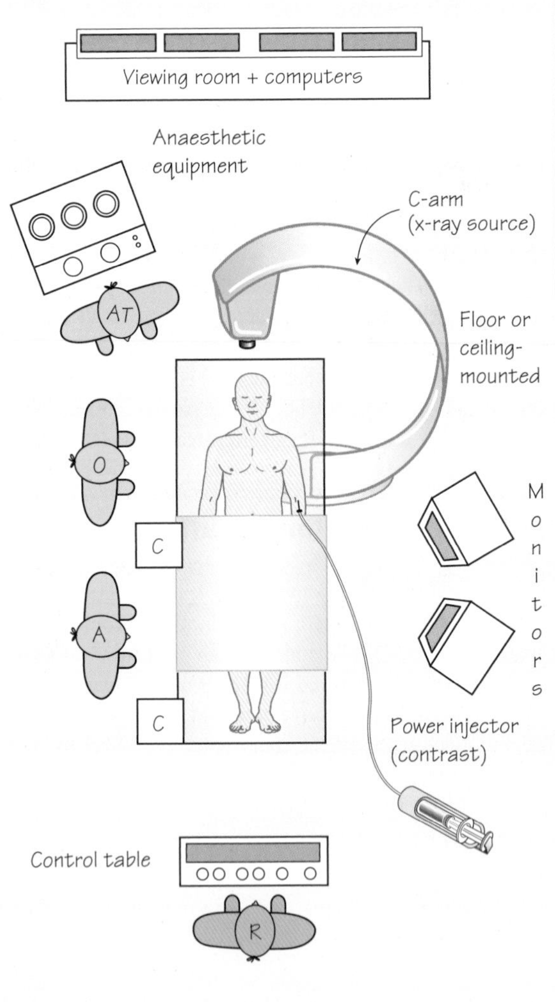

Table 20.1. Examples of commercially available contrast agents and their corresponding iodine concentration and osmolality. Ionic hyperosmolar agents give superior images (higher concentrations of iodine give 'denser' images) but have worse side effect profiles (more iodine atoms per molecule). Nonionic agents covalently bind iodine with less dissociation into component molecules, hence less side effects. In addition, nonionic compounds are more expensive.

Ionic			Nonionic		
Name	Iodine content (mg/ml)	Osmolality (mOsm/kg H_2O)	Name	Iodine content (mg/ml)	Osmolality (mOsm/kg H_2O)
Hypaque 25% (sodium distrizoate)	150	696	Ominpaque 140 (iohexol)	140	322
Hypaque 50% (sodium diatrizoate)	300	1550	Omnipaque 240 (iohexol)	240	520
Renograffin-60 (meglumine diatrizoate)	292	1549	Omnipaque 350 (iohexol)	350	884
Isopaque 370 (metrizoate)	370	2100	Visipaque 320 (iodixanol)	320	290
Hexabrix (meglumine ioxglate)	320	600	Optitray 320 (ioversol)	320	702
Conray-30 (meglamine iothalamate)	141	681	Isovue #28 (iopamidol)	128	290
			Isovue 370 (iopamidol)	370	796
			Oxilan 350 (ioxilan)	350	695
			Ultravist (iopromide)	370	774

Abbreviations: A, assistant; AT, anaesthetist (if required); C, controls (for table); O, operator; R, radiographer

Vascular and Endovascular Surgery at a Glance, First Edition. Morgan McMonagle and Matthew Stephenson.

Catheter-directed angiography is still the 'gold standard' in vascular imaging, but it is invasive (intra-arterial instrumentation) and therefore often reserved for those likely to require a simultaneous therapeutic intervention. Any stenosis identified (taken in at least two planes) is 'percentage' quantified according to the degree of luminal narrowing (50%, 75%, 90%, 100% [total occlusion]).

The angiography suite
This is a purpose-built room for diagnostic and therapeutic intervention often located in the radiology department, although in modern vascular practice the suite often doubles as an operating room (*hybrid suite*) located within the main theatre complex. The room must adhere to national radiation safety standards.

Personnel
- Operator (vascular surgeon and/or radiologist).
- Nurse assistant (scrub nurse/operating department practitioner).
- Radiology technician (radiographer).
- Anaesthetist (if anaesthesia or sedation required).

Equipment
- Fluoroscopy/X-ray equipment (with monitors).
- Angiography-compatible table.
- Power injector.
- Consumables (sheaths, wires, catheters, devices, etc.).
- Full anaesthetic equipment.

Basic steps in angiography
1 Access (vessel for instrumentation).
2 Travel (to vessel of interest).
3 Imaging.
4 Intervention.
5 Re-imaging.
6 Removal of access and haemostasis.

Radiation safety
Radiation exposure decreases proportionately by the square of the distance from the source.

The maximum permissible annual dose for adults is 5 REM (roentgen equivalent man) and is dependent on dose and exposure time with the most susceptible organs being eyes, thyroid, gonads and bone marrow.

Minimising radiation exposure
- Wear lead apparel: aprons, limb shields, neck collar, glasses, gloves.
- Maximise distance between X-ray source and operator, and aim X-ray source away from staff and close to patient to reduce 'scatter'.
- Limit the dosage and exposure time to short, intermittent 'bursts' while performing a manoeuvre or image.
- A dosimeter should also be worn by all X-ray personnel to measure annual exposure and record doses used for all procedures undertaken.

Contrast media (contrast agents)
- Iodine-based contrast agents (the most common).
- Carbon dioxide.
- Gadolinium.

Iodine-based contrast agents
Iodine-based (highly X-ray absorptive) agents are classified as ionic or non-ionic (organic). Complications are mostly due to the hyperosmolarity (290–2100 mOsm). Therefore, non-ionic hypoosmolar agents tend to be safer (e.g. Omnipaque™).

Potential side effects
- Pain on injection and 'flushed', hot feeling (due to hyperosmolarity) followed by metallic oral taste.
- Contrast-induced nephropathy (dose-related) ± cardiac overload.
- Non-dose related allergic reaction (Type 1) including rash, urticarial, bronchospasm (1/1000) and anaphylaxis (1/40,000). The risk is higher if co-existing shellfish or iodine allergy.
- Rare idiosyncratic effects: arrhythmias and pulmonary oedema.
- Lactic acidosis (rare) associated with metformin (exclusive renal clearance), especially with co-existing renal impairment. Metformin should be stopped prior to exposure (24–48 hours).

Contrast-induced nephropathy (CIN)
The risk peaks at 48–72 hours post-exposure and is defined as a rise in baseline serum creatinine >25% or 44 umol/L (0.5 mg/dL). The risk is higher in patients with pre-existing renal disease (Stage 3 chronic kidney disease [CKD] or estimated glomerular filtration rate [eGFR] <60 ml/min/1.73M^2), other co-morbidities (diabetes, dehydration, anaemia, congestive cardiac failure [CCF], hypoalbuminaemia), advanced age and addition of other nephrotoxins (ACEi [ACE inhibitor], cyclosporine, NSAIDs).

Reducing the risk of CIN
- Limit exposure and contrast volumes used (i.e. targeted images).
- Keep patients well hydrated pre- and post-procedure and stop any nephrotoxic agents (if possible).
- Use a non-ionic hypoosmolar agent (although recent evidence suggests this may not alter the incidence of CIN).
- Consider n-acetylcysteine (24 hours prior to exposure and 48 hours post-exposure).

Carbon dioxide
This alternative to contrast agents is reserved for patients with contrast allergy or severe renal impairment. It is injected manually in bolus form after which it is rapidly absorbed and exhaled by the lungs, and it is not associated with nephrotoxicity.

Although generally safe, it can cause 'air lock' in the mesenteric vessels or brain and is thus contraindicated for imaging of the aortic arch and branches or via arm access (risk of stroke). It is associated with poorer quality images, especially in small calibre vessels (e.g. tibial) because the CO_2 tends to scatter into bubbles upon hitting a stenosis as well as tending to rise (gaseous). Patients need to be positioned to allow it to flow effectively.

Gadolinium
A para-magnetic element (chiefly used in MRA) reserved for cases with previously documented contrast allergy. It is relatively safe (rarely associated with allergic reactions), but the most serious side effect is nephrogenic systemic fibrosis (NSF) (very rare).

Nephrogenic systemic fibrosis
This is a rare condition associated with gadolinium use in patients with pre-existing chronic renal impairment (especially Stage 4 or 5) or acute kidney injury (no cases have been reported with an eGFR >60 ml/min). Children <12 years are also at higher risk.

Onset can range from day of exposure up to 3 months and usually begins in the lower limbs (pain, pruritus, swelling, erythema) progressing to cutaneous and subcutaneous fibrosis (thickening) with painful contractures. It may progress to internal organ fibrosis (heart, lungs, liver and diaphragm) and death.

Figure 21.1 Basic steps and fundamental principles of angiointervention.

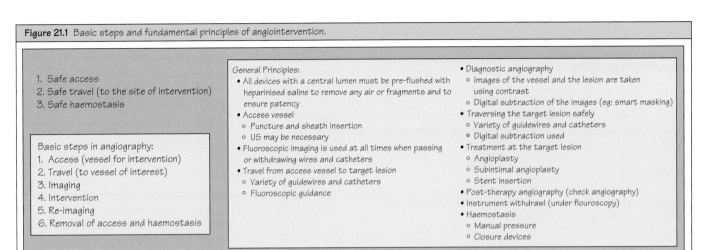

1. Safe access
2. Safe travel (to the site of intervention)
3. Safe haemostasis

Basic steps in angiography:
1. Access (vessel for intervention)
2. Travel (to vessel of interest)
3. Imaging
4. Intervention
5. Re-imaging
6. Removal of access and haemostasis

General Principles:
- All devices with a central lumen must be pre-flushed with heparinised saline to remove any air or fragments and to ensure patency
- Access vessel
  ○ Puncture and sheath insertion
  ○ US may be necessary
- Fluoroscopic imaging is used at all times when passing or withdrawing wires and catheters
- Travel from access vessel to target lesion
  ○ Variety of guidewires and catheters
  ○ Fluoroscopic guidance

- Diagnostic angiography
  ○ Images of the vessel and the lesion are taken using contrast
  ○ Digital subtraction of the images (eg: smart masking)
- Traversing the target lesion safely
  ○ Variety of guidewires and catheters
  ○ Digital subtraction used
- Treatment at the target lesion
  ○ Angioplasty
  ○ Subintimal angioplasty
  ○ Stent insertion
- Post-therapy angiography (check angiography)
- Instrument withdrawl (under flouroscopy)
- Haemostasis
  ○ Manual pressure
  ○ Closure devices

Figure 21.2 Basic steps to gain vascular access for angiography.

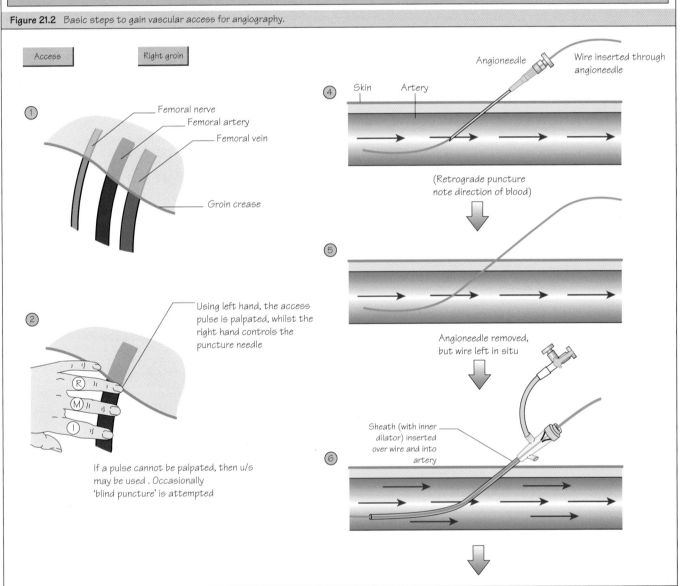

Access   Right groin

① Femoral nerve / Femoral artery / Femoral vein — Groin crease

② Using left hand, the access pulse is palpated, whilst the right hand controls the puncture needle

If a pulse cannot be palpated, then u/s may be used . Occasionally 'blind puncture' is attempted

④ Skin   Artery   Angioneedle   Wire inserted through angioneedle

(Retrograde puncture note direction of blood)

⑤

Angioneedle removed, but wire left in situ

⑥ Sheath (with inner dilator) inserted over wire and into artery

Vascular and Endovascular Surgery at a Glance, First Edition. Morgan McMonagle and Matthew Stephenson.

50 © 2014 John Wiley & Sons, Ltd. Published 2014 by John Wiley & Sons, Ltd. Companion website: www.ataglanceseries.com/vascular

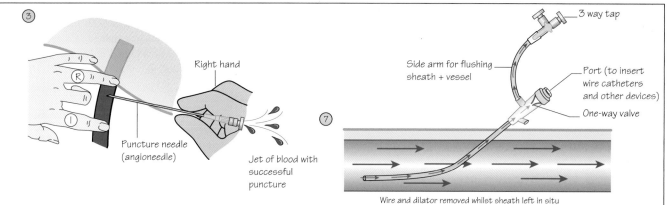

Abbreviations: ① normal arrangement of vascular anatomy in the right groin; ② the femoral artery pulse is palpated using three fingers on the left hand; ③ the middle finger is flexed to allow accurate puncturing of the femoral vessel with an angio-needle in the right hand; ④ while holding the angio-needle steady in the artery with the left hand, the guide wire is advanced into the vessel (right hand); ⑤ with the guidewire held steady in the vessel, with the left hand whilst maintaining pressure over the artery to minimise bleeding, the needle is withdrawn over the wire with the right hand; ⑥ the vascular sheath is then inserted over the wire using the right hand to gain access in the vessel. Blood should be aspirated and then the catheter flushed with heparinised saline to ensure accurate position and patency

Figure 21.3 Typical steps performed in navigating a tortuous vessel to access the diseased segment.

Wire + catheter navigation

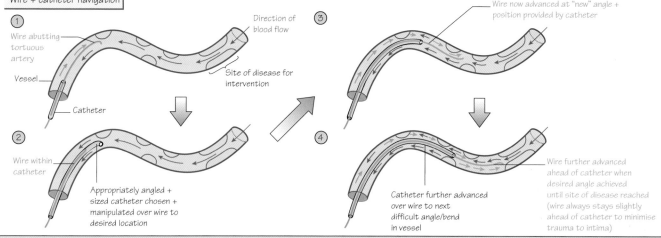

Figure 21.4 Typical steps performed to cross a diseased segment (stenosis) of artery.

Crossing the lesion

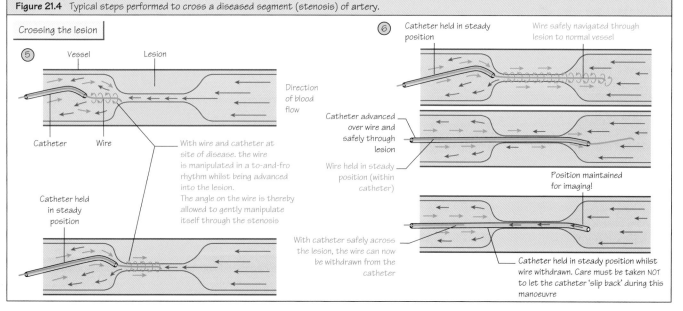

General preparation

• All previous imaging and history should be reviewed to identify the target vessel(s) for imaging as well as the access vessel.
• Identify any potential problems, especially renal failure, allergies and coagulopathy, and prepare appropriately.
• In general, antiplatelet agents do not need to be stopped.
• All devices for use should be pre-flushed with heparinised saline to remove any debris or air bubbles and to ensure patency.
• Risks of procedure include allergic reactions, haematoma, bleeding, pseudoaneurysm, dissection and limb or organ ischaemia.

Access and sheath insertion

• The access vessel is chosen (typically CFA) and manually palpated. (U/S is useful to locate an ideal puncture site if impalpable.)
• A small skin incision is created and the access vessel is punctured using a wide-bore angiography needle (use a soft part of the vessel).
• The puncture is typically *retrograde* (upwards against the flow of blood) but may also be *antegrade* (downwards in the direction of flow). Successful puncture is associated with pulsatile backflow of blood from the needle. Take care not to puncture the back wall or too high on the vessel (difficult to compress). Lower limb access is typically via retrograde puncturing of the contralateral limb.
• After successful puncture, a short semi-stiff wire (0.035 inch) is inserted through the needle into the vessel and the angio-needle removed taking care to keep the wire *in situ*.
• An appropriately sized, pre-flushed sheath (plastic access device) is then threaded over the wire and left *in situ* in the vessel for the duration of the procedure (typically 5–6 Fr sheath, 11 cm length).
• The internal 'dilator' is removed along with the wire after insertion of the entire device, but leaving the (outer) sheath within the vessel. This acts as a temporary port of entry for imaging and intervention.
• The sheath has a one-way haemostatic valve at the port site to allow wire and device insertion with a side port for flushing.

Travel to the target vessel

Travel to the target vessel is performed with a combination of guidewires and catheters to navigate tortuous angulated vessels. All manoeuvres are performed under fluoroscopy with the guidewire staying slightly ahead of the catheter to prevent vessel injury. It is also important that one or other always remains intra-luminal after crossing a stenosis until the end of the procedure.

Functions of the guidewire

• To navigate the vessel(s) to gain access to the target vessel.
• To add stiffness and rigidity for the insertion of rigid instruments.
• For 'exchanging' catheters and devices ('*over the wire*' [OTW] technique).
• To safely traverse the lesion.

Guidewire characteristics

• *Size* (diameter), *stiffness* (flexibility), *tip shape, length* and *coating*. Size is measured in inches (0.018–0.052" [mean 'working' diameter is 0.035"]) and length in centimetres (180–260 cm).
• The wire tip may be soft (floppy) and angulated ('J'-configuration) to aid navigation and prevent vessel injury (atraumatic tip).

• Hydrophilic wire coating (e.g. ePTFE) reduces friction, but makes it difficult to manoeuvre *ex vivo* (reduced *torqueability*).
• Stiffness is chosen according to the procedure and is determined by the inner core wire (*mandrel*). The mandrel is covered in an outer coil (*wrap*). Compliant wires cause less injury and are easier to manipulate, but stiffer wires are necessary for larger, stiffer devices.

Catheters

• Numerous catheters are available (depending on the intervention) that are size-matched to the wire.
• There may be one or two curves at the working end (including the primary curve [most distal] and secondary curve [more proximal]).
• The catheter is chosen according to the magnitude of difficulty (wire access in a vessel or lesion) and the specific procedure being performed. They are broadly grouped as flush catheters (for imaging), exchange catheters (exchanging wires, etc.) and selective catheters (difficult access and navigation).

Imaging

• All air bubbles must be flushed from the system and lines before administration to prevent air embolism and artefact on fluoroscopy.
• Contrast is injected using a power injector through a wide-bore flush catheter sequenced to fluoroscopy (e.g. 1000 psi at 20 ml in the aorta). Patients must remain still and a breath-hold is required for aortic imaging (diaphragmatic excursions will lead to artefact).
• Manual injection is used for targeted images close to the catheter position (smaller contrast volume (<10 ml) and low flow rates).
• A single 'mask' (non-contrast) image is taken and the X-ray source and table fixed in position. Any landmarks on the mask image serve as reference points for *digital subtraction angiography* (uses smaller contrast volumes). The mask image is 'subtracted' (faded or enhanced as required) from the contrast images to give artefact-free, sharper, contrast-only images.
• ***Road-mapping and smart masking***. Technologies allowing the 'background' contrast image to remain on screen; used in real time for visual navigation (wire + catheter) and intervention.

Sheath removal and haemostasis

Catheters and devices are removed OTW under fluoroscopy to avoid injury, followed by sheath removal. Haemostasis is achieved either *manually* or using a *closure device*.

Manual closure. Following sheath removal, manual compression is maintained for 20 minutes (activated clotting time [ACT] should be <160 s) and patients remain flat for 4 hours. In retrograde access, the arterial puncture (and compression) is higher than the skin puncture.

Closure devices. These are expensive and require training, but provide immediate haemostasis negating the need for prolonged compression, ACT measurement or bed rest. ***Non-mechanical closure devices*** apply a pro-thrombotic agent (e.g. collagen [e.g. angioseal™], polyglycolic acid [Exo Seal™]) for haemostasis. ***Mechanical closure devices*** use foreign body closure (e.g. Metal tag [Star Close™], suture [Perclose™]). They may have a lower incidence of post-procedure haemorrhage and pseudoaneurysm formation but associated complications include thrombosis, embolisation, foreign body infection, tissue adhesions (difficult surgical access) and nerve and vessel injury.

Figure 22.1 Various stents and their deployment: (a) stent deployed within vessel (b) balloon expandable stent (c) self-expanding stent partially unhoused for deployment.

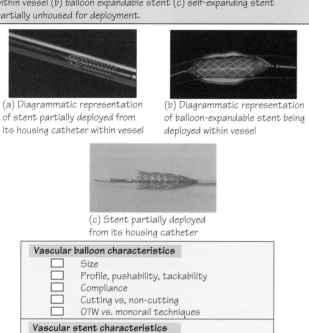

(a) Diagrammatic representation of stent partially deployed from its housing catheter within vessel

(b) Diagrammatic representation of balloon-expandable stent being deployed within vessel

(c) Stent partially deployed from its housing catheter

Vascular balloon characteristics	
☐	Size
☐	Profile, pushability, tackability
☐	Compliance
☐	Cutting vs, non-cutting
☐	OTW vs. monorail techniques

Vascular stent characteristics	
☐	Size
☐	Balloon expandable vs. self-expanding
☐	Metal framework (stainless steel, nitinol)
☐	Covered vs. uncovered
☐	BMS vs. DES

Figure 22.3 Steps in deployment of balloon expandable stents.

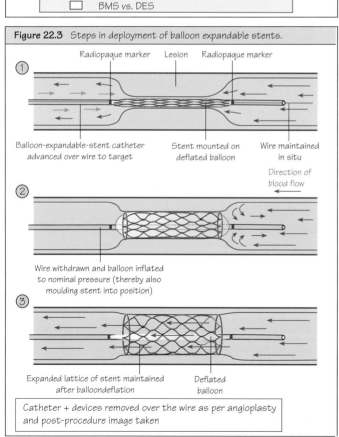

① Radiopaque marker Lesion Radiopaque marker

Balloon-expandable-stent catheter advanced over wire to target

Stent mounted on deflated balloon

Wire maintained in situ

Direction of blood flow

② Wire withdrawn and balloon inflated to nominal pressure (thereby also moulding stent into position)

③ Expanded lattice of stent maintained after balloon deflation

Deflated balloon

Catheter + devices removed over the wire as per angioplasty and post-procedure image taken

Figure 22.2 Steps in performing balloon angioplasty.

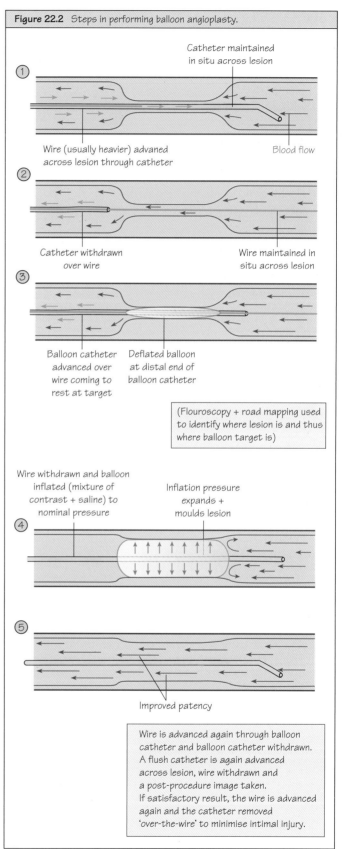

① Catheter maintained in situ across lesion

Wire (usually heavier) advanced across lesion through catheter

Blood flow

② Catheter withdrawn over wire

Wire maintained in situ across lesion

③ Balloon catheter advanced over wire coming to rest at target

Deflated balloon at distal end of balloon catheter

(Flouroscopy + road mapping used to identify where lesion is and thus where balloon target is)

Wire withdrawn and balloon inflated (mixture of contrast + saline) to nominal pressure

Inflation pressure expands + moulds lesion

④

⑤

Improved patency

Wire is advanced again through balloon catheter and balloon catheter withdrawn. A flush catheter is again advanced across lesion, wire withdrawn and a post-procedure image taken. If satisfactory result, the wire is advanced again and the catheter removed 'over-the-wire' to minimise intimal injury.

Abbreviations: BMS, bare metal stents; DES, drug eluting stents; OTW, over the wire

Vascular and Endovascular Surgery at a Glance, First Edition. Morgan McMonagle and Matthew Stephenson.
© 2014 John Wiley & Sons, Ltd. Published 2014 by John Wiley & Sons, Ltd. Companion website: www.ataglanceseries.com/vascular

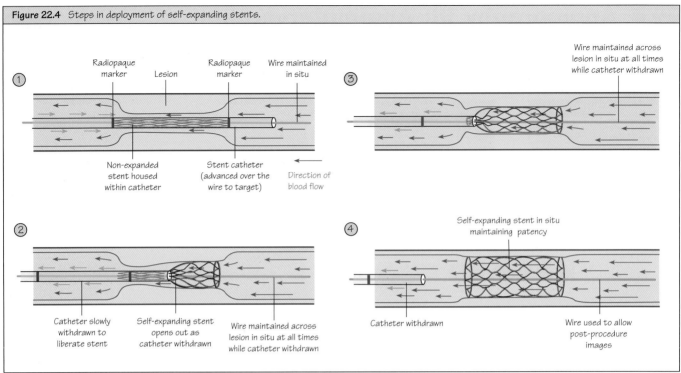

Figure 22.4 Steps in deployment of self-expanding stents.

① Radiopaque marker · Lesion · Radiopaque marker · Wire maintained in situ

Non-expanded stent housed within catheter · Stent catheter (advanced over the wire to target) · Direction of blood flow

② Catheter slowly withdrawn to liberate stent · Self-expanding stent opens out as catheter withdrawn · Wire maintained across lesion in situ at all times while catheter withdrawn

③ Wire maintained across lesion in situ at all times while catheter withdrawn

④ Self-expanding stent in situ maintaining patency · Catheter withdrawn · Wire used to allow post-procedure images

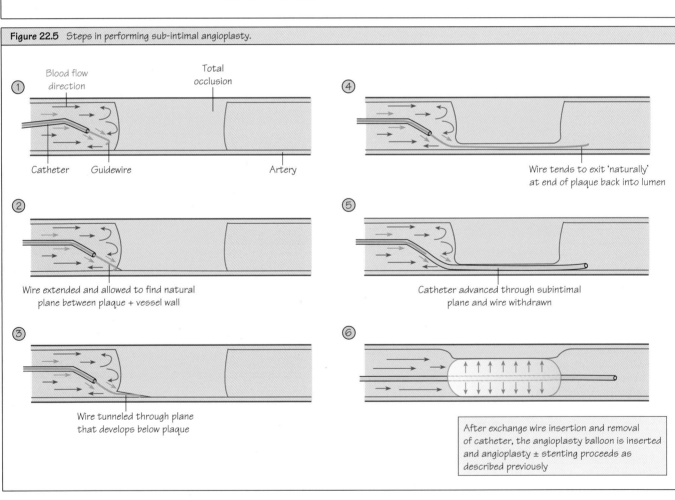

Figure 22.5 Steps in performing sub-intimal angioplasty.

① Blood flow direction · Total occlusion · Catheter · Guidewire · Artery

② Wire extended and allowed to find natural plane between plaque + vessel wall

③ Wire tunneled through plane that develops below plaque

④ Wire tends to exit 'naturally' at end of plaque back into lumen

⑤ Catheter advanced through subintimal plane and wire withdrawn

⑥ After exchange wire insertion and removal of catheter, the angioplasty balloon is inserted and angioplasty ± stenting proceeds as described previously

Preparation

Antiplatelet therapy in general should not be stopped prior to an intervention and all patients should be heparanised (e.g. 5000u i.v. bolus) during the procedure to prevent acute thrombosis. The risks are similar to catheter-directed angiography but with higher risk of acute thrombosis, dissection, haemorrhage and restenosis.

Interventions

• Angioplasty and subintimal angioplasty.
• Stent insertion (usually in conjunction with prior angioplasty).

Balloon angioplasty

• A vascular balloon is inflated inside the stenosis and the pressure physically dilates and moulds the plaque against the vessel wall thereby opening up the flow. This can be performed as a therapeutic measure alone or prior to stent insertion.
• The balloon is inflated to a pre-determined pressure using a hand-held pressure device (with manometer) and held for 30–60 seconds (repeated as necessary) followed by a check angiogram.
• Dilute contrast (25–50%) is used so that the balloon can be visualised under fluoroscopy, but pure contrast has a high viscosity requiring higher pressures to inflate and is slower to deflate.
• Sub-intimal angioplasty may be necessary in small vessels or where the stenosis cannot be crossed by the guidewire. Instead, the guidewire is allowed to find its own plane between the plaque and vessel wall, and to develop its own track after which it (usually) re-enters the lumen distal to the lesion. Angioplasty (±stenting) is then performed. There is a higher risk of rupture and pseudoaneurysm formation with this technique and patency rates are lower.
• Angioplasty is considered a *technical success* when ≤30% residual stenosis remains immediately after the intervention compared with the pre-angioplasty images. However, it is the flow below the lesion that is more important for a good functional outcome.

Vascular balloon characteristics

• Balloons are chosen according to *size, compliance, deployment method* and whether they are *cutting or non-cutting*.
• *Size* is determined by the balloon diameter when inflated, which is chosen according to the diameter of the vessel being treated. The *nominal pressure* is the application pressure required for inflation to the balloon size (3–10 ATM). Balloons also have a *rated burst pressure* (pressure at which there is a risk of rupture (e.g. 6–16 ATM)) and a *mean burst pressure* (pressure at which 50% of balloons will rupture [e.g. 10–27 ATM]).
• *Profile* describes the compatibility of the balloon around the wire (to reduce friction during vessel insertion and manipulation). *Lower profile balloons* allow easier accessibility to smaller diameters.
• *Pushability* describes the ease of advancement of the balloon catheter through the sheath, arterial tree and lesion. Hydrophilic coating enables better pushability. *Trackability* describes the ease with which the balloon catheter follows the guidewire.
• *Compliance* describes the expandability of the balloon beyond the nominal pressure diameter. Vascular balloons should have a *working pressure* labelled on them, which is applied to achieve the working diameter size. A *compliant balloon* can be inflated safely beyond the nominal pressure, is useful for moulding stents against the vessel wall after deployment (e.g. if there is a persistent leak) and therefore offers a wider range of workable diameters within a single device. However, these balloons also run the risk of overstretching and injuring the vessel wall (including rupture). *Non-compliant balloons* have the least amount of stretch beyond the nominal pressure. *Semi-compliant or controlled-compliant balloons* display intermediate compliance (linear relationship between the pressure and achievable diameter).
• *Cutting balloons* are characterised by a series of cutting blades (*atheromes*), arranged linearly along the balloon surface, which help to incise rigid, calcified plaque upon inflation.
• The majority of angioplasty balloons are *coaxial* (i.e. introduced via an *OTW technique* where the guidewire passes through the lumen of the balloon catheter). *Monorail* or *rapid-exchange catheters* are modified OTW catheters where the coaxial portion of the guidewire exits the balloon catheter somewhere along its shaft (instead of the end), with the more proximal shaft being wire-free (suitable for smaller diameter balloons in small vessels [e.g. tibial]). They have less pushability and trackability.

Vascular stents

Stents are small tubular, metallic framework structures that exert radial forces against the vessel wall to maintain patency. Usually they are deployed after initial angioplasty of the stenosis and may maintain patency over angioplasty alone (controversial!).

Vascular stent classification

Metallic framework. Numerous metals may be used in stent framework manufacture including stainless steel, nitinol (nickel-titanium alloy), tantalum, platinum and other alloys.

Coverage. *Covered stents* consist of a metal framework with interwoven synthetic material (e.g. Dacron, ePTFE). They are more expensive with poorer patency rates (in infrainguinal vessels) and are therefore used primarily in large vessels (e.g. aorta and iliacs) where flow outside the stent must also be arrested (aneurysms, pseudoaneurysms and active bleeding).

Method of deployment. Stents may be *balloon-expandable* or *self-expanding*. *Self-expanding stents* rely on their own recoil and intrinsic radial forces (after release from their constraining housing sheath [e.g. Wallstent, SMART stent]) to open a stenosis and maintain patency. *Nitinol* is the most commonly used metallic framework because it offers greater flexibility, elasticity and memory once deployed. *Balloon-expandable stents* are more *malleable*, come pre-mounted on a coaxial balloon and are deployed as the balloon is inflated within the vessel (e.g. Palmaz stent). They are more rigid and often made from stainless steel that offers superior radial force), but they are prone to crushing and fracturing if deployed in a vessel exposed to frequent mobility (e.g. popliteal).

Drug-eluting properties. *Drug-eluting stents* (DES) consist of a metallic framework coated with a polymer matrix that acts as a local reservoir for the delivery of high concentrations of an anti-proliferative agent (to reduce neointimal hyperplasia and restenosis) whereas *bare metal stents* (BMS) consist only of the metallic framework. Antiproliferative agents include rapamycin (sirolimus, arrests the cell cycle in the late G1 phase) and paclitaxel (inhibits cell replication in the G0/G1 and G2/M phases). Some specialised vascular balloons also display drug-eluting properties.

Adjuvant therapy

All patients should receive dual anti-platelet therapy after intervention (aspirin and clopidogrel). Clopidogrel may be stopped after 3 months but aspirin continued indefinitely. Occasionally long-term anticoagulation is required to enhance patency rates.

Figure 23.1 Vessel 'looping' (a) a sialastic loop (sling) is double-wrapped around the vessel above and below where surgery is to be performed. (b) the loops may be tightened by elevating them tightly. This occludes the blood flow (and hence bleeding) as well as elevating the vessel into the surgical field.

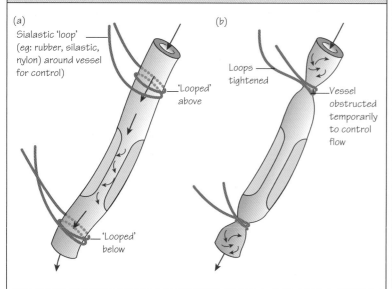

Figure 23.2 Endarterectomy. Plaque is carefully teased from vessel wall leaving smooth surface for re-endothelialisation. Typically the arteriotomy is closed with a patch graft anastomosis to reduce incidence of re-stenosis.

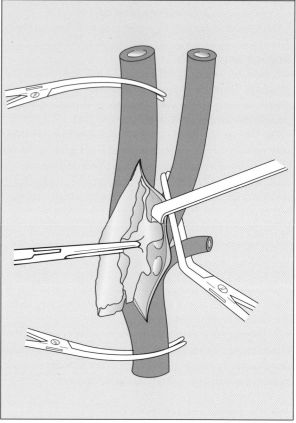

Figure 23.3 (a) Diagram of diseased segment of artery (e.g. common femoral artery) with reduced flow in the out-flow branches (i.e. 'run-off') (b) Illustration of typical bypass morphology using a reversed vein graft (note direction of venous valves). The vein graft effectively bypass the blocked segment of artery to restore blood flow distally. Note the different description for arterial anastomosis that may be used.

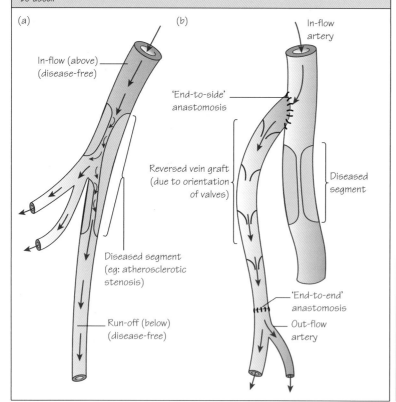

Figure 23.4 Typical arrangement of a surgical patch angioplasty. A patch (e.g. vein patch, synthetic patch) is anastomosed to the edges of an arteriotomy (opening) in the vessel, thus widening the lumen for enhanced flow and reducing the risks of re-stenosis and thrombosis.

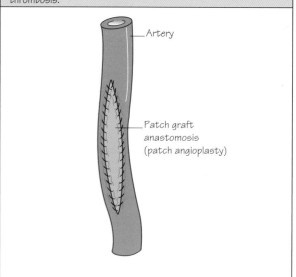

Vascular and Endovascular Surgery at a Glance, First Edition. Morgan McMonagle and Matthew Stephenson.

Successful graft function and longevity

- Good in-flow (above the disease).
- Good back-flow (i.e. run-off below the disease).
- Intermittently flush debris from vessels with heparinised saline.
- Systemic anticoagulation prior to clamping.
- Use of BMT (±anticoagulation).

Vessel dissection

- Proximal dissection and control first.
- Then distal dissection and control.
- Followed by dissection and control of the diseased segment.

Handling the vessel

- Minimally handling to reduce the risk of injury and thrombosis.
- Once vessel is opened, the intima should not be picked up with any instrument to prevent injury and thrombosis.
- For manipulation of the vessel, the adventitial layer can be gently picked up with forceps and manoeuvred.

Controlling the vessel

- A vascular 'loop' should be slung around the vessel (preferably looped twice) both above and below the diseased segment (i.e. 'looping' or 'Pottsing' the vessel).
- This allows both easy vessel manipulation and control of bleeding by lifting the vascular loops upwards, which in turn will 'snug-down' on the vessel.
- Large branches may be controlled in the same way, while smaller branches may also be looped but with a surgical tie (without actually tying a knot so as to preserve collateral supply).
- Appropriate-sized and angled vascular clamps may then be applied. Although these are atraumatic, clamp damage may still occur from fracturing the wall (especially calcified vessels) and intimal tearing.

Basic vascular surgical techniques

Anastomosis. Technique of suture repair of vessel (e.g. direct closure of vessel), graft patching a vessel (e.g. synthetic or vein) and vessel or graft sutured to vessel (vein–artery, artery–artery) to establish flow.

Endarterectomy. Technique of arteriotomy (opening a vessel [usually longitudinally]) and resecting the stenotic atherosclerotic layer from the vessel wall by developing a plane between the plaque and remaining tunica media or just leaving the adventitia. Often the arteriotomy will be closed using a patch graft to prevent restenosis.

Grafting. Technique of anastomosing a graft (e.g. vein, synthetic, patch) to a vessel to restore perfusion. This includes *interposition grafting* (graft is placed end-to-end to join two arterial segments after excision of the diseased segment) and bypass grafting.

Bypass grafting. Anastomosing and routing of a graft from above (in-flow) to below (run-off) the diseased segment (left *in situ*) to maintain perfusion below. The graft must be tunnelled in the tissues to gain access from above to below. The configuration of the anastomosis may be 'end-to-side', 'end-to-end' or 'side-to-side'.

Graft tunnelling. Bypass graft is tunnelled using specially designed instruments to create a new 'tract' within the tissues for the graft to lie in. Ideally, grafts should be tunnelled 'deep' within the tissues and

in a direct anatomical orientation (i.e. follow the same straight configuration as the normal vessel). However, they may also be tunnelled subcutaneously or sub-fascial or even non-anatomically.

Vein graft orientation. The vein graft may be *reversed* or *non-reversed*. If reversed, then the vein is harvested completely from its native bed, reversed in orientation (to overcome the valves) and tunnelled accordingly. The disadvantage of this is that there may be a size (and compliance) mismatch at the anastomosis. If non-reversed graft is used, (either left *in situ* or harvested completely but not reversed), there is less size mismatch, but the valves will need to be rendered incompetent using a *valvluotome* (risks missing a valve with increased thrombosis and restenosis rates). However, there is no convincing demonstrable difference in patency rates between reversed and non-reversed grafts.

A vein completely harvested from its natural bed has the theoretical risk of damaging its nutritional supply (risk of autolysis), whereas an *in situ* graft has a risk of AVF development (failure to ligate all tributaries that may not be apparent until maturation of the graft).

Material for grafting
Biological

Autogenous. These grafts are harvested from the patient and include vein (LSV (most common), SSV, arm (basilic or cephalic), deep vein (SFV), artery (rarely used)). Advantages include being cheap (free!) and without concerns of rejection. *Venous grafts are associated with better patency rates (LSV>SSV>arm vein) and are more resistant to infection than synthetic.*

Allografts are cadaveric harvests (cryopreserved vein or artery) and are expensive.

Xenografts (from animals) are rarely used for bypass, but bovine pericardium is frequently used in patch grafting.

Synthetic

Synthetic grafts are more expensive, but offer a good alternative when there is no autogenous availability. *Acute thrombosis rates are higher and patency rates lower with a higher incidence of graft infection in comparison to vein grafting.* Synthetic grafts may also have an external supporting framework to prevent compression.

Dacron. Multifilament polyester material, which may be 'knitted' or 'woven'. *Woven* grafts are rigid (difficult handling with reduced compliance) and prone to fraying, but with low permeability and good haemostatic properties. *Knitted* grafts (the most common) have superior handling characteristics but higher porosity levels and are therefore pre-impregnated with collagen, albumin or gelatin for superior haemostasis (older types were pre-clotted with native blood).

ePTFE (expanded polytetrafluoroethylene). An inert, hydrophobic polymer with high porosity properties. It has superior handling properties compared with Dacron but both have similar patency rates (ePTFE may have slightly lower infection rates).

Suture material

Prolene (on a vascular needle) is the most commonly used suture material (although ePTFE suture may be used with ePTFE grafts). For large vessels (aorta, iliac) use size 3–0, 5–0 for medium sized (carotid, CFA/SFA) and 6–0 or 7–0 for smaller (below knee) vessels.

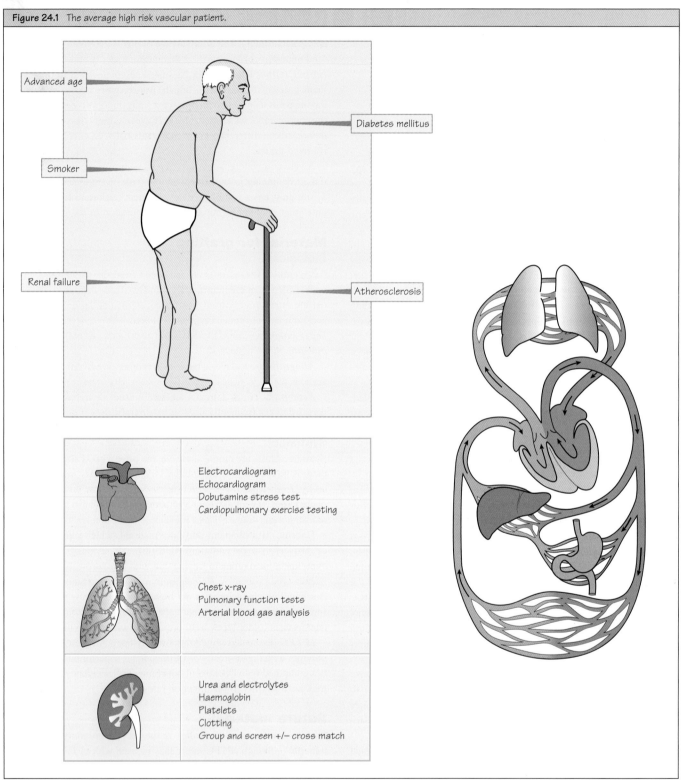

Figure 24.1 The average high risk vascular patient.

Advanced age

Diabetes mellitus

Smoker

Renal failure

Atherosclerosis

Electrocardiogram
Echocardiogram
Dobutamine stress test
Cardiopulmonary exercise testing

Chest x-ray
Pulmonary function tests
Arterial blood gas analysis

Urea and electrolytes
Haemoglobin
Platelets
Clotting
Group and screen +/- cross match

Abbreviations: ECG, echocardiogram

Vascular patients are generally **older**, more likely to **smoke**, be **diabetic** and have **generalised cardiovascular atherosclerosis**. This means they are likely to have accrued an array of co-morbidities related to these.

- Increased age:
  - higher cancer risk elsewhere
  - more frail
  - chronic kidney disease (CKD)
  - polypharmacy
  - more complicated social arrangements.
- Smoking:
  - lung cancer risk
  - ischaemic heart disease
  - chronic obstructive pulmonary disease (COPD)
- Diabetes mellitus:
  - increased risk of infection
  - visual loss (retinopathy)
  - diabetic nephropathy
  - neuropathy.
- Generalised atherosclerosis:
  - ischaemic heart disease
  - stroke
  - visceral ischaemia.

This latter point is fundamentally important to grasp – if a patient has peripheral vascular disease (PVD), they are very likely to also have coronary arterial disease and carotid artery disease. This means **your patient is at higher risk of a MI or stroke perioperatively**.

History and examination

Aside from the usual past medical history etc., be sure to focus specifically on identifying these co-morbidities preoperatively, so for instance:

Cardiac: Do you get chest pain? Do you get shortness of breath (SOB)? Do you get palpitations? Can you walk up two flights of stairs without getting chest pain or SOB (many anaesthetists consider this the most useful question)?

Carotid: Have you ever had a stroke (or TIA)?

Respiratory: Develop questioning about SOB. Do you get a cough? Do you need nebulisers? Do you need home oxygen? Have you ever been hospitalised for breathing difficulties?

Cancer risk: How is your appetite and weight? Explore a general systems enquiry.

Your examination must also focus on the heart, to identify valvular disease, cardiac arrhythmias, evidence of heart failure or cardiomegaly. Thoroughly examine the chest including oxygen saturation on air.

Investigations
Cardiac

All patients need a resting electrocardiogram (ECG), but remember you can have a completely normal resting ECG (even with three vessel coronary artery occlusion!), so it is not particularly helpful. The heart needs to be placed under strain to simulate the effects of increased physiological requirements during surgery to identify the patient's functional cardiorespiratory reserve. There are a variety of tests to do this such as:

- cardiopulmonary exercise testing
- dobutamine stress echocardiogram
- dipyridamole thallium scanning.

Most anaesthetists like to see a transthoracic **echocardiogram** preoperatively too, to assess the left ventricular function by looking at the ejection fraction (normal range 50–65%). It also helps identify valvular disease as well as regional ventricular wall motion abnormalities, which can indicate structural damage from a previous MI.

Respiratory

A **chest X-ray** is requested for all preoperative arterial cases. It identifies many pulmonary diseases and helps exclude co-morbid lung cancer, and if nothing else acts as a useful baseline for later comparison. Most anaesthetists will also want some form of **pulmonary function test** and if the patient has COPD or other chronic respiratory disease they should have a baseline **arterial blood gas**.

Laboratory

It has become standard practice to perform a range of screening tests for preoperative vascular patients. These are of varying value. The most important are:

- haemoglobin
- platelets
- clotting
- urea and creatinine
- electrolytes (mainly Na^+ and K^+)
- group and screen +/– crossmatch of packed red blood cells.

Optimisation

Maximising the patient's chances of an uneventful perioperative period requires careful planning and patient cooperation, which isn't always forthcoming particularly regarding this first point:

- **Stop smoking** – the earlier the better.
- Any co-morbid condition needs addressing (e.g. if a stress echo suggests coronary disease, a cardiological review should be requested for possible coronary revascularisation or other medical optimisation).
- **Continue antiplatelets** throughout the operative period – these patients are at high risk of perioperative coronary events and it is much easier to deal with a slightly more oozy operation than a post-operative MI. Don't miss a dose.
- Patients on **betablockers** should continue them over the perioperative period. Sudden withdrawal can result in adrenergic hypersensitivity.
- All patients should be on a **statin** and this must be continued throughout the perioperative period.
- **Blood sugars** should be well stabilised in diabetics. Knowing the HbA1C helps guide this.
- **BP** control should be maximised and all antihypertensives continued throughout the perioperative period.
- For those with respiratory disease: preoperative chest wall exercises should be taught and encouraged.
- Undernourished patients may benefit from additional **dietary support** preoperatively (e.g. with build-up drinks).
- Obese patients should ideally try to **lose weight**, but the reality is that this is rarely achieved.
- Patients should be **counselled** thoroughly about what they should expect post-operatively.
- Arrangements should be made early for **future discharge planning**, especially in elderly patients living alone. This avoids protracted hospital stays.

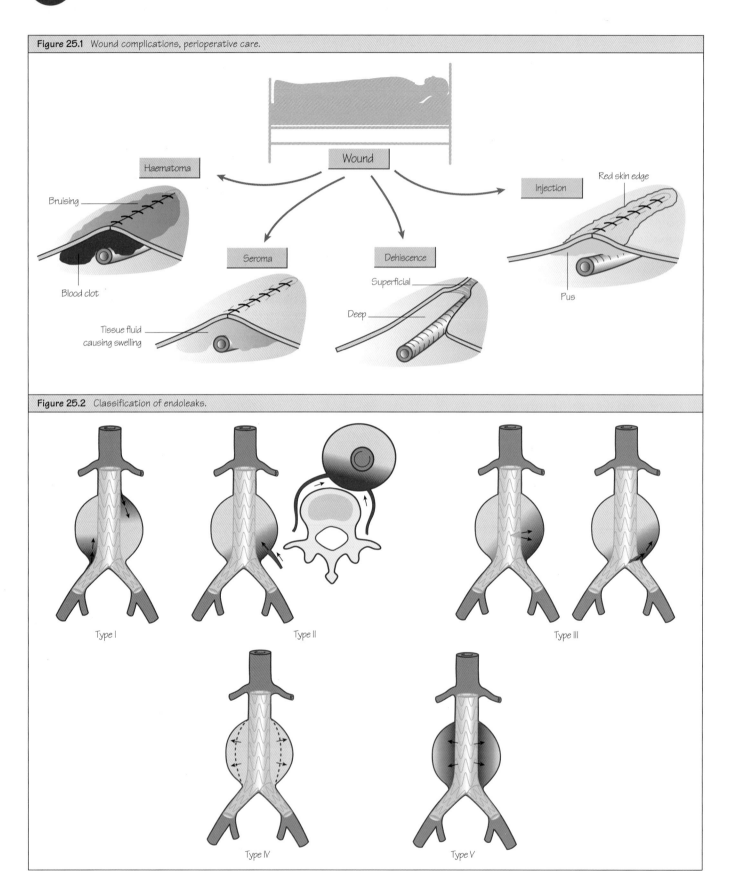

Figure 25.1 Wound complications, perioperative care.

Haematoma

Bruising

Blood clot

Wound

Seroma

Tissue fluid causing swelling

Dehiscence

Superficial

Deep

Injection

Red skin edge

Pus

Figure 25.2 Classification of endoleaks.

Type I

Type II

Type III

Type IV

Type V

Vascular and Endovascular Surgery at a Glance, First Edition. Morgan McMonagle and Matthew Stephenson.

General

As mentioned previously, vascular patients are at higher risk of post-operative MI – so take chest pain seriously. You will find the other general post-operative complications such as atelectasis, pneumonia, PE, renal failure, etc. in any other surgical textbook; here we deal with the specifics. One general risk to make a point of, though, is that vascular surgery is risky in terms of mortality: for instance, the risk during AAA repair is on average about 5%.

Wound complications

All wounds can develop these, but those at highest risk are groin wounds, particularly if made vertically.

- **Haematoma**: Essentially a blood clot, usually resolves spontaneously.
- **Seroma**: Especially groin because of injury to the abundant lymphatic tissue. Usually resolves spontaneously but may need aspiration.
- **Dehiscence**:
  - **Superficial**: Skin only.
  - **Deep**: Exposure of an underlying graft. This is very serious because the graft will become infected, which will be impossible to treat without its removal. These patients require very careful consideration if the graft is to be salvaged.
- **Infection**: Very important to treat aggressively, especially if prosthetic graft is nearby.

Specific
Open AAA repair

- **Rupture**: Leak from one of the anastomoses. Fortunately rare. Needs to be managed like any other ruptured aortic aneurysm.
- **Ileus**: Common in first few days because the bowel must be retracted.
- **Abdominal compartment syndrome**: Especially after repair of ruptured aneurysms. Occurs mainly because of bowel oedema. May require decompressive laparostomy.
- **Ischaemic legs**: Due to thrombus in the aortic sac embolising distally. May require emergency embolectomy in the post-operative period.
- **Graft infection**: More commonly occurs late (can be years later) and can present very non-specifically. Requires graft removal and revascularisation of the legs by either reconstruction of the aorta using the patient's deep leg veins or oversewing of the aortic stump and axillobifemoral bypass. Very major surgery.
- **Aortoduodenal fistula**: Another disastrous, usually late (years) complication. Always consider this in patients with gastrointestinal (GI) bleeding and previous aortic surgery. Is managed similarly to graft infection.
- **Incisional hernia**: Especially in aneurysm patients; probably due to a general collagen disorder common to both conditions.

Endovascular aneurysm repair (EVAR)

- **Endoleak**: Escape of blood around the stent into the aneurysm sac; there are five types:
  - Type 1: (A) Proximal (B) Distal. Leakage around the top or bottom of the stent. This is the most serious and needs to be treated, usually with further stenting, as soon as possible.
  - Type 2: Usually from lumbar arteries or the inferior mesenteric artery. Usually innocuous.

- Type 3: Between the various components of the graft. These usually need intervention.
  - Type 4: Leakage of blood through the stent wall. Usually innocuous.
  - Type 5: Leakage seen but source not identified.
- **Stent migration**: The stent can move or kink, which can occlude the lumen causing limb ischaemia.

Bypass graft

- **Occlusion**: three stages are often broadly considered:
  - Up to 6 weeks post-operative: technical error or poor run-off.
  - 6 weeks to 2 years: neointimal hyperplasia in the graft.
  - >2 years: progressive atherosclerosis in the native arteries.
- **Compartment syndrome**: In a leg that has been critically ischaemic pre-operatively; it can swell upon reperfusion, resulting in compartment syndrome that should be expeditiously or prophylactically managed with fasciotomies.
- **Swollen leg**: Almost all patients have a swollen leg after bypass surgery, sometimes forever. This is due to a number of factors: removal of an ipsilateral LSV, damage to lymphatic channels, especially in the groin, and improved perfusion. It is innocuous but may require elevation, especially early on to prevent wound dehiscence. If in doubt, request a venous duplex scan to exclude DVT.

Carotid endarterectomy

- **Stroke**: Usually embolic during surgery.
- **Cranial nerve injuries**:
  - XII: Hypoglossal – deviation of tongue toward side of operation.
  - X: Vagus – hoarse voice and dysphagia.
  - IX: Glossopharyngeal – dysphagia.
- **Hyperperfusion syndrome**: Rare; ipsilateral headache, seizures and neurological deficit associated with hypertension. On average 5 days post-operative. Significant mortality risk if missed.

Angioplasty

- **Arterial rupture** of the target lesion or elsewhere.
- **Complications in the puncture artery** (usually femoral):
  - Pseudoaneurysm.
  - Bleeding.
  - Dissection.
- **Embolisation**: Causing 'trashing' of the foot. Risk of limb loss.
- **Failure**: In general, angioplasty +/− stenting is less durable than open surgery.

Varicose vein surgery – open
- **Recurrence.**
- **Excessive bruising/thigh haematoma.**
- **Nerve injury** (especially SSV ligation).

Varicose vein surgery – endovenous
- **Recurrence.**
- **Bruising.**
- **Initial thrombophlebitis.**
- **Skin burns.**
- **Pigmentation of skin** over course of vein.

Figure 26.1 Signs and symptoms of stroke by vascular territory.

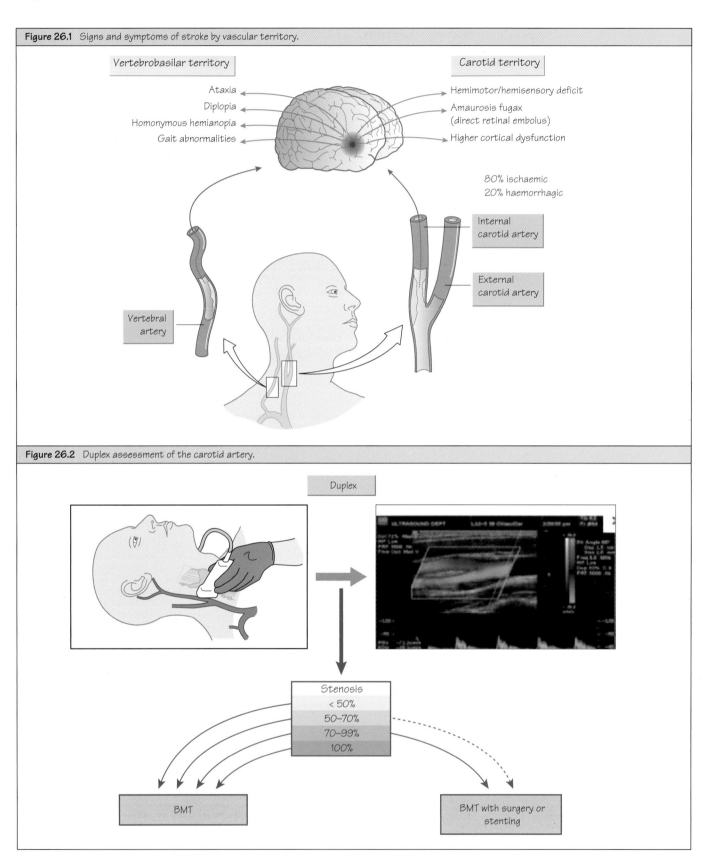

Vertebrobasilar territory

Carotid territory

Ataxia
Diplopia
Homonymous hemianopia
Gait abnormalities

Hemimotor/hemisensory deficit
Amaurosis fugax
(direct retinal embolus)
Higher cortical dysfunction

80% ischaemic
20% haemorrhagic

Internal carotid artery

External carotid artery

Vertebral artery

Figure 26.2 Duplex assessment of the carotid artery.

Duplex

Stenosis
< 50%
50–70%
70–99%
100%

BMT

BMT with surgery or stenting

Abbreviations: BMT, best medical therapy

Vascular and Endovascular Surgery at a Glance, First Edition. Morgan McMonagle and Matthew Stephenson.

Overview

After heart disease then cancer, stroke is the third leading cause of death in the Western world. 20% of strokes are haemorrhagic, 80% are ischaemic – mostly due to embolus but some due to small vessel disease in the brain and occasionally from prothrombotic disorders such as myeloma or sickle cell. Main sources of emboli:

- Left atrium or ventricle ('cardiogenic').
- Aortic arch.
- Middle cerebral artery.
- Carotid artery.
- Vertebral artery.

It is disease in the carotid artery that has relevance to vascular surgery. A stenosis in the carotid causes problems because there is potential debris that could embolise to the cerebral circulation (the reduced flow to the brain from the stenosis is of relatively little significance because there is good collateral supply).

The anterior and posterior cerebral circulation

The carotids serve the anterior part of the brain whereas the vertebral arteries serve the posterior part of the brain. It is crucial to establish if the patient's symptoms are from the anterior circulation (or carotid territory) or posterior circulation (or vertebrobasilar territory), because surgery may be offered for the carotid but not the vertebral.

Anterior circulation features

1 Hemimotor/hemisensory deficit.
2 Monocular visual blindness (amaurosis fugax).
3 Higher cortical dysfunction (e.g. dysphasia or visuospatial neglect).

Posterior circulation features

- Dysarthria.
- Diplopia/vertigo/nystagmus.
- Homonymous hemianopia.
- Ataxia/gait abnormalities.
- Bilateral blindness.

Lastly there are other features sometimes erroneously ascribed to carotid territory disease. These are non-specific:

- Collapse/loss of consciousness.
- Seizures.
- Headaches.
  So to summarise, it's essential to clarify that:
- the presentation is with carotid territory symptoms
- the symptoms are on the appropriate side to the stenosis:
  - **opposite** side for hemimotor/sensory deficit
  - **same** side for monocular visual loss
  - **dominant** side for higher cortical dysfunction (left if right handed, usually still left if left handed but may be right).

Investigations

All patients presenting with a stroke or TIA should have Duplex U/S of their carotid arteries within 24 hours (as an aside, a carotid bruit is of little clinical significance because it has low sensitivity and low specificity). This indicates the % stenosis.

- <50% – no indication for surgery.
- 50–70% – moderate benefit from surgery.
- 70–99% – significant benefit from surgery.
- 100% (occluded) – no benefit from surgery, because there is no flow to carry emboli to the brain.

All patients with a stroke or TIA should also have a computed tomography (CT) scan of the brain. Rarely, where doubt exists about the carotid Duplex, a CT angiogram can help, and where doubt exists about the nature of the cerebral symptoms or CT brain findings, an MRI of the brain may help.

Treatment

All patients should have BMT as a minimum, but those with a 70–99% stenosis should also undergo surgery, which is explained in more detail in Chapter 27. There is some debate about those with a 50–70% stenosis. You would need to do 13 carotid endarterectomies to prevent one stroke in this group (NNT = 13), compared with 6 in the 70–99% group (NNT = 6).

Non-surgical

- BMT (for all):
  - Stop smoking.
  - Antiplatelet agent (usually aspirin or clopidogrel).
  - Statin (irrespective of baseline cholesterol).
  - Control of hypertension (aim for BP < 140/90).
  - Control of blood glucose in diabetics.
  - Exercise.

Surgical

- Carotid endarterectomy.
- Carotid stenting.
  For details of the surgical options, see Chapter 27.

Asymptomatic carotid stenosis

In people over 65, up to 10% have a significant asymptomatic carotid stenosis. These patients are usually identified because of a chance finding of a cervical bruit, a private health check or when a stenosis is found following a stroke on the non-stroke side. There is considerable debate about the best management of these patients. The Asymptomatic Carotid Surgery Trial and the Asymptomatic Carotid Atherosclerosis Study broadly identified a small benefit, mainly in men and minimal in women (no benefit in women over 75). It is largely left to individual clinician and patient choice as to whether or not to offer surgery in addition to BMT.

27 Carotid surgery

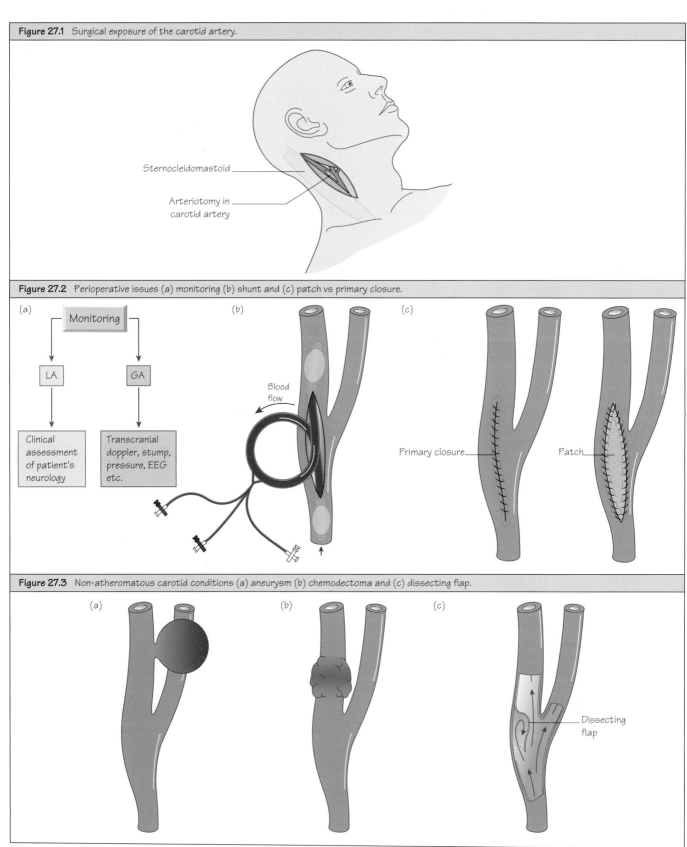

Figure 27.1 Surgical exposure of the carotid artery.

Sternocleidomastoid

Arteriotomy in carotid artery

Figure 27.2 Perioperative issues (a) monitoring (b) shunt and (c) patch vs primary closure.

(a)

Monitoring

LA

GA

Clinical assessment of patient's neurology

Transcranial doppler, stump, pressure, EEG etc.

(b)

Blood flow

(c)

Primary closure

Patch

Figure 27.3 Non-atheromatous carotid conditions (a) aneurysm (b) chemodectoma and (c) dissecting flap.

(a)

(b)

(c)

Dissecting flap

Abbreviations: EEG, electrocardiogram; GA, general anaesthetic; LA, local anaesthetic; pt, patient

Vascular and Endovascular Surgery at a Glance, First Edition. Morgan McMonagle and Matthew Stephenson.

Overview

By far the most common operation for carotid disease is for a significant carotid stenosis in the context of a stroke. Non-atheromatous carotid disease is briefly discussed at the end of this chapter.

Context

Carotid endarterectomy or stenting is indicated following a stroke or TIA affecting the carotid territory of the appropriate side. Carotid surgery is now considered an urgent treatment because it has become clear that a TIA can be a warning sign of impending further TIAs or major stroke; hence, in general, the sooner the carotid surgery, the bigger the risk reduction benefit. Within 2 weeks is considered acceptable. Beyond this the benefit reduces weekly, especially in women.

Carotid endarterectomy
Procedure

- An incision is made in the neck along the anterior border of the sternocleidomastoid muscle.
- The incision is deepened through platysma and fascia. The internal jugular vein is mobilised posterolaterally and its branches divided.
- The common, external and internal carotid arteries are dissected.
- The arteries are clamped and the patient's cerebral function is monitored.
- The artery is opened longitudinally (arteriotomy).
- The plaque, along with the intima and media, is dissected out of the artery, leaving only the thin adventitia.
- The artery is thoroughly inspected for loose debris.
- The artery is closed with or without a patch.
- The wound is closed.

Controversies

For a common operation with a huge amount of scientific data behind it, there is still considerable debate in carotid surgery. The principal controversy is how do you **monitor** the patient's cerebral function while the internal carotid is clamped? The vast majority tolerate this clamping without any ill effect because of collateral supply from the contralateral side via the circle of Willis; however, not all.

- **Option 1**: *Local anaesthetic (LA)* – the whole operation is performed under local anaesthetic with an awake patient.
  - *Pros*: allows gold standard continual monitoring of cerebral function because you can converse with the patient.
  - *Cons*: can be uncomfortable for long periods; doesn't suit all patients (or surgeons).
- **Option 2**: *General anaesthetic (GA)* – alternative arrangements are made to monitor cerebral blood flow/function; however, none are perfect:
  - Cerebral oximetry.
  - Stump pressures.
  - Transcranial Doppler.
  - Electroencephalogram (EEG) monitoring.
    - *Pros*: the patient has no intraoperative discomfort and some surgeons find it less stressful.
    - *Cons*: no continual monitoring of cerebral function.

The General Anaesthesia versus Local Anaesthesia (GALA) trial identified no overall benefit to either approach – it is up to individual surgeons and patients.

So what if there is intraoperative evidence of cerebral dysfunction during clamping? A **shunt** must be immediately deployed to restore flow from the common carotid artery to the internal carotid artery. This can be used selectively in patients under LA, but some surgeons use a shunt on all patients under GA to make up for the lack of a perfect intraoperative monitoring device; others trust their intraoperative monitoring and deploy shunts selectively.

- *Pros*: allows continued blood flow to brain throughout operation.
- *Cons*: can occlude or cause injury (e.g. dissection); makes the endarterectomy more difficult because it is in the way.

The last area of contention is the use of a **patch** to close the arteriotomy after the endarterectomy. If you close the artery with a line of sutures (primary closure), you necessarily narrow the artery slightly because you have to bring the sutured edges together. The alternative is to stitch a patch (usually bovine pericardium or Dacron) into the defect, which keeps it widely open. Some patch all carotids; some never; some selectively, based on size of the artery.

- *Pros*: reduces risk of restenosis and thrombosis, and may reduce stroke risk.
- *Cons*: operation takes longer and prosthetic material may get infected, which would be a disaster because it would need to be removed.

Complications

- Stroke or death: 5%.
- Cranial nerve injury: 5–10% (IX, X and XII resulting in dysphagia, hoarse voice or deviated tongue).
- Restenosis.
- Patch infection.

Carotid stenting

Angioplasty with stenting of carotid stenoses is still relatively in its infancy; however, a few centres have adopted it. It is still perceived by most to have a higher stroke risk. The femoral artery is cannulated, the catheter advanced to the carotid artery and a stent placed through the stenosis, usually with a cerebral protection device *in situ* (which prevents emboli that are dislodged from travelling to the brain). The procedure has a more mainstream role in carotid restenosis because re-do open carotid surgery is very hazardous and difficult.

Non-atheromatous carotid disease

- **Aneurysm:** rare. No agreed consensus about size at intervention. Presents most commonly with pulsatile mass, dissection or embolisation.
- **Dissection:** more common in younger patients and may cause a stroke. May be associated with head or neck pain and cranial nerve palsy. Can be spontaneous, traumatic or iatrogenic (during angioplasty). Vast majority managed medically by BP control and anticoagulation (to prevent thrombosis and stroke).
- **Tumour:** carotid body tumour, or chemodectoma. Rare. Presents with pain/compression symptoms/pulsatile mass/cranial nerve palsy; 5% bilateral, 5% locally malignant, 5% systemically malignant. Treatment – excision. Conservative if in elderly patient and benign.
- **Fibromuscular dysplasia:** very rare. Resection and interposition graft or angioplasty.
- **Arteritis:** as part of a large vessel arteritis such as Takayasu's. Treatment – steroids.

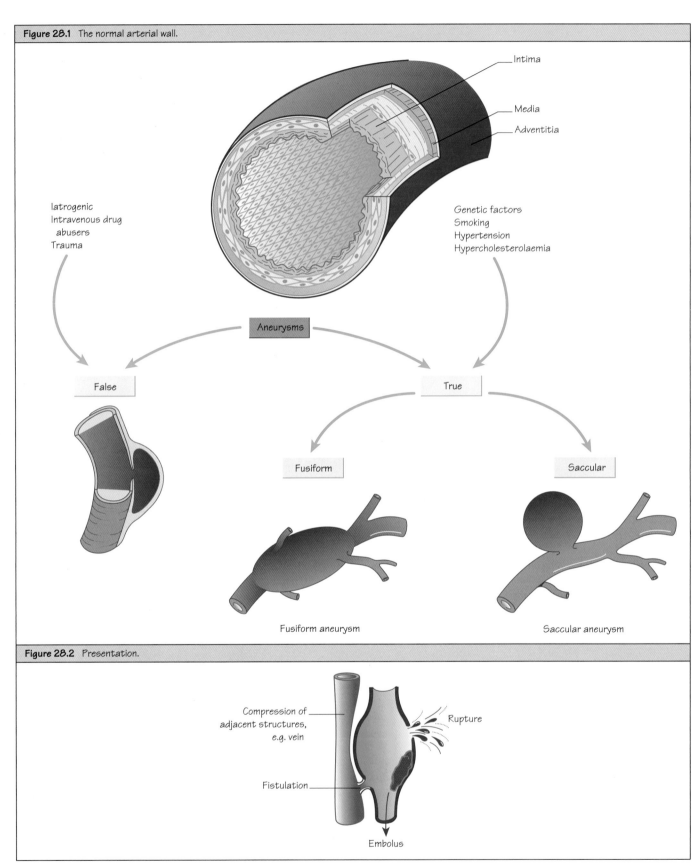

Figure 28.1 The normal arterial wall.

Intima

Media

Adventitia

Iatrogenic
Intravenous drug
 abusers
Trauma

Genetic factors
Smoking
Hypertension
Hypercholesterolaemia

Aneurysms

False

True

Fusiform

Saccular

Fusiform aneurysm

Saccular aneurysm

Figure 28.2 Presentation.

Compression of
adjacent structures,
e.g. vein

Rupture

Fistulation

Embolus

Vascular and Endovascular Surgery at a Glance, First Edition. Morgan McMonagle and Matthew Stephenson.

Definitions

An aneurysm is a localised dilatation of an artery by **greater than 50%** of the original diameter.

An increase of arterial diameter by less than 50% is termed 'ectasia'. Aneurysms can be either **true** or **false**:

• A **true aneurysm** is a localised dilatation of an artery including all three layers (intima, media and adventitia).

• A **false aneurysm** (pseudoaneurysm) is a contained sac containing flowing arterial blood communicating with the lumen of the artery through a defect in its wall. It is usually surrounded by haematoma and contained by surrounding tissues. It doesn't have any arterial wall layers.

True aneurysms

True aneurysms can also be divided into type:

• **Fusiform:** Wide in the middle and tapers at both ends, classically an abdominal aortic aneurysm.

• **Saccular:** May be almost spherical and projects from one point on the arterial wall; classically an intracerebral aneurysm, but still contains all three wall layers.

Common locations

Aortoiliac segment
• Thoracic.
• Abdominal.
• Iliac.
• Thoracoabdominal.
• Aortoiliac (abdominal aorta and iliac).

Neck and trunk
• Carotid.
• Splenic.
• Rarely: renal or mesenteric arteries.

Limbs
• Popliteal.
• Femoral.

Head
• Intracranial.

Aetiopathogenesis

Broadly speaking, aneurysms develop due to **degeneration** in the arterial wall as a result of metabolic disturbances of elastin and collagen, the full details of which are as yet undetermined. The most important known enzymes implicated are **matrix metalloproteinases** (MMPs), which are zinc-dependent endopeptidases. They are capable of degrading extracellular matrix.

Histopathological assessment of aneurysms also shows a **chronic inflammatory infiltrate** in the arterial wall.

A unifying hypothesis does not yet exist but it is likely to include a combination of polygenetic anomalies in MMPs with resultant degraded proteins in the arterial media, which might result in an inflammatory response, compounded by **local haemodynamic stresses**. This latter point is exemplified by the higher rates of aneurysmal degeneration in hypertensives. The principal modifiable risk factors are:

• smoking
• hypertension
• hypercholesterolaemia.

Presentation

• Mostly asymptomatic – discovered coincidentally.
• Presence of a pulsatile mass.
• Rupture (especially aortic and intracerebral).
• Thrombosis (especially popliteal).
• Embolism (especially from aortic and popliteal).
• Pressure on other structures.
• Inflammation (approximately 5–10% of AAAs have periaortic inflammation that may result in ureteric obstruction and/or pain).
• Fistulation (e.g. AAA into IVC or duodenum).

Management

The management of aneurysms depends on the site, size and morphology but essentially consists of:

• management of risk factors (especially hypertension and stopping smoking)
• surveillance of small aneurysms
• elective prophylactic operative repair for larger aneurysms:
  • open surgical
  • endovascular.
• emergency repair for symptomatic aneurysms.

False aneurysms

False aneurysms have a fairly unpredictable risk profile. With arterial pressure flowing through them, they have only the surrounding tissues to prevent massive blood loss. By far the most common causes are iatrogenic or related to drug misuse.

Iatrogenic

• **Angiography** following radiological or cardiological procedures. Risk factors include if the femoral artery wasn't compressed sufficiently following catheter withdrawal, if the artery was heavily diseased with calcium/plaque, or if the sheath used was large.

• **Central lines**, which may have been inadvertently inserted into the artery instead of an intended vein, or from arterial lines. Occur mainly because insufficient pressure has been applied following withdrawal.

Intravenous drug abusers (IVDUs)

When IVDUs have run out of available veins, they may try to inject an artery (with potentially catastrophic embolic consequences) or they may inadvertently hit an artery next to a vein. The femoral artery is the most common. The added complication is that these are frequently infected (because of poor hygiene and unclean needles) resulting in an infected pseudoaneurysm that can make the patient extremely unwell. Always beware a groin abscess in an IVDU – do Duplex U/S to confirm no communication with the femoral artery. The surgical management of these is generally ligation of the femoral artery because the infection destroys the artery, making repair impossible. These patients therefore have a risk of limb ischaemia post-operatively if arterial reconstruction was not possible, although it is surprising how many still have a pink foot despite ligation of the femoral artery!

Figure 29.1 Aneurysmal development and complications.

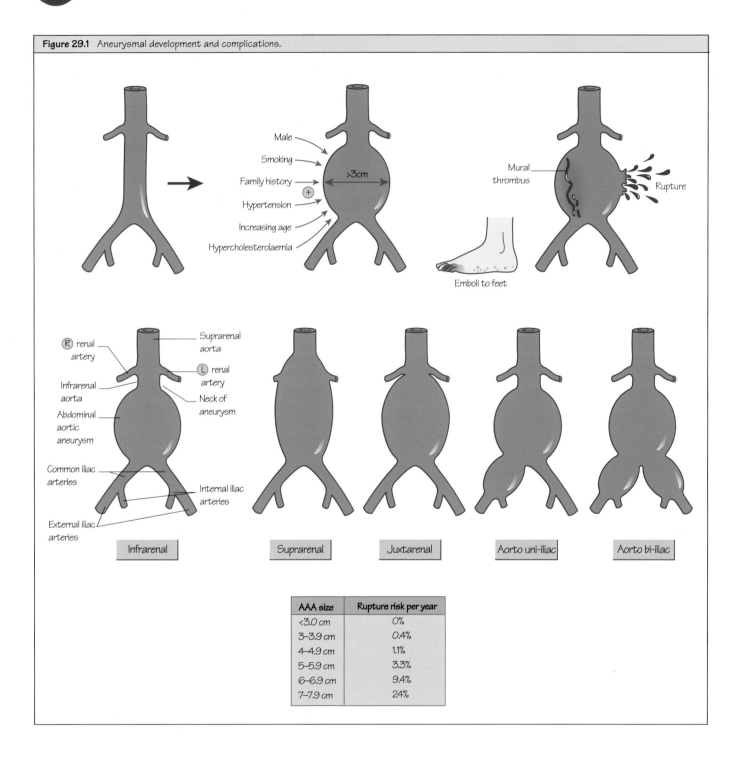

AAA size	Rupture risk per year
<3.0 cm	0%
3–3.9 cm	0.4%
4–4.9 cm	1.1%
5–5.9 cm	3.3%
6–6.9 cm	9.4%
7–7.9 cm	24%

Vascular and Endovascular Surgery at a Glance, First Edition. Morgan McMonagle and Matthew Stephenson.

The most common aneurysm in general vascular practice is the abdominal aortic aneurysm (AAA). The normal maximum aortic diameter is about 2 cm, so 3 cm is taken to be the minimum size for it to be aneurysmal; 2–3 cm is ectatic.

Key facts:
- Approximately 8% of men over the age of 65 have an AAA.
- Men are affected 6 times more often than women.
- Caucasians are affected more than Asians or Africans.
- Five per cent of people with an AAA also have a popliteal aneurysm.
- The vast majority of AAAs are infrarenal (i.e. below the renal arteries). Fewer than 10% involve the suprarenal aorta and these are much more difficult to treat. Juxtarenal AAAs are technically infrarenal; however, they are aneurysmal right up to the renal arteries with no normal diameter neck.
- AAAs may extend into the iliac arteries.
- Five to ten per cent of AAAs have an inflammatory wall and are called 'inflammatory aneurysms', characterised by marked thickening of the aneurysmal wall and often retroperitoneal fibrosis.

Aetiology/risk factors
For pathogenesis, see Chapter 28.
- Male.
- Increasing age.
- Family history.
- Smoking.
- Hypertension.
- Hypercholesterolaemia.

Presentation
Occasionally a thin patient will self-diagnose an AAA after discovering a pulsatile lump in their abdomen, or during examination or investigation for something else by their doctor. These are effectively asymptomatic and this accounts for the vast majority of AAA presentations. Occasionally, however, AAA may present with:
- **low back pain**/vague abdominal discomfort; this is more common if the aneurysm is inflammatory
- **emboli** to feet (thrombus in the aortic sac), also called '**trashing**'.

But the real risk is of **aneurysm rupture** resulting in severe abdominal pain radiating to the back with massive blood loss and collapse of the circulatory system resulting in unconsciousness. If the aneurysm ruptures posteriorly, this may then be followed by a period of relative calm as the surrounding tissues tamponade the leak. However, this inevitably fails eventually within a few hours and the patient exsanguinates. If the aneurysm ruptures anteriorly, there is little to contain the leak and the patient usually dies within minutes with no opportunity for treatment.

It is during the golden moments when the posterior rupture is temporarily tamponaded that the situation may be salvageable with immediate surgery.

Uncommonly, AAAs can fistulate into the duodenum or IVC. However, this is usually following repair of an AAA with a graft that becomes infected.

Investigation
In the elective setting where the AAA is asymptomatic or causing mild symptoms, an **abdominal U/S** will allow the maximum size to be assessed. When the AAA is greater than 5.5 cm and surgery is considered, a **CT aortogram** will allow accurate morphological assessment to plan surgery. No other investigations are required specifically for the AAA; other investigations are directed at assessing fitness for surgery.

Surveillance
Small aneurysms (<5.5 cm) can be managed expectantly by repeat U/S usually on a 6-monthly basis unless they are enlarging rapidly, in which case they are followed 3 monthly. The annual aneurysm rupture risk is shown in Table 29.1.

Because the operative mortality risk of AAA repair is roughly 5%, 5.5 cm has been arbitrarily defined as the threshold at which the intended benefits of operation outweigh the risks of leaving it. The UK Small Aneurysm Trial and US Aneurysm Detection and Management Trial have shown no benefit in repairing small aneurysms. The only indications for operative repair of small AAAs are:
- rapid expansion in size (>1 cm in 1 year)
- symptomatic
- occasionally when the AAA has a more saccular morphology because these are more likely to rupture (they are usually fusiform)
- emboli.

Screening
The Multicentre Aneurysm Screening Study showed evidence that aneurysm-related death could be reduced by screening people aged between 65 and 74. Screening for AAA in the UK is now being rolled out nationwide by the NHS. Men aged 65 or over are eligible. When men turn 65, they are invited for a one-off U/S scan.
- If they have no AAA, they are not invited back. They are unlikely to develop a significantly sized one over the rest of their lives.
- If they have a small AAA, they enter a local surveillance program.
- If they have an AAA >5.5 cm, they are referred for surgical consultation.

Patients aged between 65 and 74 who feel they have missed out can also attend screening if they wish.

Treatment
Non-ruptured
- Non-surgical: in those too unfit for surgery or who decline it.
- Surgical:
  - Open repair.
  - EVAR.

Ruptured
- Palliative: in those too unfit to contemplate surgery.
- Surgical:
  - Open repair.
  - EVAR.

For further details of aneurysm repair, see Chapter 30.

Figure 30.1 AAA management.

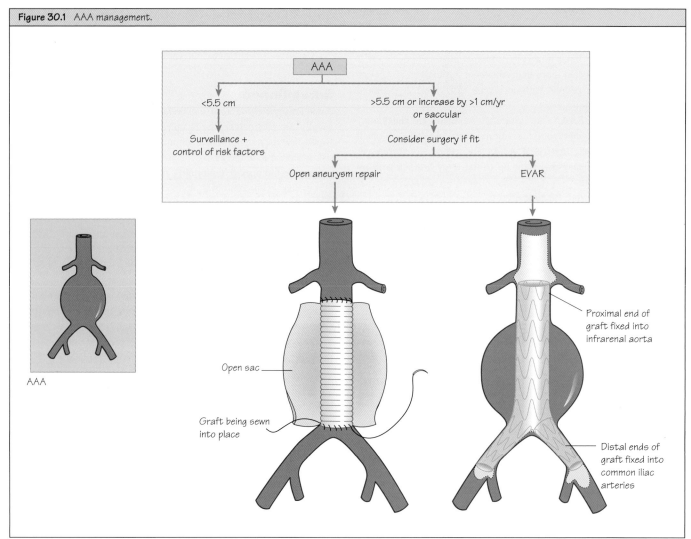

Abbreviations: AAA, abdominal aortic aneurysm; EVAR, endovascular aneurysm reapir

Vascular and Endovascular Surgery at a Glance, First Edition. Morgan McMonagle and Matthew Stephenson.

70   © 2014 John Wiley & Sons, Ltd. Published 2014 by John Wiley & Sons, Ltd. Companion website: www.ataglanceseries.com/vascular

The management of AAA has changed dramatically particularly following the first successful attempt at EVAR by Parodi in 1991. EVAR has now become the first-line surgical option in many vascular units and has been the subject of two large famous British multicentre randomised controlled trials. While there were several drawbacks and caveats to these studies, these are the principal points:

- **EVAR-1 Trial:** 1082 fit patients with AAA suitable for either open repair or EVAR; 30-day mortality was 4.7% versus 1.7% respectively, although there was a higher rate of late complications (mainly stent related) with EVAR. Although aneurysm-related mortality was slightly lower in the EVAR group, over time, all-cause mortality was no different.
- **EVAR-2 Trial:** 338 medically unfit patients with AAA who were suitable for either open repair or EVAR but not fit for open repair. The patients were therefore randomised between EVAR and BMT. There was no difference in mortality between the groups. See Chapter 66 for more on these.

Elective versus rupture

An **elective** repair should generally be planned when the AAA is larger than 5.5 cm with a CT aortogram to assess the morphological suitability for EVAR. The patient should also be assessed for physiological fitness with the usual preoperative tests but also assessment of cardiac and respiratory function with investigations such as:

- cardiopulmonary exercise testing (CPEX)
- echocardiogram
- lung function tests.

In the **ruptured** setting, attention is directed to confirming the diagnosis and stabilising the patient for immediate surgery. Often the diagnosis is made clinically without any specific tests. If the patient is too unstable, they should not have a CT scan but proceed directly to theatre. If the patient is stable, a CT aortogram confirms the diagnosis and assesses suitability for emergency EVAR, when available. Management should proceed with the help of the anaesthetic staff to commence invasive arterial monitoring and venous access. Resuscitation should allow **permissive hypotension** (i.e. do not try to restore normal BP with i.v. fluids because this may burst the tamponaded leak). Blood transfusion is usually saved until the AAA is clamped in theatre and ideally is performed using autologous blood transfusion (i.e. the blood that is suctioned out of the abdomen is filtered and transfused back).

Open surgical repair
Procedure
- The patient is supine under GA.
- A long midline laparotomy is made.
- The small bowel is mobilised to the right.
- The duodenojejunal flexure is mobilised to the right.
- The AAA is dissected at the neck superiorly and the iliacs inferiorly.
- The AAA is clamped superiorly and inferiorly.
- A longitudinal arteriotomy is made and the sac thrombus removed.
- The graft is sutured in superiorly then distally with end-to-end anastomoses.
- The sac is closed over the graft.
- The abdomen is closed.

Recovery and long term
- Physiologically challenging operation and recovery.
- Average post-operative stay 7–10 days.

- Following surgery, the AAA is effectively cured with usually only one follow-up appointment necessary; no further imaging.

Complications
- Immediate:
  - Haemorrhage.
  - MI.
  - Death.
- Early:
  - Haemorrhage.
  - Ileus.
  - Ischaemic colitis.
  - Cardiorespiratory complications including MI.
  - Renal failure.
  - Wound infection.
- Late:
  - Incisional hernia.
  - Late graft infection (can be years after).

EVAR
Procedure
- The patient is supine under GA, epidural or even LA.
- Two small groin wounds are made.
- The common femoral arteries are dissected out and clamped proximally and distally.
- The femoral arteries are cannulated with the Seldinger technique and a sheath and catheter inserted into the thoracic aorta.
- An angiogram is taken of the AAA.
- The main body of the stent is passed up one side on a delivery system.
- The opposite limb of the graft is inserted through the contralateral artery and negotiated into the main body of the stent.
- The graft is usually moulded into place with a balloon.
- A completion angiogram is taken to confirm position and no leak.
- The wires, sheaths and delivery system are withdrawn.
- The femoral arteries are closed.

Recovery and long term
- Quick recovery with less physiological burden.
- Usually home the next day or the day after.
- Back to usual activities quickly.
- However, because the stent may move resulting in leakage into the sac (endoleak) – requires lifelong surveillance with regular imaging +/– revision of the stent.

Complications
- Immediate:
  - Aneurysm rupture with conversion to open (rare).
  - Haemorrhage.
  - Stent misplacement (e.g. covering renal artery).
  - MI.
  - Death.
- Early:
  - Contrast nephropathy.
  - Endoleak (see Chapter 25 for more details).
- Late:
  - Endoleak.
  - Stent migration.
  - Infection.

Figure 31.1 Non-aortic aneurysms.

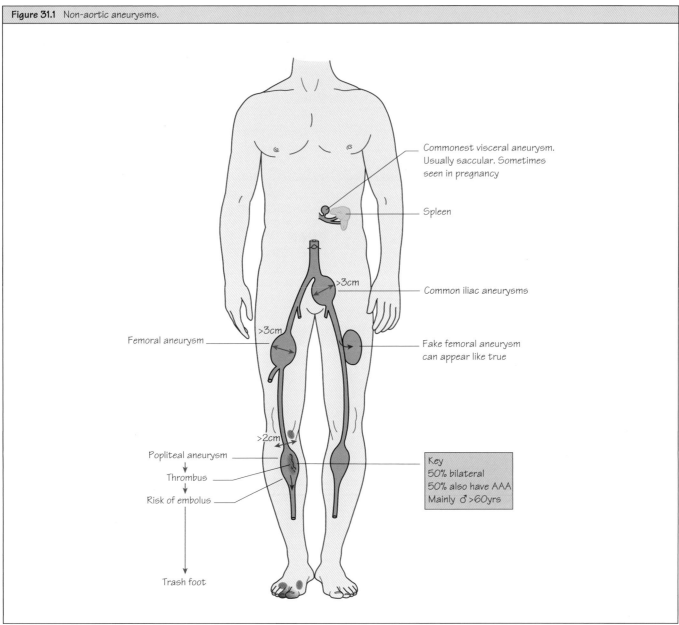

Commonest visceral aneurysm. Usually saccular. Sometimes seen in pregnancy

Spleen

Common iliac aneurysms

>3cm

Femoral aneurysm

>3cm

Fake femoral aneurysm can appear like true

>2cm

Popliteal aneurysm
↓
Thrombus
↓
Risk of embolus

Key
50% bilateral
50% also have AAA
Mainly ♂ >60yrs

↓

Trash foot

Abbreviations: AAA, abdominal aortic aneurysms

Vascular and Endovascular Surgery at a Glance, First Edition. Morgan McMonagle and Matthew Stephenson.

Thoracic and thoracoabdominal aortic aneurysms will be discussed in Chapter 33 and carotid aneurysms were discussed in Chapter 27.

Popliteal
Key facts
- The most common peripheral aneurysm.
- Fifty per cent are bilateral.
- Fifty per cent also have an AAA.
- Mainly men in their 60s.

Presentation
The key thing to understand is that popliteal aneurysms rarely rupture: they thrombose acutely, resulting in a severely ischaemic foot that requires emergency bypass. They may also present with:
- a pulsatile mass behind knee
- emboli to foot (trashing).

Investigation
- Duplex U/S to size.
- CT or MR angiogram.

Treatment
- No definite consensus on size before intervention but most say >2 cm diameter because the risk of thrombosis becomes higher the larger the aneurysm.
- For small aneurysms or while awaiting repair, antiplatelets or even anticoagulation to reduce risk of thrombosis.
- Repair electively is either by ligation of the aneurysm above and below with femoral–popliteal/distal bypass or to open the aneurysm and insert an interposition graft, like an AAA.
- Increasingly popliteal aneurysms are being treated with stents by an endovascular approach; however, the natural flexion and extension of the knee places great stresses on such a stent.
- Repair in emergency for acute thrombosis – femoral–popliteal/distal bypass.

Iliac
Key facts
- Usually in association with aortic aneurysm but occasionally in isolation.
- No definite consensus on size before intervention but most say >3 cm.
- Usually affects common iliac or internal, rarely external.

Investigation
- Duplex may not visualise well if overlying bowel gas.
- CT angiogram shows morphology and size accurately.

Treatment
- When combined with aortic aneurysm, managed as part of the treatment for that.
- When isolated, usually amenable to EVAR.

- When treated with EVAR, the internal iliac origin may be covered although this is best avoided, especially if bilateral, because the internal iliac supplies the pelvis and gluteal region.

Common femoral
Key facts
- By far the most common femoral aneurysm is the false aneurysm, which is usually iatrogenic; true aneurysms are relatively uncommon.
- Two per cent of patients with AAA have a femoral artery aneurysm.
- Mainly elderly men (M:F = 30:1).
- Often bilateral.
- No definite consensus on size before intervention but most say >3 cm.

Presentation
- Pulsatile mass in groin.
- Leg swelling if compresses adjacent femoral vein.
- Rupture is rare.
- Emboli to foot.

Treatment
- Usually best managed by opening and inserting a short interposition graft.

Visceral
Key facts
- Uncommon aneurysms that can affect a variety of visceral vessels but mainly (60%) the splenic artery; the hepatic artery is the second most common.
- Splenic artery aneurysms are associated with pregnancy and may rupture in the third trimester.

Presentation
- Usually asymptomatic.
- Can form thrombus in the sac that can embolise and cause gut ischaemia.
- No definite consensus on size before intervention; managed on case-by-case basis.

Treatment
- Usually by endovascular approach with stenting or coiling of the aneurysm (because these aneurysms are mostly saccular).

Other
- **Subclavian aneurysms** are uncommon and usually caused by thoracic outlet compression with resultant post-stenotic dilatation. Generally managed by open surgery.
- Other upper limb aneurysms are extremely rare.
- **Renal artery aneurysms** are rare, usually asymptomatic, frequently associated with hypertension and commonly treated by endovascular coiling because they are usually saccular.
- **Intracranial aneurysms** are managed by neurosurgeons and are therefore not discussed further here.

32 Thoracic aortic disease I: Dissection

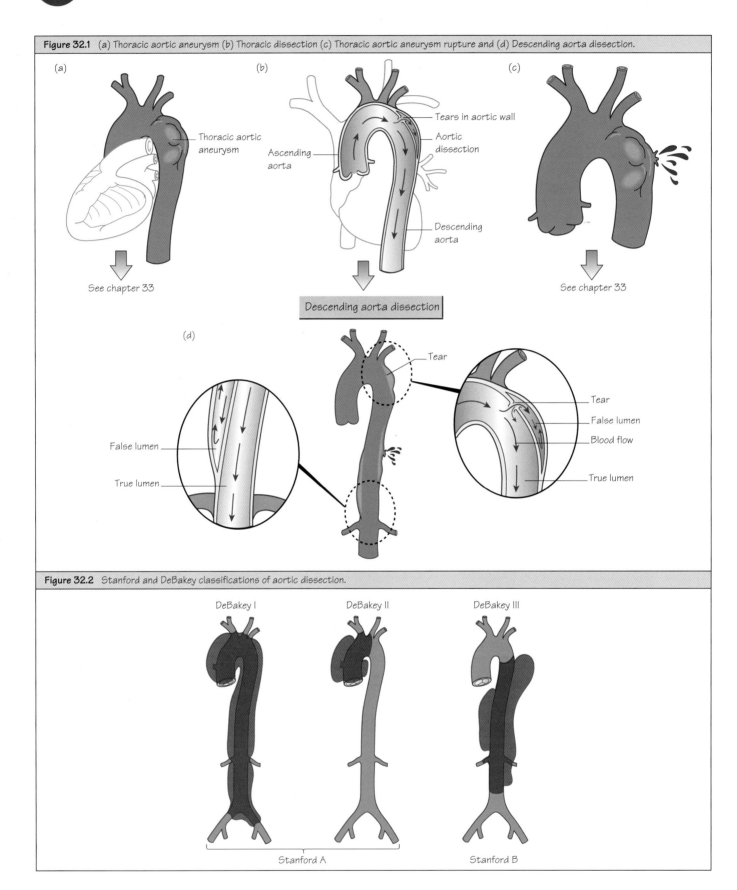

Figure 32.1 (a) Thoracic aortic aneurysm (b) Thoracic dissection (c) Thoracic aortic aneurysm rupture and (d) Descending aorta dissection.

(a) Thoracic aortic aneurysm · See chapter 33

(b) Tears in aortic wall · Aortic dissection · Ascending aorta · Descending aorta · Descending aorta dissection

(c) See chapter 33

(d) Tear · False lumen · True lumen · Tear · False lumen · Blood flow · True lumen

Figure 32.2 Stanford and DeBakey classifications of aortic dissection.

DeBakey I · DeBakey II · DeBakey III · Stanford A · Stanford B

Vascular and Endovascular Surgery at a Glance, First Edition. Morgan McMonagle and Matthew Stephenson.

Overview

Cardiothoracic surgeons tend to manage the thoracic aorta where the disease process includes any part of the aorta proximal to the origin of the left subclavian artery. Distal to the left subclavian artery origin is vascular surgeon territory.

There are three principal disease processes affecting the thoracic aorta that present to vascular surgeons:
1 Thoracic **dissection**.
2 Thoracic **trauma**.
3 Thoracic **aneurysm**:
  • Thoracic.
  • Thoracoabdominal.

Thoracic dissection will be dealt with in this chapter, trauma in Chapter 39 and aneurysmal disease in Chapter 33.

Thoracic dissection

A tear in the thoracic intimal lining allows blood to track into the aortic wall itself where it may create a false channel, usually between the inner 2/3 of the media and the outer 1/3. The flowing blood in the false channel can:
• recirculate back through the same defect
• continue down the aorta (antegrade) for a variable length and then re-enter the lumen through secondary tears in the flap
• continue down the aorta and rupture out of the aorta resulting in aortic rupture
• track back up the aorta (retrograde), theoretically ending in the pericardium with subsequent tamponade or coronary ischaemia.

The blood flowing in the usual way through the normal lumen is called the '**true lumen**'. The blood flowing under the flap is the **false lumen**. The aortic branches (e.g. to the kidneys and gut) of course arise from the true lumen, and not the false. If the dissecting flap occludes the true lumen, then the visceral branches may occlude with resultant hypoperfusion and **end-organ ischaemia**.

The dissection flap can start anywhere from aortic root downwards and can then extend distally. Dissections are classified according to the **Stanford Classification** or the **DeBakey Classification**, which overlap somewhat:
• Stanford A: Involves the ascending aorta (cardiothoracic territory).
• Stanford B: Does not involve the ascending aorta, this is generally the remit of vascular surgeons if surgery is necessary.
• DeBakey I: From the ascending aorta to at least the aortic arch or beyond (cardiothoracic territory).
• DeBakey II: Isolated to the ascending aorta (cardiothoracic territory).
• DeBakey III: From the descending aorta and may extend distally (vascular surgery territory).

Aetiology and risk factors

• Hypertension.
• Connective tissue disorders (e.g. Marfan's).
• Bicuspid aortic valve (creates abnormal flow in the ascending aorta).
• Turner syndrome.
• Blunt trauma.

Presentation

Severe thoracic back pain, which is tearing in nature and may move distally as the dissection progresses. It is often confused with an MI and for this reason diagnosis and treatment is often delayed. In addition to this pain, patients may present with any of the features of these potential sequelae:
• Organ ischaemia:
  • Stroke (carotid).
  • Ischaemic arm (subclavian).
  • Ischaemic gut (visceral vessels).
  • Paraplegia (lumbar/intercostal arteries).
  • Renal failure (renal arteries).
  • Ischaemic leg (iliac/femoral artery).
• Pericardial tamponade.
• Rupture, with profound shock resulting in rapid death.

Acute and chronic

The timing of the symptoms is important. Acute dissections (<2 weeks' history) generally require surgical intervention. Chronic (>2 weeks, e.g. late presentations) tend to be managed medically.

Complicated and uncomplicated

Complicated dissections are those that include organ ischaemia or other sequelae as listed earlier. Uncomplicated refers to the presence of the dissection *per se*.

Investigations

• **Chest X-ray (CXR):** Non-specific in acute dissections; there is no significant mediastinal widening because the aortic calibre is not changed; it is not aneurysmal disease unless this is a chronic dissection that has caused aneurysmal degeneration (see Chapter 33).
• **CT aortogram:** An excellent test to identify the detail of the dissection and any affected branches.
• **MR angiogram:** Also highly accurate but limited availability.

Treatment
Stanford A

Stanford A dissections always need surgical intervention to replace the aortic root. Such dissections are almost always acute in presentation because survival is unlikely to last to permit chronicity. Type A dissections have a 1% per hour mortality due to rupture or tamponade.

Stanford B

Open surgery is very rarely considered for any Type B dissections; where necessary, surgery is in the form of an endovascular repair by inserting a stent into the thoracic aorta to cover the original tear, thus redirecting blood into the true lumen.
• **Acute:** Stanford B dissections are treated surgically. There is some debate about whether both complicated and uncomplicated acute Type B dissections should be managed in this way.
• **Chronic:** Stanford B dissections are treated surgically only if they are complicated or progressing. The majority are uncomplicated and are treated medically, principally by rigorous control of BP. This latter group comprises the majority of thoracic dissections; thus thoracic dissection is most commonly considered a medical condition.

Figure 33.1   Descending thoracic aortic aneurysms.

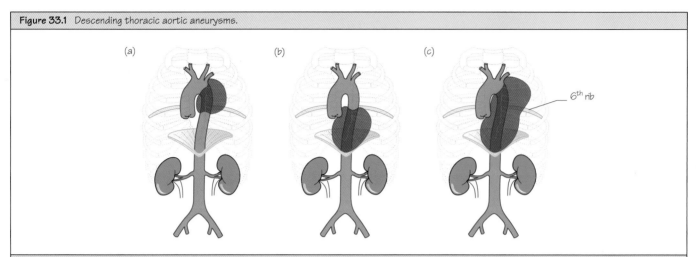

Figure 33.2   Thoracoabdominal aortic aneurysms - Crawford classification.

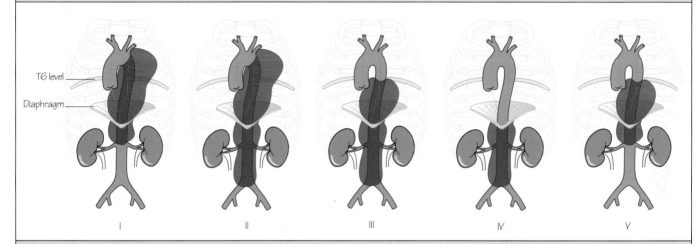

Figure 33.3   Example of hybrid repair. The entire thoracoabdominal aneurysm has been excluded by an endovascular stent and the visceral vessels are perfused by a retrograde graft from the iliac artery which has been sewn in using an open technique.

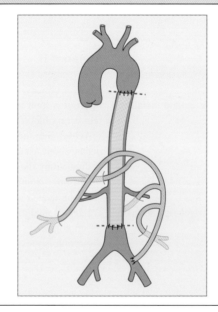

Vascular and Endovascular Surgery at a Glance, First Edition. Morgan McMonagle and Matthew Stephenson.

Aneurysms can affect the thoracic aorta in isolation (**thoracic aortic aneursysm [TAA]**) or can extend into the abdominal aorta (**thoraco-abdominal aortic aneurysms [TAAA]**).

Thoracic aortic aneursym

The most common location for TAAs is the descending thoracic aorta. Where the ascending aorta or aortic arch is involved, this is the domain of the cardiothoracic surgeon. TAAs in the descending aorta are classified into:
• Type A: Upper half (above sixth intercostal space)
• Type B: Lower half (below sixth intercostal space)
• Type C: Entire descending TAA.

Key facts
• Usually fusiform in shape but may be saccular – for instance, in infective (mycotic) aneurysms.
• More common in men (M:F = 3:1).
• Increasing incidence with increasing age.

Aetiology
Risk factors of smoking, hypertension and hypercholesterolaemia, but also particularly related to:
• connective tissue disorders (e.g. Marfan's, Ehlers-Danlos).
• syphilis (rare now).
• chronic dissections.
• infection.
For more on the aetiology of aneurysms, see Chapter 31.

Presentation
• Usually asymptomatic and diagnosed incidentally.
• Chest or back pain.
• Compression symptoms:
  • Superior vena cava (SVC) syndrome.
  • Dysphagia.
  • Stridor.
  • Hoarse voice.
• Rupture: inevitable mortality without intervention.

Investigations
• **CT aortogram** is the mainstay of diagnosis and assessment for suitability of surgery. A diameter of 6 cm is generally considered to be the threshold size for intervention. Smaller TAAs should be kept under surveillance like AAAs, but there is less evidence in this area.
• **CXR** may be performed for patients with chest and back pain, but lacks sensitivity and specificity for TAA.

Treatment
• *Open surgery*: Rarely performed now because of endovascular alternative. Requires left thoracotomy, clamping of the aorta and insertion of a graft from normal-sized artery above to normal-sized artery below. Very high risk.

• *Endovascular surgery*: Now the mainstay of treatment – thoracic endovascular aneurysm repair (TEVAR). A stent is inserted via the femoral artery. It requires a 'landing zone' for the stent of reasonably normal calibre aorta above and below the aneurysm.

Complications
Open surgery has a high morbidity and mortality principally from cardiovascular problems and the large painful thoracotomy. Endovascular surgery has a much faster recovery time and reduced physiological stress. Both, however, have the potential for paraplegia (due to occlusion of the intercostal arteries at the back from the aortic circulation, which in turn contribute to the spinal cord circulation. The risk is in the order of 5%, higher with open repair. Like AAA repair, endoleak is a potential complication and drawback of thoracic EVAR.

Thoracoabdominal aortic aneurysm

These are generally the most complex aneurysms presenting to the vascular surgeon. Unlike most other aneurysmal pathology, they tend to be symptomatic, especially causing back pain. They are often associated with chronic thoracic dissection. Because of the variety of major arterial branches from the thoracoabdominal aorta, operating on these is highly complicated requiring rapid anastomosis and re-implantation of the major branches into the graft. They are classified by the **Crawford Classification** (see Figure 33.1):
• Type I: Distal to the left subclavian to the renal arteries.
• Type II: Distal to the left subclavian to below the renal arteries.
• Type III: From T6 level to below the renal arteries.
• Type IV: T12 to the aortic bifurcation.
• Type V: From T6 to above the renal arteries.

Treatment
Open surgical repair
Usually requires a left thoracotomy for the thoracic aorta with extension over the abdomen and exposure of the abdominal aorta through the retroperitoneum. Very major surgery with high morbidity and mortality risk. Paraplegia rates are roughly 5–10%.

Endovascular repair
Also very complex because the stent must have branches or fenestrations that must be manipulated into the aortic branches. Still relatively in its infancy and still long major surgery.

Hybrid repair
A combination of open and endovascular repair. Essentially a long stent is inserted in the aorta to exclude the whole of the aneurysm – this of course would occlude all the arteries and be disastrous, so via open surgery all the major vessels (renal, celiac, superior mesenteric artery [SMA], etc.) are anastomosed to the iliac arteries distally and blood flows to those organs retrogradely (see Figure 33.1).

Figure 34.1 Illustration of the pattern of intermittent claudication on history taking: ischaemic muscle pain coming on with exercise and relieved with rest and reproducible at the same claudication distance.

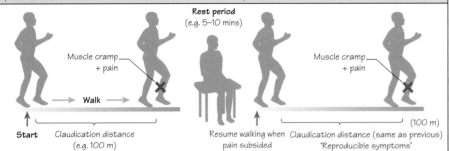

Rest period (e.g. 5–10 mins)

Muscle cramp + pain

Muscle cramp + pain

Start
Walk

Claudication distance (e.g. 100 m)

Resume walking when pain subsided

(100 m)

Claudication distance (same as previous) 'Reproducible symptoms'

Figure 34.2 Scope of clinical presentations of critical and subcritical limb ischaemia.

Subcritical → Night pain

Critical ischaemia

Pain at rest (forefoot)

Sunset foot

Tissue loss (ulceration)

Gangrene
• Dry
• Wet

Figure 34.3 Lower limb arterial anatomy.

Internal iliac artery
Groin crease

Common iliac artery
External iliac artery
Common femoral artery
} In-flow (proximal)

Profunda femoris artery — Most important vessel for chronic development of collaterals

Superficial femoral artery — Commonest site of stenosis

Knee crease

Popliteal artery — Typically behaves like end-artery (limited collaterals)

Tibia-peroneal trunk
Peroneal artery

Posterior tibial artery

Anterior tibial artery

} Run-off (distal)

Table 34.1 Fontaine classification of severity of PAD.

Fontaine stage	Clinical description	Definition	Typical ABPI
I	Asymptomatic	Incidental finding with no symptoms	0.9–1.2
II	Intermittent claudication	Cramp-like pain in muscle brought on by exercise and relieved with rest (IIa=mild, IIb=moderate to severe)	0.5–0.7
III	Rest pain	Constant pain in forefoot (worse at night)	<0.4
IV	Tissue loss	Arterial ulceration/gangrene (wet/dry)	<0.3

Table 34.2 Rutherford classification of PAD.

Category	Clinical	Objective findings	Fontaine equivalent
0	Asymptomatic	Normal treadmill test	I
1	Mild claudication	Symptoms on treadmill, but AP>50 mmHg at end (but <20 mmHg compared to resting AP)	IIa
2	Moderate claudication	(between 1 and 3)	IIa–IIb
3	Severe claudication	Cannot complete treadmill test/ AP<50 mmHg at end	IIb
4	Rest pain	Resting AP<40 mmHg/TP<30 mmHG	III
5	Minor tissue loss	Resting AP<60 mmHg/TP<40 mmHG	IV
6	Major tissue loss/ gangrene	Resting AP<60 mmHg/TP<40 mmHG	IV

Figure 34.4 'Sunset foot' with characteristic rubor of cold, ischaemic forefoot. Note small patch of dry gangrene at tip of great toe.

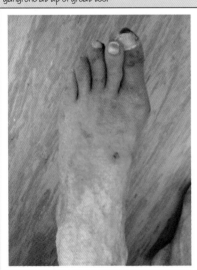

Figure 34.5 Trash foot. Foot is viable, but note skin discolouration (ischaemic skin).

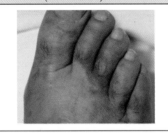

Figure 34.6 Dry gangrene of left foot requiring forefoot amputation and restoration of perfusion.

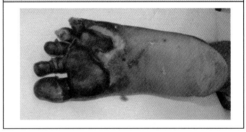

Figure 34.7 Pressure ulceration over medial aspect of first metatarsal head in a neuropathic foot (diabetic).

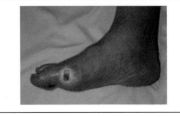

Figure 34.8 Severe ischaemic ulceration of heels (pressure areas) with superimposed infection.

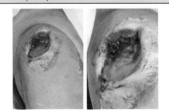

Vascular and Endovascular Surgery at a Glance, First Edition. Morgan McMonagle and Matthew Stephenson.

Peripheral vascular disease (PVD) is arterial disease that may lead to limb ischaemia.

Pathophysiology

The normal resting oxygen demand in the lower limb is 130–150 mL/min. In symptomatic PVD, there is an imbalance between limb perfusion supply and demand. During exercise the increased metabolic demand by muscle cannot be met, leading to anaerobic metabolism and by-product formation (e.g. lactate) causing 'cramp-like' pain.

In critical disease, even the *resting oxygen demand* cannot be met and tissue necrosis ensues. Perfusion pressures are severely reduced (<50 mmHg tibial pressure [<30 mmHg toe pressure]).

Aetiology

- Atherosclerosis (>95%).
- Rare causes (<5%):
  - Cystic adventitial disease.
  - Popliteal entrapment syndrome.
  - Persistent sciatic artery.
  - Fibromuscular dysplasia.
  - Buerger's disease.

Epidemiology

PVD affects ~10% of the general population and predominantly affects smokers and/or people with diabetes with a male preponderance. It is also an independent surrogate marker for both coronary and carotid artery disease (i.e. systemic atherosclerosis).

Risk factors

These are the same as for atherosclerosis (see Chapter 9) and include smoking, diabetes, hypercholesterolaemia, advancing age, hypertension and hyperhomocystinaemia.

Clinical presentation

- Presentation may be *symptomatic* or *asymptomatic* and *chronic (non-critical)* versus *acute* (often *critical*).
- *Pain is the predominant presenting symptom.*
- Symptom development is dependent on the number and distribution of the atherosclerotic plaques, which may occur as isolated, localised lesions or diffuse and multilevel (especially in diabetes).
- The most common artery affected is the SFA, although the profunda artery is also commonly affected (especially in diabetes).
- The clinical severity may be broadly classified according to the *Fontaine Classification* (see Table 34.1).

Asymptomatic disease

Usually picked up incidentally and does not require treatment other than risk factor modification and BMT (which also provides coronary protection).

Symptomatic disease

- **Chronic:** Usually presents as intermittent claudication over a variable distance. Arterial stenosis >70% is required for symptoms (variable depending on collateral supply and rapidity of onset).
- **Acute:** Represents an acute deterioration in vascular supply (usually on a background of chronic PVD) proceeding to critical ischaemia.

Non-critical limb ischaemia

Intermittent claudication (IC) is muscular pain on exercise that is relieved with rest.

The distance walked before the onset of symptoms is referred to as the *claudication distance*, which is *reproducible* on resumption of walking (sometimes slightly longer because of vasodilatation). IC typically affects the calf muscle (SFA occlusion), but proximal (in-flow) occlusions (i.e. iliac) will have more proximal symptoms (e.g. thigh and buttock claudication). As PVD and ischaemia progress, the claudication distance shortens (*deterioration of claudication distance*).

Sub-critical versus critical limb ischaemia

This is pain at rest (*rest pain*) but covers a spectrum of clinical presentations. It typically starts in the toes and forefoot (most distal perfusion) and is not related to exercise (little muscle in the foot). It represents 'all-tissue ischaemia' due to inability to meet even the resting oxygen demand and it is the precursor to tissue necrosis.

Typically rest pain begins as *night pain* (lower perfusion pressures due to absence of gravitational enhancement of perfusion upon lying horizontal in combination with nocturnal reduced cardiac output and vasodilatation [warm bed] causing a local 'steal' effect to the skin). The pain is often relieved by hanging the foot over the edge of the bed (this cools it and aids perfusion by gravity). This is sub-critical ischaemia and the precursor to persistent (not relievable) rest pain.

Critical limb ischaemia is persistent rest pain and/or tissue loss.

Pain should be present for at least 2 weeks' duration for a reliable diagnosis. Further deterioration will lead to ulceration (epidermal tissue loss) and gangrene (full tissue necrosis).

The sunset foot (ischaemic rubor)

The term 'sunset foot' is used to describe a critically ischaemic foot where there is accompanying maximum compensatory vasodilatation. The foot is cold, pulseless, mottled and painful with an erythematous hue, cyanosed toes and a prolonged capillary refill time.

Foot trash

Small emboli from a proximal source (e.g. AAA, popliteal aneurysm, cardiac) lodging in the small vessels of the feet usually affecting the toes and skin (ischaemic patches). The vessels may fibrose over time as a result of the small emboli showering into them.

Treatment is usually with anticoagulation and treatment of the source. It may be self-limiting but patchy skin necrosis and ulceration may develop as well as digital gangrene.

Gangrene

Gangrene is necrotic (dead) tissue and may be wet or dry.

Dry gangrene is necrosis in the absence of infection. The tissues are hard, mummified and often insensate. Dry gangrene is not managed as an emergency and may be excised non-emergently or allowed to 'auto-amputate' as healing by secondary intention occurs below the gangrenous tissue.

Wet gangrene is necrosis in the presence of infection. The infection is often polymicrobial; it may occur as a result of critical ischaemia or gangrene may develop secondary to infection itself (micro-thrombosis in the tissue vessels). It is moist and strongly malodourous, and it should be excised as an emergency (wide excision and debridement back to healthy, bleeding tissue). Antibiotics are indicated if there is systemic involvement or cellulitis.

Figure 35.1 Algorithm for the assessment of peripheral arterial disease according to its clinical presentation: asymptomatic intermittent claudication and critical ischaemia.

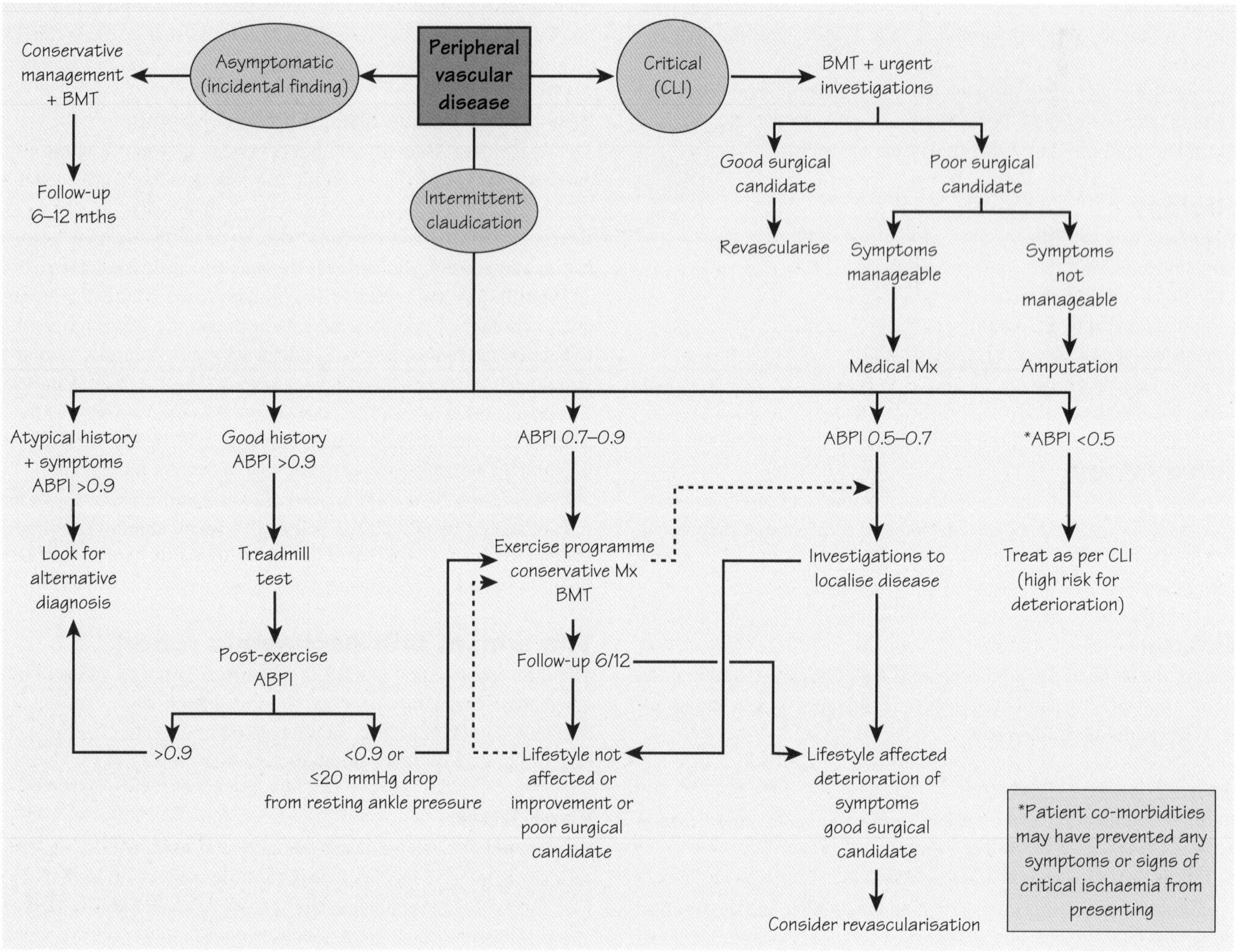

Abbreviations: ABPI, ankle-brachial pressure index; BMT, best medical therapy; CLI, critical limb ischaemia

Vascular and Endovascular Surgery at a Glance, First Edition. Morgan McMonagle and Matthew Stephenson.

The assessment and investigation of the patient with PVD is aimed at establishing whether or not the symptoms warrant further interventional treatment, as well as assessing the patient's cardiorespiratory fitness for invasive management.

Clinical history and examination

• A full cardiovascular and respiratory history should be taken to assess fitness to withstand treatment (particularly if invasive).
• Documentation of the claudication distance and its evolution.
• Documentation of any rest pain and tissue loss or gangrene.
• Palpate and document all pulses. Pedal pulses present at rest should be palpated post-exercise (patient may have significant in-flow disease).
• Measure Buerger's angle and perform Buerger's test.
• Full peripheral neurological examination.

Laboratory investigations

Ankle brachial pressure index (ABPI)

• Should be performed in a rested patient in a warm environment.
• The *highest pedal pressure* (DP or PT) is divided by the *highest brachial pressure* and gives an objective measurement of ischaemia.
• ABPI <0.7 → claudication, <0.3 → rest pain.
• The Doppler signal should be used in conjunction with Buerger's test. The angle of signal disappearance corresponds to the ischaemic angle!

Exercise ABPI

• Useful in proximal (aorto-iliac) disease where pulses are present at rest but disappear on exercise.
• ABPIs should be measured at rest and after supervised treadmill exercise (alternatively, allow the patient to walk until pain appears, then remeasure!).
• A drop of >20 mmHg suggests a haemodynamically significant lesion.

Segmental pressure studies

This is akin to the ABPI but measured segmentally along the lower limb (mid-thigh, distal thigh, popliteal and pedal), using an appropriately sized BP cuff. It may be useful in determining if the perfusion pressure after an AK reconstruction will correspondingly also elevate the BK pressure (e.g. in non-reconstructable BK disease) or if below-knee amputation (BKA) is likely to heal (popliteal pressure >70 mmHg is required for the healing of a BKA). A pressure drop of >20 mmHg (or segment:brachial ratio difference >0.2) is considered significant.

Toe pressures

In heavily calcified vessels (diabetes, chronic renal failure), ABPIs are often falsely elevated because of loss of vessel wall compliance. Digital arteries are resistant to calcification and may be used to record perfusion pressures similar to the ABPI. A specially adapted digital cuff (2–3 cm wide) is placed around the great toe and the digital pressure is measured using a photoelectric cell (photoplethysmography or laser Doppler). The toe pressure is divided by the brachial to calculate the ratio. Toe pressures are normally slightly lower than pedal pressures, with a normal toe pressure ratio of 0.8–0.9, and critical ischaemia occurs with toe–brachial pressure <0.3 (absolute pressure <30 mmHg).

Transcutaneous oximetry

A probe is placed on the skin to measure the partial pressure O_2 in the surrounding 'penumbra' of an ulcer to indicate if a reperfusion procedure is necessary.

Imaging

Arterial duplex ultrasound

Duplex assesses the severity of a stenosis as well as in-flow and run-off with a sensitivity and specificity of 92–95% and 97–99% respectively. At 50% stenosis the waveform is biphasic with a doubling of the peak flow velocity (cross-lesion ratio of 2.0). At >70% stenosis the waveform is monophasic with a cross-lesion ratio of 2.5–3.0 (*critical ratio*). More information is contained in Chapters 17–19.

CT angiography/MR angiography

CT angiography is a relatively non-invasive test (save for contrast and radiation) and gives accurate images of vascular disease and anatomy including the level and severity of disease, the number of lesions and assessment of the in-flow and run-off. MR angiography gives the same information, but small-calibre, heavily calcified vessels are difficult to assess accurately. Digital subtraction with vessel reconstruction enhances the attraction of these modalities as the investigations of choice in many institutions (see Chapter 20).

Catheter-directed angiography

Catheter-directed angiography is considered the gold standard investigation. However, it is invasive and in general is reserved for patients undergoing a simultaneous intervention.

An aorto-bifemoral angiogram, starting with the catheter placed at renal artery level, is performed. The catheter is then placed at the aortic bifurcation and images performed of the limbs in stages (varying the volume and contrast injection speed accordingly on moving distally down the limbs). Selective catheterisation of an individual vessel is performed for more accurate images and to limit the contrast volume used. The angle of the X-ray tube can be altered to improve views of vessels that are obscured (e.g. internal iliac vessels, vessels). It gives accurate views of the in-flow and run-off, collateral vessels, number and site of lesions, and vessel size, and assesses anatomical suitability for intervention (see Chapters 21–22).

Complications of catheter-directed angiography

• Contrast-related (renal failure, allergic reaction).
• Puncture site haematoma and pseudoaneurysm formation.
• Vessel occlusion.
• Puncture site infection.
• Arteriovenous fistula.
• Distal embolisation ± occlusion.
• Retroperitoneal haemorrhage (high femoral puncture).

Figure 36.1 DSA angiogram of treatment of RCIA critical stenosis. (a) DSA angiogram displaying the RCIA stenosis. (b) Aorto-bi-iliac DSA angiogram (angiography catheter within the aorta and inserted from right femoral artery). (c) Balloon expandable stent deployed (with balloon inflated) within the RCIA with successful re-moulding of iliac stenosis (note road mapping (vessel displayed as white) used for accurate navigation and deployment.(d) Successful deployment and position of iliac stent (balloon deflated) with little residual stenosis and preservation of prograde flow in artery.

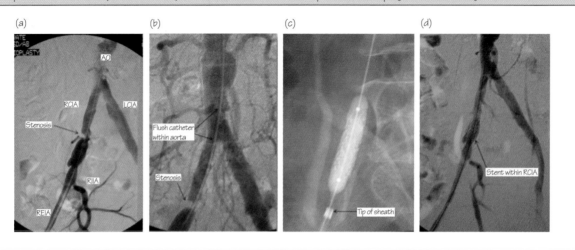

(a) (b) (c) (d)

Figure 36.2 Fem-fem cross over graft. The graft is tunneled under the skin of the lower abdomen.

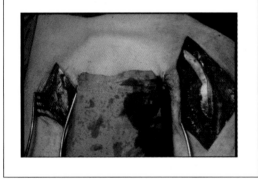

Figure 36.3 Critical SFA stenosis on angiogr.am at level of adductor hiatus (arrow) (a) and mage taken immediately post-angioplasty demonstrating successful treatment (b).

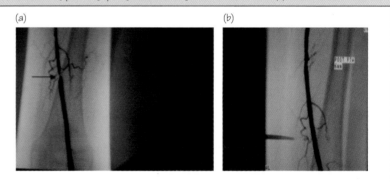

(a) (b)

Abbreviations: AO, aorta; DSA, digital subtraction angiogram; RCIA, right common iliac artery; REIA, right external iliac artery; RIIA, right internal iliac artery; SFA, superficial femoral artery

Vascular and Endovascular Surgery at a Glance, First Edition. Morgan McMonagle and Matthew Stephenson.

82 © 2014 John Wiley & Sons, Ltd. Published 2014 by John Wiley & Sons, Ltd. Companion website: www.ataglanceseries.com/vascular

Conservative (non-surgical) management

All patients with PVD should be managed with conservative management and BMT, including those who have also undergone an intervention (endovascular and/or surgery). As a guide, for those undergoing conservative management alone, *about a third of patients will improve, a third will stay the same and about a third will suffer symptomatic deterioration over a 6-month period.*

Lifestyle adjustment

- Smoking cessation (nicotine replacement and counselling enhances compliance!).
- Hypertension management (<140/90) and lipid optimisation.
- Diabetic control and treatment of renal failure.
- Exercise (supervised classes enhances compliance!).
- Weight loss and healthy diet.

Best medical therapy

- Antiplatelet agent (APA).
- Statin therapy (regardless of baseline lipid profile).
- BP and glucose control.
- Low dose ACEi (regardless of BP).
- Cilostazol (+/− other vasodilators).

Revascularisation

This includes angiointervention or open surgery. The decision to proceed will depend on numerous factors:

- General health versus risks of procedure (30% mortality <5 years!).
- Vessel suitability (length and number of lesions).
- Is there a suitable access site (angiointervention)?
- Is there a suitable distal target vessel for anastomosis (surgery)?
- Is amputation a better option (poor health/non-reconstructable)?

Indications for intervention

Absolute indications
- Critical ischaemia:
  - Ischaemic rest pain.
  - Tissue loss/gangrene.

Relative indications
- Short-distance claudication (<50 M).
- Symptoms interfering with work/lifestyle.
- Failure to improve despite conservative therapy.
- Worsening symptoms despite conservative treatment.

Angiointervention

This includes *angioplasty* (including subintimal), *stenting* and *atherectomy*. It is less invasive than surgery without the risk of GA with less cardiac stress, fewer wound complications, and earlier recovery and ambulatory periods.

Small calcified or occluded vessels may require a *subintimal* approach if the guidewire fails to safely navigate the lesion. *Atherectomy* is a catheter-directed technique of 'debulking' non-calcified atherosclerotic lesions either by mechanical forces (*directional atherectomy*) or laser (*laser atherectomy*).

Patency rates are dependent on *site*, *length* and *number* of lesions.

Treatment success rates are higher in the iliac system and SFA compared with popliteal and tibial vessels (smaller calibre, often calcified). In addition, lesions longer than 3–4 cm are associated with poorer patency rates (but may temporise the ischaemia prior to further treatment). Often a single surgical procedure is preferable to a whole multitude of endovascular procedures (e.g. multilevel disease).

Surgery

Open surgery is still considered the gold standard but carries higher risks; therefore, the *risk:benefit ratio* must be considered on an individual patient basis with surgery generally reserved for those with adequate cardiorespiratory reserve in whom the lesions are considered unsuitable for or have previously failed angiointervention.

Endarterectomy and patch angioplasty. Longitudinal arteriotomy and removal of the stenotic plaque (plane created between plaque and vessel wall) followed by closure using a vein or synthetic patch (e.g. iliac/femoral endarterectomy, profundaplasty).

Bypass. An occluded vessel is bypassed using either vein or synthetic conduit. Examples include aorto-bifemoral (iliac disease), ilio-femoral (isolated iliac disease), femoral-femoral crossover, axillo-bifemoral bypass, femoral-popliteal bypass (above or below knee) and femoral-distal bypass (anterior tibial artery [ATA], PTA, peroneal or dorsalis pedis). A successful bypass depends on good in-flow and run-off, graft quality (preferably vein), anticoagulation during clamping, disease-free anastomosis and long-term BMT.

Vein grafts offer superior patency rates over synthetic (especially below knee) and are associated with lower rates of infection, but they should be of an adequate size (>3 mm) with no fibrosis or varicosities and free of numerous branches or repairs. There is no demonstrable patency outcome difference between *in-situ* vein grafting (*valvotomised*) and *reversed vein* grafting. If possible, grafts should be tunnelled 'anatomically' to maintain in-line flow (e.g. sub-sartorial tunnel, popliteal tunnelling). In addition, if using a BK synthetic graft, then a vein patch (e.g. Taylor patch) or extension cuff (Miller cuff) should be fashioned between graft and artery (associated with superior patency rates and easier revision surgery (re-do surgery)).

Hybrid techniques

This combines surgery and endovascular techniques at the same sitting. Examples include femoral endarterectomy with patch angioplasty followed by an antegrade puncture and SFA stenting of a more distal lesion, or retrograde puncture and iliac stenting.

Other treatments

Amputation. Indications include extensive necrosis and unreconstructable critical disease. A brief operation is often preferable in patients in poor health than being subjected to a prolonged revascularisation procedure that is doomed to fail!

Sympathectomy. This may be *open* (division of the lumbar sympathetic chain) or *chemical* (translumbar injection of sclerosant [e.g. alcohol] to chemically ablate the chain); it may be useful in non-reconstructable disease by eradicating vasoconstriction, but is probably of little benefit with autonomic neuropathy (e.g. diabetes).

Spinal cord stimulation attempts to achieve the same outcome, but has failed to show convincing benefit. There has been some success for wound healing using **calf and foot compression** therapy.

Table 37.1 Causes of acute arterial.

Cause of arterial occlusion	Examples
Thromboembolism	Cardiac (A. fib, dilated chamber, valve disease), AAA, TAA, mycotic, aneurysm, idiopathic embolism, hypercoagulopathy, tumour (marantic) embolism
Thrombosis (in situ)	Atherosclerotic plaque, aneurysm thombosis (e.g. popliteal), hypercoagulopathy, acute dissection
Trauma	see Hard signs of Vascular injury (Chapter 41)

Table 37.2 The 6 P's of the acute limb ischaemia.

1. *Pain* (ischaemic pain at rest)
2. *Pulselessness* (occluded inflow)
3. *Paraesthesia* (ischaemic sensory neuropathy)
4. *Paralysis* (ischaemic motor neuropathy)
5. *Pallor* (poor skin perfusion)
6. *Poikilothermia* (cold)

Table 37.3 Categorisation of the severity of acute limb ischaemia and the expected findings on hand-held Doppler and clinical examination and its treatment.

Category	Viability	Sensation	Motor	Skin	Arterial Doppler signal	Venous Doppler signal	Treatment
I	Viable	Normal	Normal	Normal	Audible with ABPI >30 mmHg	Audible	Delayed treatment while investigations undertaken
IIa	Threatened	Normal or slightly decreased (forefoot)	Normal	Cool with prolonged capillary refill	Not audible	Audible	Investigations before treatment, but treatment soon
IIb	Immediately threatened	Decreased	Decreased	Cold with non- fixed mottling	Not audible	Audible	Emergency reperfusion
III	Irreversible ischaemia	Insensate	Complete paralysis	Fixed mottled appearance or gangrene	Not audible	Not audible	Amputation likely

Figure 37.1 Critically ischaemic (mottled appearance).

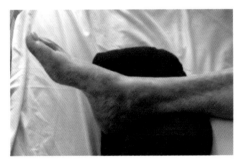

Table 37.4 Table of typical distinguishing features between acute-on-chronic ischaemia and true acute ischaemia. The distinguishing features are not always this clear cut.

Acute-on-chronic ischaemia (thrombosis)	Acute ischaemia (embolism)
History of peripheral vascular disease (intermittent claudication)	No history of peripheral vascular disease
No source of embolism identified	Source of embolism identified (e.g. A. fib)
Long history (days to weeks) of worsening symptoms	Sudden onset (hours to days)
Signs of chronic peripheral vascular disease in the affected limb	No signs of chronic peripheral vascular disease in the affected limb
Signs of chronic peripheral vascular disease in the contralateral (unaffected) limb	No signs of chronic peripheral vascular disease in the contralateral (unaffected) limb

Abbreviations: AAA, abdominal aortic aneurysm; ABPI, ankle-brachial pressure index; TAA, thoracic aortic aneurysm

Vascular and Endovascular Surgery at a Glance, First Edition. Morgan McMonagle and Matthew Stephenson.

The acute limb describes the sudden deterioration in the blood supply to a limb leading to acute ischaemia and threatened viability.

Aetiology
- Acute arterial occlusion (>95%):
  - Thromboembolism (e.g. cardiac source, aneurysm).
  - Thrombosis (e.g. atherosclerosis, popliteal aneurysm).
  - Trauma (see Chapter 41).
- Acute venous occlusion with ischaemia (<5%).

Common sites of occlusion
This occurs at the sites of branching vessels:
- Aortic bifurcation.
- Common femoral artery.
- Below-knee trifurcation (not a true trifurcation!).

Symptoms and signs
The salient feature of the acute limb is pain!

It can be difficult to decide between pain from an acute limb and pain from deteriorating PVD (see Table 37.1), but in general the acute limb will have:
- Short history
- Sudden presentation
- The 6 Ps of acute limb ischaemia (see Table 37.2).

Rest pain coupled with neurology (decreased sensation or motor function) mandates emergency treatment!

Complications of the acute limb
- Irreversible necrosis and gangrene (note: 'ischaemic window').
- Tissue loss and ulceration (especially digits).
- Ischaemic neuropathy (motor/sensory).
- Painful ischaemic neuritis.
- High rate of limb loss (amputation).
- Septicaemia and acute kidney injury (wet gangrene).

Ischaemic window
This is the time from onset of acute ischaemia before irreversible tissue necrosis occurs, which in the lower limb is about 4–6 hours. The amputation rate rises exponentially after this time. However, the ischaemic window is variable depending on numerous factors including history of PVD and collateral supply, acuteness of onset and whether systemic hypoperfusion (shock) is also present. Reperfusion should be re-established as soon as possible after onset of ischaemia.

Investigations
Most of the decision making for treatment can be made on clinical grounds alone. However, further investigations may be necessary if the diagnosis is not clear, including:
- Duplex U/S (variable availability out of hours)
- CT angiogram (good screening tool if diagnosis in doubt)
- MR angiogram (usually not available out of hours)
- Catheter-directed angiogram (gold standard but invasive, so best reserved if endovascular treatment is also planned)
- On-table angiogram (adjunct to surgery before and after treatment)
- Other investigations to look for source of embolism (e.g. CT aorta, U/S aorta, echocardiogram, ECG) may be carried out but should not delay emergency treatment.

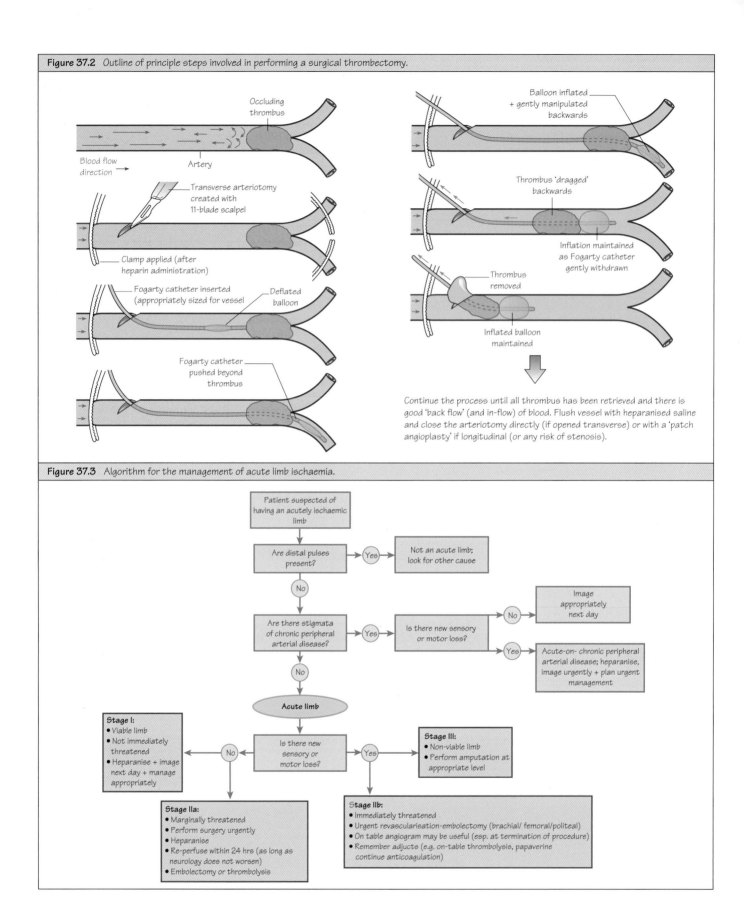

Figure 37.2 Outline of principle steps involved in performing a surgical thrombectomy.

Occluding thrombus

Blood flow direction →

Artery

Transverse arteriotomy created with 11-blade scalpel

Clamp applied (after heparin administration)

Fogarty catheter inserted (appropriately sized for vessel

Deflated balloon

Fogarty catheter pushed beyond thrombus

Balloon inflated + gently manipulated backwards

Thrombus 'dragged' backwards

Inflation maintained as Fogaranised catheter gently withdrawn

Thrombus removed

Inflated balloon maintained

Continue the process until all thrombus has been retrieved and there is good 'back flow' (and in-flow) of blood. Flush vessel with heparanised saline and close the arteriotomy directly (if opened transverse) or with a 'patch angioplasty' if longitudinal (or any risk of stenosis).

Figure 37.3 Algorithm for the management of acute limb ischaemia.

Patient suspected of having an acutely ischaemic limb

Are distal pulses present? — Yes → Not an acute limb; look for other cause

No

Are there stigmata of chronic peripheral arterial disease? — Yes → Is there new sensory or motor loss? — No → Image appropriately next day

Yes → Acute-on-chronic peripheral arterial disease; heparanise, image urgently + plan urgent management

No

Acute limb

Is there new sensory or motor loss? — No → **Stage I:**
- Viable limb
- Not immediately threatened
- Heparanise + image next day + manage appropriately

Yes → **Stage III:**
- Non-viable limb
- Perform amputation at appropriate level

Stage IIa:
- Marginally threatened
- Perform surgery urgently
- Heparanise
- Re-perfuse within 24 hrs (as long as neurology does not worsen)
- Embolectomy or thrombolysis

Stage IIb:
- Immediately threatened
- Urgent revascularisation-embolectomy (brachial/ femoral/politeal)
- On table angiogram may be useful (esp. at termination of procedure)
- Remember adjucts (e.g. on-table thrombolysis, papaverine continue anticoagulation)

Management

- General patient resuscitation, analgesia and anticoagulation.
- Angiointervention:
  - Catheter-directed thrombolysis.
  - Catheter-directed thrombectomy.
- Surgery (open embolectomy):
  - Femoral or popliteal approach.
  - Brachial (acute upper limb).

Anticoagulation

This does not dissolve thrombus but will limit its propagation (into collaterals) and is a bridge to further treatment. Use either i.v. heparin (activated partial thromboplastin time [APTT] × 2–3 normal) or LMWH (more predictable response).

Angiointervention

This is most useful in the high-risk, frail and elderly patient.

Catheter-directed thrombolysis. Catheter is navigated to the site of occlusion and thrombolytic agent (e.g. alteplase) is injected directly into the thrombus (low-dose infusion over several hours or a pulsed spray), with or without an initial bolus. Heparin is also given to counteract the prothrombotic state after release of clot by-products.

Thrombectomy. Numerous devices are available (e.g. Trellis) that mechanically disrupt the thrombus followed by removal/aspiration or further thrombolysis until thrombus has been cleared.

Surgery

Open embolectomy is the gold-standard treatment that in the lower limb may be performed via a femoral or BK-popliteal approach. The vessel is dissected and controlled as described in Chapter 23, and an arteriotomy (transverse or longitudinal) is created.

A balloon-embolectomy (Fogarty) catheter is passed into both the proximal and distal vessel, inflated and the thrombus removed with a dragging action. This is continued until the vessels are clear of thrombus with good in-flow and back-flow (of blood), following which the vessel is flushed with heparinised saline. The arteriotomy is then closed directly (if transverse) or patched (if longitudinal). The advantage of the popliteal approach is that the tibial vessels may be individually embolectomised of thrombus.

Adjuncts to surgical repair

- Intra-arterial injection of thrombolytic agent (e.g. urokinase, tPA) to lyse smaller clots (if poor back-flow). Half-life is short (20–30 minutes) thus limiting any systemic absorption.
- Intra-arterial injection of vasodilator (e.g. papaverine) to treat spasm in small vessels. Systemic absorption (hypotension) may occur but is usually transient.
- Copious flushing of vessel with heparinised saline.
- On-table angiogram at completion of surgery (to look at in-flow and run-off).
- Fasciotomy (if there has been a prolonged ischaemic time).

Complications following reperfusion

- Acute compartment syndrome (do an urgent fasciotomy!).
- Rhabdomyolysis with hyperkalaemia and acidosis.
- Myoglobinuria and acute kidney injury (see Chapter 42).

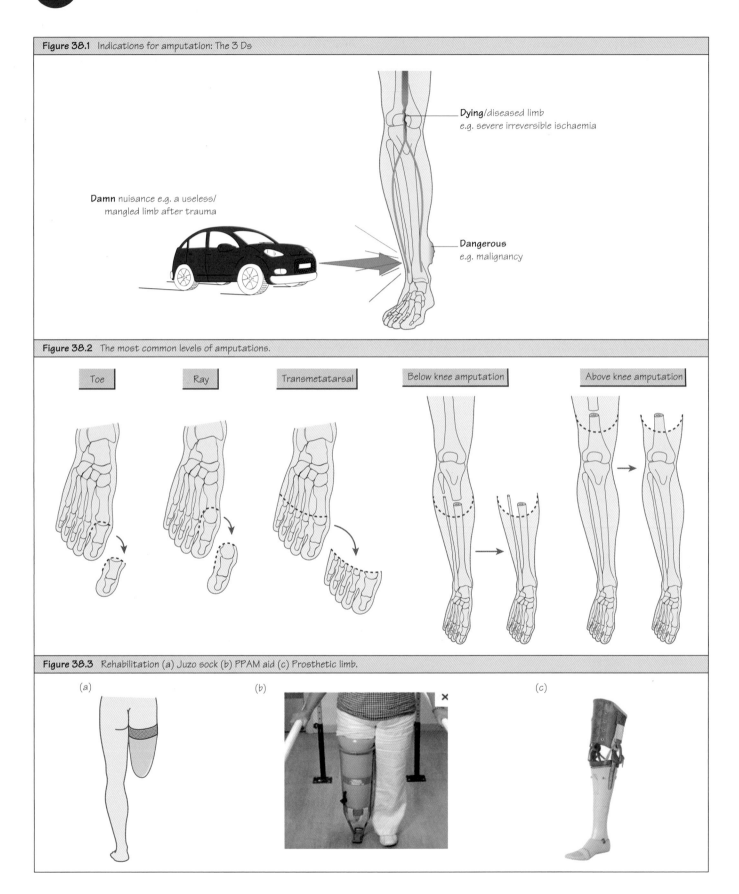

Figure 38.1 Indications for amputation: The 3 Ds

Damn nuisance e.g. a useless/ mangled limb after trauma

Dying/diseased limb e.g. severe irreversible ischaemia

Dangerous e.g. malignancy

Figure 38.2 The most common levels of amputations.

Toe

Ray

Transmetatarsal

Below knee amputation

Above knee amputation

Figure 38.3 Rehabilitation (a) Juzo sock (b) PPAM aid (c) Prosthetic limb.

(a)

(b)

(c)

Vascular and Endovascular Surgery at a Glance, First Edition. Morgan McMonagle and Matthew Stephenson.

Definition

The intentional surgical removal of a limb (almost always part of the foot or leg in the vascular context).

Epidemiology

Eighty per cent in the UK due to vascular disease, 25% of which are diabetic.

Indications

The 3 Ds:.
• **D**ying/**D**iseased limb (e.g. irreversible ischaemia).
• **D**angerous (e.g. malignancy or severe foot sepsis).
• **D**amn nuisance/useless (e.g. severe malformation or following trauma).

Levels of amputation

Proximal to distal:

• Toe/digit (through proximal phalanx or metatarsophalangeal joint [MTPJ]).
• Ray (through one metatarsal).
• Transmetatarsal (through all transmetatarsals).
• Chopart's (midtarsal, very rare now).
• Syme's (through ankle joint, very rare now).
• BK (transtibial, either skew flap or long posterior flap).
• Through knee.
• Gritti Stokes (a particular technique of through-knee amputation).
• AK (transfemoral).
• Hip disarticulation (rare, more for malignancy).

Choosing the level of amputation

As a general principle, the more distal the amputation the better the chances of walking on a prosthetic limb at a cost of slower wound healing; the opposite is true for more proximal amputations. Most crucially, there must be a good supply to the amputation site if it is to heal. If it is expected that the patient will walk afterwards, every attempt should be made to keep the knee joint.

It should always be remembered that an amputation will not heal if it doesn't have a good blood supply. There is no sense in doing a BKA if the patient has an occluded SFA and profunda artery, for instance: it won't heal and will inevitably need revision to an above-knee amputation (AKA).

Consider also an ischaemic foot in which there is a necrotic toe. The toe should never be amputated until the foot has been revascularised by one of the means described in Chapter 36. Otherwise the wound will not heal (the only exception is in deep foot sepsis, which should be drained urgently (and this may include a toe amputation) with revascularisation as soon as possible afterwards!).

For patients whom you know will never walk (e.g. very elderly and frail), there is no sense in trying to preserve the knee joint, which will just become contracted and a nuisance. Therefore, either do a through-knee amputation or a long AKA to improve the patient's sitting balance and provide a 'lever' to help them be nursed in bed.

It should be remembered that, just because a patient has a dead leg, it doesn't necessarily mean they should have an amputation. The very elderly, frail, demented, co-morbid patient, for example, may be far better saved an amputation and instead be offered palliative treatment. This of course, should be considered carefully in conjunction with the patient and their family.

Rehabilitation

If it is expected that the patient will walk afterwards, then a successful amputation should provide a stump that will support a prosthetic limb.

The rehabilitation process is a very multidisciplinary team approach involving surgeons, rehabilitation doctors, nurses, physiotherapists, occupational therapists, prosthetists and psychologists.

An average recovery flow rate process without any complications in an otherwise fit and healthy patient is now described – it can of course be highly variable.

Week 1:
• Recovery from surgery.
• Upper limb exercises.
• Stump exercises.
• Learning to transfer and use the wheelchair (will be needed at least temporarily by all patients).
• Attention to pressure areas.

If the decision has not already been made, decide whether the patient is a candidate for rehabilitation.

Week 2:
• If healing, placement of a stump shrinker sock (e.g. Juzo® sock) to reduce swelling.

Week 3:
• Ambulation on a PPAM (pneumatic post-amputation mobility) aid.

Week 4:
• Continued ambulation

Weeks 6–8:
• Fitting for bespoke prosthesis.

Week 8 onwards:
• Ongoing physiotherapy.

It is considerably easier to walk on a BK prosthesis than an AK one. For bilateral amputees, the energy required to ambulate is substantially higher, and with bilateral AKAs, the energy requirement is 280% higher. Very few bilateral AK amputees walk unless young and motivated: most simply find it easier to use a wheelchair.

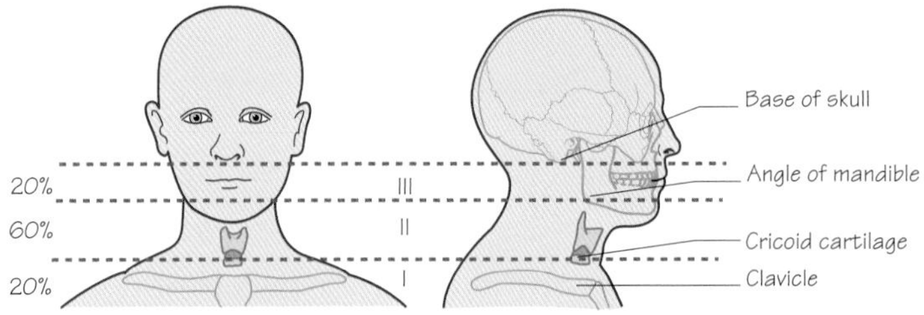

Figure 39.1 Illustration of the Zones of the Neck and the percentage prevalence of involvement of each zone after penetrating injury.

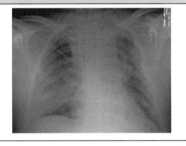

20%

III

60%

II

20%

I

Base of skull

Angle of mandible

Cricoid cartilage

Clavicle

Table 39.1 Injury grade, stroke rate, mortality and description of blunt carotid artery injury (Source: Adapted from Biffl, W.L. et al. (1999) *Journal of Trauma*, 47, 845-853. Reproduced with permission from LWW).

Injury grade	AIS-90		Stroke rate (%)		Mortality (%)		Description
	Intracranial	Extracranial	Carotid	Vertebral	Carotid	Vertebral	
I	3	3	3	19	11	31	Intimal tear/dissection <25% lumen narrowing
II	3	3	11	40	11	0	Intimal tear/dissection mural haematoma, lumen thrombus >25% lumen narrowing
III	3	3	33	13	11	13	Pseudoaneurysm
IV	4	4	44	33	22	11	Occlusion
V	5	5	100		100		Transection with free haemorrhage

Figure 39.2 Chest X-ray displaying widened mediastinum with blunting of aortic angle consistent with traumatic aortic transection. Note there is also extensive bilateral lung contusions.

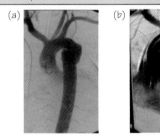

Figure 39.3 Management of traumatic aortic transection as seen on aortogram, (a) Irregular outline of descending aorta just distal to the origin of the left subclavian artery. Flush catheter is in situ within the ascending aorta for aortogram, (b) Thoracic aortic stent is aligned within the descending aorta, (c) Successful deployment of thoracic aortic stent with stabilisation of transected segment of aorta.

(a)   (b)   (c)

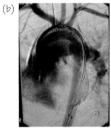

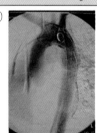

Figure 39.4 Classification of grade of traumatic aortic injury.

Grade I
intimal tear

Grade II
intramural
haematoma

Grade III
pseudoaneurysm

Grade IV
rupture

Intima

Media

Adventitia

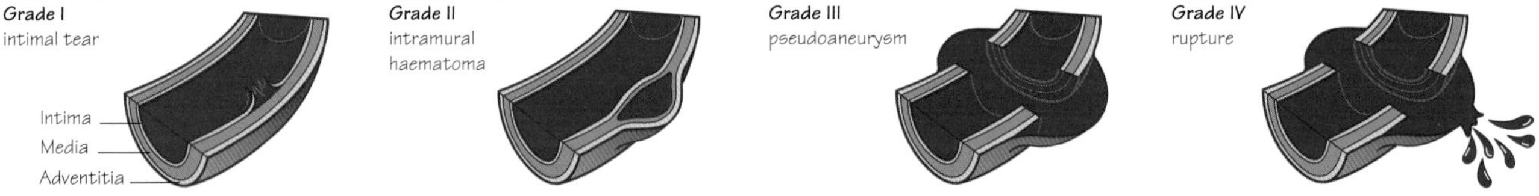

Figure 39.5 Illustration of various incisions that may be used to gain access to the chest and neck in the management of vascular injury. These incisions may be extended and joined for adequate access as needed.

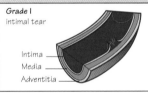

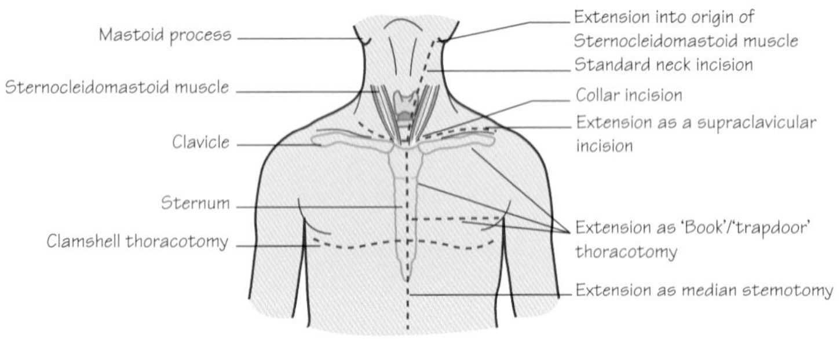

Mastoid process

Sternocleidomastoid muscle

Clavicle

Sternum

Clamshell thoracotomy

Extension into origin of Sternocleidomastoid muscle

Standard neck incision

Collar incision

Extension as a supraclavicular incision

Extension as 'Book'/'trapdoor' thoracotomy

Extension as median sternotomy

Table 39.2 Comparisons of the complications associate with open and endovascular repair of traumatic aortic Injury.

Open surgery vs. endovascular management		
	Open surgery	Endovascular
Mortality	20%	9%
Acute kidney injury	8%	3%
Paraplegia	10%	3%
Stroke rate	3%	3%

Abbreviation: AIS, abbreviated injury score

Vascular and Endovascular Surgery at a Glance, First Edition. Morgan McMonagle and Matthew Stephenson.

Carotid, vertebral and subclavian vessels

Carotid and subclavian artery injuries (blunt or penetrating) account for less than 2% of vascular trauma, but carry a high mortality and morbidity. The neck is divided into three distinct anatomical zones but more than one zone may be involved.

All patients should be managed initially as per the advanced trauma life support (ATLS) guidelines. Blunt injury is associated with multiple competing injuries requiring treatment. If the patient is physiologically well, then a CT with contrast (arterial and portal venous phase) is the investigation of choice.

Blunt carotid trauma

These carry a high mortality and stroke rate and are associated with a high incidence of c-spine and head injuries (contributing to the high mortality and morbidity). Often the neurological injury has already occurred by the time of presentation (head trauma or embolic stroke).

Management

- Surgery has not been shown to alter either the mortality or stroke rates although free haemorrhage should undergo surgical control.
- Anticoagulation (heparin or LMWH) has been shown to improve both mortality and stroke outcomes. However, this is often contraindicated in trauma (especially head injury).
- Angiointervention may be used but its role has not been well scrutinised to date.
- A post-hanging carotid injury with intimal tear (although a blunt injury) should be repaired if grade II or greater. A grade I injury may be treated with antiplatelet therapy (e.g. aspirin).

Penetrating carotid trauma

- Operative management is mandatory and the approach will depend on the zone involved. The thorax should be prepared within the operative field. Acute ligation of the ICA (if *in extremis*) carries a 15–20% risk of stroke.
- *Zone I*: Proximal control must be gained from within the chest via median sternotomy (or 'Clamshell' thoracotomy if *in extremis*). The incision may be extended further into the neck as per zone II or supraclavicular for an SCA approach as necessary.
- *Zone II*: Standard carotid incision along the anterior border of the sternocleidomastoid muscle. Repair may be with patch grafting (if only anterior wall involved), direct anastomosis (if tension free) or with an interposition graft.
- *Zone III*: Challenging access, but the approach is similar to the incision for zone II. If inaccessible and *in extremis*, a balloon catheter may be inserted into the ICA, inflated, clipped and cut, and left *in situ*.

Subclavian artery and vertebral artery (VA) injury

SCA: May be approached with a combination of supraclavicular and infraclavicular incisions with removal of the clavicle as required followed by direct repair with interposition grafting. Proximal control may need to be from within the chest. Endovascular management is an option (well patient with contained haematoma).

VA: Rare because of its deep position in the neck. Endovascular coiling is now the treatment of choice (antegrade and retrograde [by crossing the basilar artery from the contralateral VA]). Open repair is reserved for active bleeding that has failed endovascular treatment.

Thoracic aortic transections (TATs)

Patients presenting to hospital alive with a TAT DO NOT present with hypotension!

The majority of TATs occur as a result of blunt trauma (10–15% of road traffic fatalities) and 70–90% of these patients will die before reaching hospital from rapid exsanguination and associated injuries. TAT results from rapid deceleration at relatively 'fixed' points:
- Ascending aorta (fixed by the large branches [15%]).
- Descending aorta (fixed just distal to the left SCA origin by the ligamentum arteriosum [75%]).
- Junction of the thoracic and abdominal aorta (as it passes through the diaphragmatic arcuate ligament [10%]).

Survivors will have a contained leak and will be either normotensive (unless there are other sources of bleeding) or even hypertensive (aortic wall baroreceptor stretch reflex). There may be a difference in the systolic BP between the upper limbs (>20 mmHg) and decreased femoral pulse volume ('pseudocoarctation').

Investigations

Specific investigations and management for a TAT may have to be delayed as more life-threatening injuries are prioritised.
- *CXR*. CXR findings suggestive of TAT include: 1. widened mediastinum (>8 cm on erect PA film); 2. loss of aortic contour; 3. obliteration of aorto-pulmonary angle; 4. splitting of aortic wall calcium (if present); 5. left apical 'capping' (blood tracking over apex of lung); 6. left main stem bronchus pushed downwards (by haematoma); 7. trachea pushed to the right (by haematoma); 8. paravertebral stripe (blood tracking into paravertebral space); and 9. left haemothorax. It is a poor screening tool with high false positive findings. Up to 10–15% of patients with TAT will have a normal-looking CXR.
- *CT angiography*. This is the best screening modality and should be multisliced with reconstructed views looking for evidence of both aortic injury (irregular dilated appearance) and peri-aortic mediastinal haematoma (rarely pseudoaneurysm).
- *Transoesophageal echocardiography*. This is useful with the patient already in theatre to look for an intimal flap. Transthoracic echocardiography is not sensitive enough to rule out a TAT.
- *Catheter-directed angiography*. This is still considered the gold standard test, but it is an invasive tool and should be reserved for those patients with a positive finding on CT scanning who are to undergo further endovascular management.

Management

- *Assessment and resuscitation*. As per ATLS principles. Life-threatening injuries (active bleeding) should be prioritised.
- *Medical (critical care) management*. Patients should have induced hypotension (SBP 100 mmHg) and bradycardia (heart rate < 60 beats per minute) using a combination of i.v. nitrate and β-blockade to reduce both the luminal pressure and aortic wall shear stress (pulsatile pressure per heart beat). Parameters may have to be altered to prevent renal and mesenteric ischaemia as the patient's condition changes.
- *Surgical/endovascular repair*. Up to 50% of non-operated cases will die (usually due to associated injuries!). In selected cases, patients may undergo safe, delayed repair of the TAT. Open repair of TATs is via a posterolateral thoracotomy (direct repair or grafting). Endovascular stenting is associated with superior outcomes and is now the preferred management. These patients will require lifelong surveillance because there is a trend towards re-intervention for stent complications.

Figure 40.1 Zones of the retroperitoneum.

Zone I is the 'central' retroperitoneum and consists of the aorta and IVC, pancreas, lesser sac and duodenum (D2–D4). Operative exploration is mandatory for injuries in this zone.

Zone II is lateral to zone I (flanks) and consists of the kidneys (and their hilar vessels), ureters and psoas muscle. The majority of zone II injuries can be managed non-operatively, unless there are signs of active arterial bleeding (expanding or pusatile haematoma or contrast extravasation on CT angiogram). All zone II penetrating injuries should be explored.

Zone III consists of the pelvic complex, the iliac vessels and its organs. Management of injuries here is more complex. 80% of bleeding is venous in origin and is typically managed non-operatively. Arterial bleeding (20%) is best managed with angiointervention. Pelvic extraperitoneal packing is used to control bleeding in combination with bony stabilisation of the pelvic ring. Penetrating injuries should be explored.

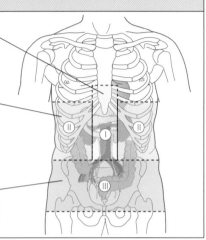

Figure 40.2 Right medial visceral rotation: (a) The right peritoneal reflection line is mobilised and the caecum and ascending colon brought forward and mobilised towards and midline to expose the psoas muscle, right psoas muscle, right kidney, inferior vena cava and aorta. Often the retroperitoneal haematoma creates a natural dissection plane and lifts the colon forward. (b)This dissection can be carried further cephalad and combined with a Kocher manoeuvre of the duodenum for wider exposure of zones I and II of the retroperitoneum including the anterior and posterior aspects of the duodenum and head of pancreas. The right kidney may be left in situ in its bed or also mobilized forward depending on injury findings.

(a)

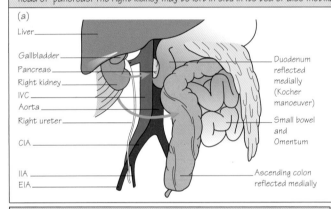

Liver
Gallbladder
Pancreas
Right kidney
IVC
Aorta
Right ureter
CIA
IIA
EIA
Duodenum reflected medially (Kocher manoeuver)
Small bowel and Omentum
Ascending colon reflected medially

(b)

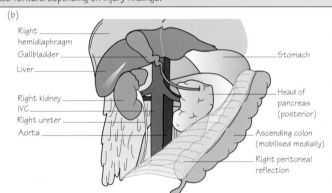

Right hemidiaphragm
Gallbladder
Liver
Right kidney
IVC
Right ureter
Aorta
Stomach
Head of pancreas (posterior)
Ascending colon (mobilised medially)
Right peritoneal reflection

Figure 40.3 Left Medial Visceral Rotation: The left lateral peritoneal reflection is divided and the descending colon, spleen and tail of pancreas mobilised medially. The left kidney may be mobilised or left in situ depending on the injury and exposure required. The visceral branches (coeliac, SMA and renals) are best exposed in this way.

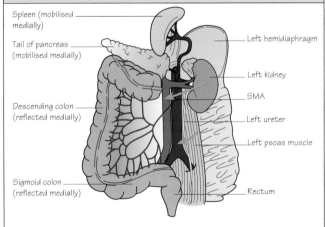

Spleen (mobilised medially)
Tail of pancreas (mobilised medially)
Descending colon (reflected medially)
Sigmoid colon (reflected medially)
Left hemidiaphragm
Left kidney
SMA
Left ureter
Left psoas muscle
Rectum

Figure 40.4 Exposure of IVC with haemostatic control above and below the injury.

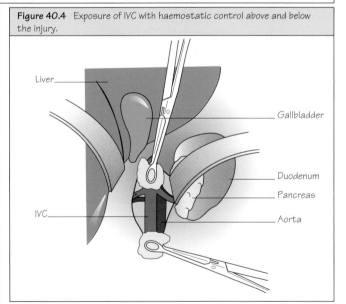

Liver
IVC
Gallbladder
Duodenum
Pancreas
Aorta

Abbreviations: CIA, common iliac artery; CT, computer tomography; EIA, external iliac artery; IIA, internal iliac artery; IVC, inferior vena cava; SMA, superior mesenteric artery

Vascular and Endovascular Surgery at a Glance, First Edition. Morgan McMonagle and Matthew Stephenson.

92 © 2014 John Wiley & Sons, Ltd. Published 2014 by John Wiley & Sons, Ltd. Companion website: www.ataglanceseries.com/vascular

Retroperitoneal (RP) injuries

These are associated with a very high mortality and morbidity (including pancreatic, biliary and duodenal injuries), mostly due to massive haemorrhage. Management is dependent on which of the three distinct anatomical zones is involved (see Figure 40.1).

Investigation versus immediate management

• The decision to surgically manage RP injuries emergently or to investigate further is dependent on physiology at presentation.
• If physiologically unwell, then immediate surgery is mandatory because of the high mortality from exsanguination.
• Damage control surgery is often necessary to limit haemorrhage and to avoid physiologic and metabolic exhaustion.

Investigations

• *Bedside abdominal U/S*. May rule in an intra-abdominal bleed, but is not sensitive for RP bleeding.
• *Contrast-enhanced CT scan*. This is the most sensitive and specific investigation (arterial and portal venous phase).

Zone 1 RP injury

Zone 1 haematoma (adjacent to the great vessels) on CT scanning or intra-operatively mandates further operative exploration!

Abdominal aorta

This carries a very high mortality (>80%) with most dying before reaching hospital! Proximal control of the aorta can be performed via a *transperitoneal* (infrarenal) or *supracoeliac* approach (through the lesser sac). Although quickest for control, supracoeliac clamping >60 minutes in trauma has a near 100% mortality! If *in extremis*, proximal control should be via a left lateral thoracotomy. During surgery, the best exposure is with a left medial visceral rotation.

Small aortic tears may be sutured directly for rapid haemostasis. However, more often an interposition graft is required. Endovascular stent grafting may be used for smaller contained injuries seen on CT scanning, although this is unusual because patients are usually critically shocked. Small intimal tears may be managed expectantly.

Aortic visceral branches

Exposure and control of the visceral segment is best achieved with supracoeliac clamping followed by a left medial visceral rotation.

The inferior mesenteric artery (IMA) may be ligated (small risk of sigmoid ischaemia and re-look surgery is recommended. The coeliac artery may be ligated if the SMA is uninjured, but a dual coeliac-SMA injury is associated with >90% risk of bowel infarction. The level at which the SMA or its branches branch may be ligated is dependent on the *Fullen zone* involved (zones I and II are proximal to the middle colic artery branch and should be repaired). Shunting may be used for damage control and definitive repair delayed (24–48 hours). If the vessel origin is involved, then perform ligation with bypass. Renal artery injuries may be ligated (+nephrectomy) as long as the other kidney is intact!

Inferior vena cava (IVC)

IVC injuries are associated with a high mortality (50–90%) because very high energy transfers are required to injure it (as a result of its well-protected position). In addition, 15% of liver injuries will also have an IVC injury! Patients who have survived to theatre have often self-tamponaded.

The IVC has four anatomically distinct segments; infrarenal, suprarenal, retrohepatic and suprahepatic (abdominal and thoracic components). Exposure is best via a combined right medial visceral rotation and Kocher Manoeuvre, but access is most difficult for the retrohepatic and suprahepatic injuries that carry the highest mortality. Suprahepatic injuries can be managed in combination with a right-sided thoracotomy (or clamshell thoracotomy) with division of the right hemi-diaphragm. For retrohepatic injuries, the liver will need to be mobilised forward (divide the right and left triangular ligaments). However, this often destabilises a contained haematoma with rapid exsanguination! Therefore, if possible, leave a retrohepatic haematoma undisturbed! Pack it with large abdominal packs for tamponade and re-look in 24–48 hours.

The IVC should be controlled using direct pressure (sponge-forceps above and below the injury) and not clamping because the vessel tears easily. Posterior wounds are repaired via an anterior venotomy and direct suturing of the back wall (inside the vessel) followed by anterior wall repair. If *in extremis* the IVC may be ligated, but this is associated with massive leg oedema and acute venous hypertension necessitating fasciotomies. Veno-veno bypass may be required, but the use of an atrio-caval shunt carries a very high mortality and is no longer recommended.

Portal vein injuries

These carry >50% mortality and are associated with severe injuries to other structures including pancreas, duodenum and visceral branches. If possible, the portal vein should be preserved to avoid severe small bowel oedema, venous ischaemia and abdominal compartment syndrome associated with ligation (which is reserved for patients in extremis). Occasionally the neck of the pancreas must be divided to gain access to the bleeding portal vein (followed by distal pancreatectomy).

Trauma in Zone 2

The renal complex is surrounded by Gerota's fascia which often provides a natural haemostatic barrier to low-pressure (venous) bleeding. Therefore, a haematoma in this region should be left undisturbed, unless it is *expanding* or *pulsatile* (i.e. arterial bleeding). A contrast extravasation 'blush' seen on CTA is an equivalent radiological sign of active arterial bleeding mandating exploration.

A bleeding kidney should be repaired (±meshed) leaving the kidney intact where possible. Renal artery bleeding is more difficult to manage and may require a nephrectomy (ensure contralateral kidney present!) with vessel ligation. The injured renal vein may be ligated.

Trauma in Zone 3

Do not open a contained non-expanding pelvic haematoma!

Eighty per cent of pelvic bleeding is venous which may be controlled using a combination of pelvic packing and pelvic fracture reduction (external pelvic binder and/or pelvic fixation) to reduce pelvic volume for bleeding. Pelvic packing may be extraperitoneal (safest) via a lower mid-line incision or intraperitoneal (if laparotomy in progress).

Endovascular management by embolising or coiling actively bleeding internal iliac branches is preferable if patient suitable (not if shocked!). Use a covered stent for common / external iliac artery bleeding, but failure to control haemorrhage will mandate surgical control (repair/ligation/bypass or shunting for damage control).

Table 41.1 Clinical signs of vascular injury (any patient presenting with hard signs of vascular injury mandates immediate surgical exploration).

Hard signs of arterial injury	Soft signs of arterial injury

• Pulsatile (arterial) bleeding
• Expanding haematoma
• Palpable thrill/audible bruit
• Loss of distal pulses (+/− signs of the acute limb)
  o Pain
  o Pallor
  o Paralysis
  o Poikilothermia (coolness)
	• History of bleeding at scene
	• Proximity of wound/bleeding/trajectory to artery
	• Diminished (but not absent) pulse
	• Non-pulsatile haematoma
	• Neurologic deficit
	• Abnormal ankle-brachial index (<0.9)
	• Abnormal waveform on duplex ultrasound

Table 41.2 Typical vascular injury patterns and associations.

Injury	Associated arterial injury
Posterior knee dislocation	Politeal artery
Femur fracture	Superficial femoral artery
Supracondylar fractures	Brachial artery
Elbow dislocation	Brachial artery
Clavicular fracture	Subclavian artery
Anterior shoulder dislocation	Axillary artery

Figure 41.1: Left SFA dissection with vessel looping for control.

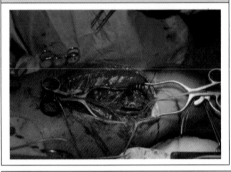

Figure 41.2: Steps of opereative approach to management of peripheral vascular injury.

- Control the haemorrhage
  - o Proximal control first
  - o Distal control second
  - o Open the haematoma and visualise the injury last
- Manage ischaemia
  - o Shunt the vessel across the injury if physiologically unwell or there are multiple competing injuries
  - o More definitive repair if physiology/time allows
    - −Vein graft from the contralateral (uninjured) limb
    - −Synthetic graft
- Perform a fasciotomy

Figure 41.3: Selection of 'Argyle' shunts.

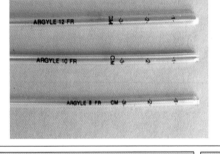

Figure 41.4: Repair of SFA using reinforced PTFE after GSW to thigh.

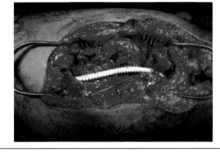

Figure 41.5: Vascular shunt in SFA.

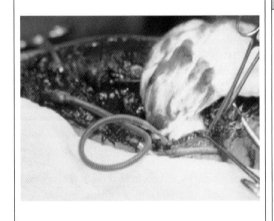

Figure 41.6: Angiogram of right lower limb (post-GSW) demonstrating occlusion of distal SFA with active bleeding.

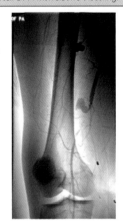

Figure 41.7: Factors associated with higher limb loss rates after vascular trauma.

- Treatment delay (>6 hours)
- Shock
- Blunt mechanism of injury
- Lower extremity >upper extremity
- Associated injuries
  - o Nerve (most predictive of amputation)
  - o Bone
  - o Vein
  - o Soft tissue
- High velocity gun-shot wound
- Pre-existing disease (esp. PAD)
- Failure/delay in performing fasciotomy

Abbreviations: GSW, gun-shot wound; PAD, peripheral arterial disease; PTFE, polytetrafluoroethylene (Teflon); SFA, superficial femoral artery

Vascular and Endovascular Surgery at a Glance, First Edition. Morgan McMonagle and Matthew Stephenson.

Aetiology
- *Penetrating* (e.g. gunshot [GSW], shotgun, stabbings, IVDU).
- *Blunt* (e.g. direct contusion, displaced fracture, joint dislocation (e.g. posterior dislocation of knee).
- *Iatrogenic* (e.g. arteriography, cardiac catheterisation, balloon angioplasty, inadvertent arterial puncture, aortic balloon pump).

Physical examination
- Vascular (hard and soft signs).
- Neurological (evidence of nerve damage).
- Bone and joint (fractures or joint dislocation).
- Soft tissue (bruising and degloving injuries).

Vascular examination: Hard versus soft signs
The clinical signs of vascular injury are divided into hard and soft signs. **Hard signs** have a >98% sensitivity for the presence of arterial injury. **Soft signs** have a low sensitivity.

The presence of hard signs of vascular injury mandates surgical exploration.

Further diagnostic work-up is usually unnecessary (save for an on-table angiogram). All pulses must be palpated and comparison can be made with the contralateral (uninjured) limb.

The absence of hard signs in an injured extremity effectively excludes the presence of significant vascular injury!

Minimal vascular injury (MVI)
This describes radiological evidence of arterial injury in the absence of hard signs of which there are four types:
1 Focal segmental narrowing.
2 Intimal flap/irregularity.
3 Small pseudoaneurysm.
4 AVF.

More than 90% of MVI injuries will heal spontaneously with the remainder deteriorating and requiring intervention (without an increase in morbidity or mortality!). Small pseudoaneurysms (<2 cm) picked up incidentally can be safely monitored, although 40–50% of larger pseudoaneurysms will become symptomatic and require intervention.

Investigations
In the absence of hard signs, further diagnostic imaging may be carried out, but it offers little over physical examination!
- ABPI or ankle-ankle pressure index (AAPI).
- Duplex ultrasonography.
- CT angiography.
- Catheter-directed angiography.

An ABPI reading >0.9 effectively rules out significant vascular injury, but has a comparable diagnostic accuracy to physical examination alone. Catheter-directed angiography is the gold standard investigation, but it is invasive and has now been superseded by CT angiography as a screening tool with catheter angiography being reserved for endovascular treatment of injuries.

Management
Non-operative management
Most MVIs and injuries in the absence of hard signs may be managed non-operatively, but frequent physical examination is advised. MVI may be treated with an antiplatelet agent, but its utility in young trauma patients has not been well established.

Endovascular management
This is useful for the physiologically well patient (if available). However, mandatory surgical exploration should not be delayed awaiting the endovascular service!

Operative management
- The operating suite should be warm and well-lit, with full vascular capabilities including endovascular facilities.
- Management follows the same sequence as described in Chapter 23 with proximal and distal control followed by opening of the haematoma to expose the area of vessel injury. Anticoagulation should be avoided in trauma.
- An on-table angiogram may be useful to locate the injury, but is best reserved for a post-operative confirmatory image.
- Interposition grafting or ligation and bypass may be used. Native vein is best because of its superior longevity, but infection rates are similar for both native and synthetic graft in the trauma patient.
- If vein grafting is used, harvest from the contralateral (uninjured) limb to preserve the superficial drainage on the injured side (if the deep system is also injured) to reduce post-operative swelling and reduce venous hypertension in the injured limb.
- A vascular shunt should be used as part of damage control in the physiologically unwell patient or while other surgery is undertaken (e.g. orthopaedic manipulation of a fracture). Definitive repair may then be delayed, but regular physical examination is mandatory.
- Where possible, the deep vein should be repaired (or shunted). This will reduce post-operative swelling, acute venous hypertension and blood loss (especially after fasciotomy). This is particularly important in the first few days after repair, although up to 60% will thrombose within 2 weeks (with 30% re-canalising in the future). Limb salvage and function rates are higher with preservation of venous flow (especially popliteal).
- Perform a *fasciotomy*! Especially with; shocked patient, delay in repair (>1–2 hours), dual arterial-venous injury or vessel shunt is being used.

Factors associated with higher amputation rates
- Treatment delay (>6 hours).
- Shock (the 4–6 hour ischaemic window may be 1–2 hours after trauma (for limb loss and good functional outcomes).
- Blunt injury leading to ischaemia.
- Lower extremity (compared with upper extremity).
- Associated injuries (nerve [most important], bone, vein, soft tissue).
- High velocity GSW.
- Pre-existing disease (especially PVD).
- Failure/delay in performing fasciotomy.

Figure 42.1 Calf fasciotomies.

(a)

Lateral incision: In the natural muscle groove about half way between anterior tibial spine and the fibula, (to decompress anterior and lateral compartments

Medial incision: About 1cm behind the tibia (to decompress deep and superficial posterior compartments)

(b)
- Anterior compartment
- Lateral compartment
- Deep posterior compartment
- Superficial posterior compartment

(c)
- 1cm
- Medial incision
- Lateral incision Half way
- Deep fascia

(d)
- Long saphenous vein
- Saphenous nerve
- Fascia

Soleus muscle which must be dissected off the underside of the tibia (avascular plane) to access the deep compartment

(e)
- Facia between comppartments incised

Raise skin flaps to directly expose fascia overlying anterior and lateral compartment

All four compartments must be decompressed

Table 42.1 Compartments of the calf muscle group.

Compartments	Contents
1 Anterior compartment	Anterior tibial vessels
	Deep peroneal nerve
	Anterior muscle group
2 Lateral compartment	Superficial peroneal nerve
	Peroneal muscle group
3 Posterior deep compartment	Posterior tibial vessels
	Peroneal vessels
	Soleus muscle
4 Posterior superficial compartment	Gastrocnemius muscle group

- **Medial longitudinal incision:** Fingers breath below the medial spine of the tibia (care not to injure the LSV) to access the deep and superficial posterior compartments.
- **Lateral longitudinal incision:** Half way between the anterior spine of the tibia and the fibular bone in the muscle groove to access the anterior and lateral compartments. Care must be taken not to injure the deep or superficial peroneal nerve (drop foot).
- Skin flaps are raised over the fascial compartments.
- Separate longitudinal incisions are made in the fascia overlying each compartment and then joined by a 'T-shaped incision across the fascial septum.
- The soleus muscle must be dissected off the back off the tibia (avascular plane) to access the deep posterior compartment.
- Viable muscle will contract on stimulation (pinching/diathermy) and only gangrenous muscle should be debrided. If the viability is in doubt, plan a re-look in 24–48 hours.
- Aim to close the fasciotomies within 5–7 days. Otherwise a skin graft may be necessary.

Figure 42.2 Thigh fasciotomy.

- Medial (adductor) compartment
- Anterior (quadriceps) compartment
- Posterior (hamstring) compartment

(a) lateral-only incision will usually suffice in thigh compartment syndrome with decompression of the anterior and posterior compartments. (b) Skin flaps are raised and separate longitudinal incisions made over each compartment with a joining 'T-shaped septal incision. (c) If necessary, a separate medial incision may be made to decompress the adductor compartment, but is often unneccessary.

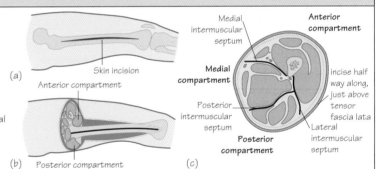

(a) Skin incision — Anterior compartment

(b) Posterior compartment

(c)
- Medial intermuscular septum
- Anterior compartment
- Medial compartment
- Posterior intermuscular septum
- Posterior compartment
- incise half way along, just above tensor fascia lata
- Lateral intermuscular septum

Figure 42.3 Hand-held manometer device for measuring compartment pressures.

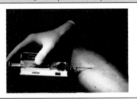

Figure 42.4 Images of completed calf fasciotomies. (a) Medial incision and (b) lateral incision.

(a) 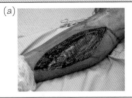 (b)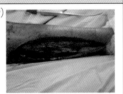

Figure 42.5 Urinary catheter bag with dark coloured urine consistent with myoglobinuria.

Table 42.2 Causes, complications and management of compartment syndrome.

Causes	Complications		Management
	Limb complications	Systemic complications	
Vascular (ischaemia-reperfusion injury)	• Limb ischaemia	• Rhabdomyolysis	Treat the underlying cause
Trauma and crush injury	• Neuropathy	• Myoglobinuria	Optimise fluid resuscitation (do not over-resuscitate)
Fractures (50% of compartment syndrome, e.g.: tibial plateau)	• Painful neuritis	• Acute renal failure	Correct coagulopathy
Haemorrhage into a compartment	• Loss of limb function	• Hyperkalaemia	Perform fasciotomy
Shock and over-resuscitation (swelling of compartment)	• Need for amputation	• Acidosis	Treat the rhabdomyolysis and acute renal failure
Drug injection into a limb		• Acute cardiac arrhythmia	Treat hyperkalaemia
Prolonged compression (e.g. during surgery)			Manage acidosis

Abbreviations: F, fibula; T, tibia

Vascular and Endovascular Surgery at a Glance, First Edition. Morgan McMonagle and Matthew Stephenson.

Compartment syndrome (CS)

This is an elevated and sustained pressure within a fascial compartment.

The inelastic fascia lacks the necessary compliance to accommodate tissue swelling with a resultant increase in the absolute pressure. Affected compartments include calf (the most common), thigh, buttocks, forearm, hands and feet (rare).

Aetiology

- Vascular (acute limb ischaemia-reperfusion injury).
- Trauma and crush injury.
- Fractures (50% of CS; e.g. tibial plateau).
- Haemorrhage into a compartment.
- Shock and over-resuscitation (swelling).
- Drug injection (intra-arterial or inadvertent tissue infusion).
- Prolonged compression (e.g. during surgery).

Symptoms and signs

The dominant early symptom is pain but all the Ps of an acute limb may be present (see Chapter 37). The pain is often described as 'out of proportion' to the clinical findings, but this is a variable finding. There is pain on passive stretch of the muscle (e.g. flexing the toe, which causes stretch within the calf muscle). Patients will also have pain on active movement of the muscle within the compartment. A tender compartment is a sign of muscle ischaemia.

Complications
Tissue ischaemia

This is a direct result of the high compartmental pressure leading to venous ischaemia and capillary congestion. A loss of arterial pulses is a very late (often irreversible) sign. There is a high rate of limb loss (amputation) associated with missed (untreated) CS.

Neuropathy

A combination of ischaemia and pressure on peripheral nerves can lead to both a sensory (earliest sign) and motor neuropathy (e.g. foot drop) as well as a chronic painful ischaemic neuritis. Complete paralysis is a late (often irreversible) finding.

Myoglobinuria, hyperkaelemia and acute kidney injury

Ischaemia leads to muscle necrosis and breakdown (rhabdomyolysis). CK levels, although not toxic *per se* serve as a useful marker for the severity and progress of rhabdomyolysis. *Rhabdomyolysis* leads to a release of intracellular cations (H^+ and K^+) into the blood stream leading to *acidosis* and *hyperkaelemia* respectively (with risk of cardiac arrest). Released myoglobin (from ischaemic muscle) is filtered by the kidneys giving rise to myoglobinuria, which precipitates out in an acidic (urine) environment and is toxic to the renal tubules leading to *acute kidney injury*.

Diagnosis

A high clinical suspicion is key to the diagnosis and management!

Compartment pressures

These can be measured directly using a Stryker needle attached to a pressure gauge, inserted directly into the compartment. Most clinicians will use >30 mmHg as diagnostic criteria, but lower pressures in the *symptomatic* patient are also diagnostic. However, the technique has a significant false negative rate and therefore adds little above clinical examination alone with a high index of suspicion!

Management

- **Treat the underlying cause.** This includes treating any ischaemia (e.g. embolectomy, revascularisation), fixation of fractures, evacuation of haematoma, etc.
- **Optimise coagulation and fluid resuscitation,** but do not over-resuscitate with fluids.
- **Perform a fasciotomy.**
- **Manage the rhabdomyolysis and its complications**.

Fasciotomy

The biggest risk in performing a fasciotomy is not adequately decompressing all compartments!

A fasciotomy is best done as a *prophylactic* procedure in the high-risk patient, because of the high morbidity associated with a delayed diagnosis, but it is also an emergency therapeutic procedure for any patient with a clinical suspicion of CS.

It involves widely opening the fascia to decompress the compartment and restore perfusion, or as prophylaxis in high-risk cases to prevent a pressure rise. Often swollen muscle is seen to 'bulge' through the wound upon opening the fascia. Calf and thigh fasciotomy are covered in the figure. A forearm fasciotomy is covered in Chapter 44.

Ischaemic time

The lower limb has a 4–6 hour ischaemic window before irreversible damage occurs, although this timeframe can be variable depending on collateral supply, presence of shock, acuteness of the ischaemia and amount of tissue trauma. The ischaemic window is greatly shortened if there is underlying shock, and it may be as short as 2 hours for amputation and <1 hour for a good functional outcome!

Treatment for rhabdomyolysis

- Calcium (e.g. Ca^{2+} gluconate or chloride) i.v. to stabilise the hyperkaelemia-induced myocardial irritability.
- Aggressive fluid hydration to ensure good diuresis and reduce myoglobinuria-induced acute kidney injury.
- Sodium bicarbonate ($NaHCO_3$) and insulin-dextrose infusion to drive the K^+ ions intracellularly along with oral and rectal resonium to reduce K^+ absorption from the GIT (reduce the hyperkalaemia).
- Renal replacement therapy to treat acutely life-threatening hyperkaelemia and acidosis.
- Alkalinisation of the urine with $NaHCO_3$ (urinary pH > 6.5) to prevent myoglobinuria precipitation in the renal tubules. This is cumbersome to achieve and may not offer any great benefit over hydration alone. Intravenous $NaHCO_3$ also carries side effects including venous thrombosis and risk of alkalosis.
- Forced diuresis (e.g. mannitol) may be used in resistant cases but offers little benefit over adequate hydration alone.

Figure 43.1 Typical clinical findings in the groin and lower limb associated with chronic IVDU.

Left leg

Groin crease

Fistula/sinus (repetitive trauma from needles

Abscess (tender, pulsatile mass) ± mycotic aneurysm)

Surrounding cellulitis

Old scarring (repetitive IVDU or old I + D of abscess)

Chronic lymphoedema ± Peau d'Orange (chronic trauma from IVDU ± repeat infection)

Signs of chronic venous hypertension from recurrent venous thrombosis 2° proximal IVDU (varicose veins are usually NOT present due to chronic superficial thrombophlebitis and fibrosis)

There may also be signs of chronic arterial ischaemia if fibrosis or micro-thrombosis from IVDU

Figure 43.2 Chronic skin sinus in the groin from IVDU.

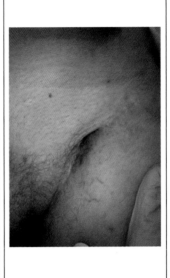

Figure 43.3 Right groin wound with healing by secondary intention after mycotic aneurysm rupture and ligation.

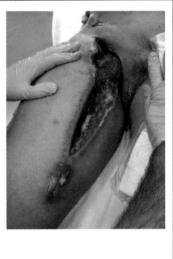

Figure 43.4 Algorithm for the management of suspected mycotic peripheral vascular aneurysm.

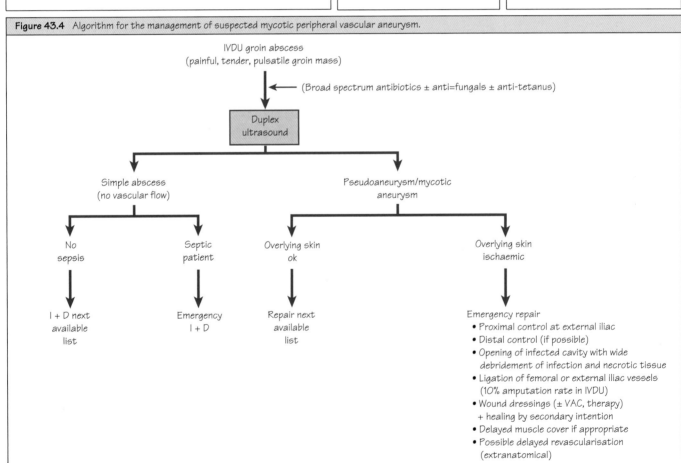

IVDU groin abscess
(painful, tender, pulsatile groin mass)

(Broad spectrum antibiotics ± anti=fungals ± anti-tetanus)

Duplex ultrasound

Simple abscess (no vascular flow)

Pseudoaneurysm/mycotic aneurysm

No sepsis

Septic patient

Overlying skin ok

Overlying skin ischaemic

I + D next available list

Emergency I + D

Repair next available list

Emergency repair
• Proximal control at external iliac
• Distal control (if possible)
• Opening of infected cavity with wide debridement of infection and necrotic tissue
• Ligation of femoral or external iliac vessels (10% amputation rate in IVDU)
• Wound dressings (± VAC, therapy) + healing by secondary intention
• Delayed muscle cover if appropriate
• Possible delayed revascularisation (extranatomical)

Abbreviations: IVDU, intravenous drug use; VAC, vacuum assisted closure

Vascular and Endovascular Surgery at a Glance, First Edition. Morgan McMonagle and Matthew Stephenson.

Management of complications in the chronically traumatised and infected groin are especially challenging. The IVDU groin will have chronic scarring and fibrosis with fistula formation from repeated arterial and venous puncture.

Complications in the IVDU groin
- Oedema and lymphoedema (chronic trauma and infection).
- Scar tissue (chronic trauma and recurrent infection).
- Infection:
  - Abscess formation (may be prevascular).
  - Cellulitis.
  - Necrotising fasciitis.
- Pseudoaneurysm formation:
  - Infected (mycotic) versus non-infected.
  - Ruptured (massive haemorrhage) versus non-ruptured.
- Fistula formation (chronic traumatic injection).
- Venous thrombosis (proximal DVT):
  - Chronic venous fibrosis.
  - Valve destruction and chronic venous reflux.
  - Venous hypertension.
- Arterial thrombosis (acute, chronic, acute-on-chronic).
- Arterial stenosis.
- Distal embolisation (mycotic material, thrombus from aneurysm).
- Necrosis of overlying skin.

Microbiology
- The IVDU groin contains challenging and unusual microflora due to repeated trauma weakening tissue defences, use of unsterile needles, unsterile injected substance and repeated injection through unclean skin.
- Growth is often polymicrobial with unusual bacteria and fungi that can disseminate to distant sites (e.g. liver abscess, brain abscess and endocarditis).
- Gram negative anaerobic bacteria predominate (including bacteroides, E.coli and tetanus subspecies), but peptostreptococcus (G+ve) is also common.
- There is also a high prevalence of blood-borne viral infections including hepatitis B, C and HIV.
- Tuberculosis is more common amongst drug users.

Broad spectrum antibiotics should be prescribed empirically for the complicated IVDU groin to cover both gram negative and positive bacteria as well as extended range organisms. Anti-fungal agents should be considered as well as empirical anti-tetanus vaccination.

Management
Cellulitis and groin abscess
- Broad spectrum antibiotics should be started empirically.
- Simple abscesses may be treated with incision and drainage with debridement of any infected, necrotic tissue.
- The surgeon needs to be aware that the abscess may be an infected pseudoaneurysm (perform a preoperative Duplex U/S to confirm).

Always perform a Duplex U/S of a groin abscess in the IVDU patient to rule out an infected pseudoaneurysm!

Acute ischaemia from intra-arterial injection
Intra-arterial injection of illicit substance is often non-sterile and particulate in nature, not fully dissolved with vasoconstrictive properties (e.g. cocaine). This directly injures the endothelium with an intense inflammatory reaction and acute thrombosis (with ischaemia). Revascularisation is not a safe option in these patients because of the chronically infected and scarred tissue planes.

Management is aimed at *damage limitation* by prevention of further clot propagation and preservation of collateral perfusion:
- Pain relief (remember higher doses of opiates may be necessary in chronic IVDU users). Nerve blocks may be useful.
- Elevation of extremity.
- Intravenous steroids (e.g. dexamethasone) to reduce inflammation.
- Anticoagulation (unfractionated heparin or LMWH) with the addition of Dextran-40 i.v. if no improvement.
- Thrombolysis may have a role if the thrombus is very proximal.
- Vasodilators including iloprost to maintain open collaterals.
- Sympathectomy may have a role in chronic management (e.g. if a complex regional pain syndrome develops).
- Physiotherapy and mobilisation as pain allows.
- Allow any ischaemic tissue to demarcate before undertaking debridement or amputation (unless there is wet gangrene).

Mycotic pseudoaneurysm
Infected pseudoaneurysm (rarely true aneurysm) presenting as a painful, red, tender pulsatile mass in the groin that is often difficult to distinguish from a simple skin abscess! Do a Duplex if in doubt!

Poor viability of overlying skin mandates surgical exploration (regardless of the aetiology of the pseudoaneurysm!) because free rupture and rapid exsanguination may occur as the overlying skin ulcerates.

Immediate management includes direct groin pressure, intravenous access (often central because of a lack of available peripheral veins!) and administration of warmed blood and blood products as necessary. These patients should be allowed to remain slightly hypotensive (SBP 80–100 mmHg) to reduce further blood loss until surgical haemostasis is achieved.

Surgical options. Dissection of the groin vessels is too hazardous in the hostile groin because of the risk of uncontrollable haemorrhage through difficult, scarred tissue planes. Therefore, proximal control should be achieved via an RP approach onto the iliac vessels. If actively bleeding, the vessels (external iliac artery [EIA]) should be ligated at this level. Distal control may not be necessary because these vessels are often chronically thrombosed! Reconstruction after ligation is not recommended because of the chronic infection and risk of further 'blow out'.

The amputation rate after ligation of the EIA in an IVDU is 10–15% (30–50% in non-IVDU population), due to the rich collateral circulation from chronic microthrombi giving rise to chronic ischaemia! All patients should also undergo four-quadrant calf fasciotomies to minimise the limb loss rate. Haemostasis from the fasciotomies is often troublesome because of the marked lower limb oedema and chronic venous hypertension (chronic DVT and venous fibrosis). Usually the groin cannot be closed primarily, but the surgeon should achieve good muscle coverage (e.g. sartorius or rectus flap) and allow secondary healing over this.

Revascularisation. Very short distance claudication may be an indication for revascularisation (performed months later after complete healing of the skin and infection). An extra-anatomical reconstruction is safest to avoid the hostile, fibrotic groin (e.g. obturator bypass [internal iliac to SFA or profunda tunnelled via obturator foramen]). All vascular repairs must ensure healthy tissue (muscle) coverage.

Figure 44.1 Steps in performing an upper limb fasciotomy.

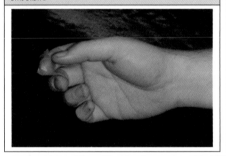

(a)

(b)

Forearm fasciotomy	Brachial embolectomy
• Two incisions are needed, one on the volar aspect of the forearm and the other on the dorsum. • The flexor compartment (anterior/ volar) contains the most muscle as well as two arteries (radial and ulnar) and two nerves (median and ulnar). • The volar compartment also crosses two joints (elbow and wrist). • Volar compartment is decompressed in a 'lazy-S' fashion from the medial aspect above the elbow and following in a loose wavy pattern across the forearm coming back to the midline at the centre of the wrist, crossing the wrist joint and into the palmar fascia for about 2 cm (beware median nerve here!). • The dorsal incision is a single semi-lunar incision on the dorsum of the forearm and does not cross any joints.	• Artery is exposed in the proximal arm in the natural groove between the biceps and triceps. • The vessel should be followed distal along the arm with a lazy 'S' incision across the antecubital fossa to expose the brachial bifurcation (radial and ulna arteries). • After heparinisation and clamping, a transverse arteriotomy is made in the brachial artery. • An appropriately sized Fogarty embolectomy catheter is passed proximal and distal (incl. the exposed forearm vessels) and thrombus retrieved. • This is followed by flushing with heparinised saline. • There should be good in-flow and back-bleeding from the vessels post-embolectomy. • The arteriotomy is then closed with interrupted prolene.

Figure 44.2 Ischaemic right hand (pale, pulseless and paraesthetic): hand secondary to brachial artery embolism.

Figure 44.3 Anatomy relevant to upper limb vascular occlusion. Note the close association between the brachial artery and median nerve. In addition the brachial vein is often paired and adherent to the brachial artery. If visualised, the basilic vein is typically the largest vein in the upper limb.

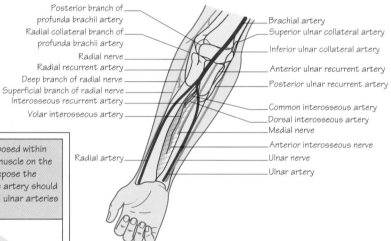

Posterior branch of profunda brachii artery
Radial collateral branch of profunda brachii artery
Radial nerve
Radial recurrent artery
Deep branch of radial nerve
Superficial branch of radial nerve
Interosseous recurrent artery
Volar interosseous artery
Radial artery

Brachial artery
Superior ulnar collateral artery
Inferior ulnar collateral artery
Anterior ulnar recurrent artery
Posterior ulnar recurrent artery
Common interosseous artery
Dorsal interosseous artery
Medial nerve
Anterior interosseous nerve
Ulnar nerve
Ulnar artery

Figure 44.4 Exposure of the brachial artery. The artery is exposed within the 'natural groove' palpated between the biceps and triceps muscle on the median aspect of the upper arm. The incision is deepened to expose the brachial artery, taking care not to injure the median nerve. The artery should be followed down to its bifurcation so that both the radial and ulnar arteries may be individually embolectomised.

Biceps brachii muscle
Bicipital aponeurosis divided and reflected upwards to expose vessel
Brachialis muscle
Brachioradialis muscle
Pronator teres muscle

Brachial artery
Median nerve

Figure 44.7 Diagrammatic representation of subclavian steal syndrome. (a) Note the normal flow in the BCA but occluded LSCA. (b) During left arm exercise, blood 'steals' from the posterior circulation and flows retrograde down the LVA to meet the demand of the ipsilateral upper limb. CSCA bypass also demonstrated.

Figure 44.5 DSA angiogram demonstrating a 'Bovine arch' where both common carotid arteries arise from the same common origin on the aortic arch. There is also an aberrant origin of the RSCA along the aortic arch just distal to the origin of the left SCA. Both RVA and LVA's respectively arise from the normal position, This aberrant RSCA is at risk of aneurysmal degeneration over time. In this particular case, the RSCA passed between the oesophagus and trachea with mild symptoms of dysphagia lusoria.

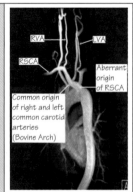

RVA
LVA
RSCA
Aberrant origin of RSCA
Common origin of right and left common carotid arteries (Bovine Arch)

Figure 44.6 Diagrammatic representation of a left carotid-subclavian bypass.

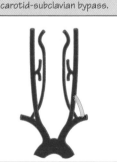

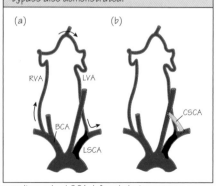

(a)
(b)
RVA
LVA
BCA
LSCA
CSCA

Abbreviations: BCA, brachiocephalic artery; CSCA, carotid-subclavian artery bypass; DSA, digital subtraction andiography; LSCA, left subclavian artery; LVA, left vertebral artery; RSCA, right subclavian artery; RVA, right subclavian artery

Vascular and Endovascular Surgery at a Glance, First Edition. Morgan McMonagle and Matthew Stephenson.

Aetiology of upper limb vascular disease

- Atherosclerosis:
  - Asymptomatic.
  - Arm claudication.
  - Acute thrombosis.
- Thromboembolism (acute limb).
- Subclavian steal syndrome.
- Kommerall's diverticulum.
- Trauma (see Chapter 41).
- Thoracic outlet syndrome (see Chapter 45):
  - Arm claudication.
  - Post-stenotic aneurysm with embolization.
  - Secondary Raynaud's phenomenon.
- Raynaud's (see Chapter 48).
  - Primary.
  - Secondary.
- Vasculitis (see Chapter 46–47).
- Complications of renal access (steal syndrome, ischaemia, gangrene, aneurysmal degeneration of fistula, occlusion/thrombosis).

Upper limb atherosclerosis

The upper limb is resistant to ischaemia partly because of the generous collateral supply around the shoulder girdle and the collateral-rich profunda brachii branching very proximal from the brachial artery in the upper arm. The most commonly affected vessel is the SCA, but more distal vessels may also be involved (especially in diabetes and chronic renal failure).

Asymptomatic arterial occlusion does not require treatment (e.g. absent radial pulse found on routine examination). Symptomatic disease often presents as arm fatigue or forearm claudication on exercise (e.g. arms working above shoulder level) that is well tolerated, and treatment is only indicated if affecting work or lifestyle. Critical ischaemia is rare. Treatment includes BMT, balloon angioplasty, stenting, open bypass (e.g. carotid-subclavian bypass, SCA-axillary bypass).

Subclavian steal syndrome

This is an uncommon cause of vertebrobasilar insufficiency because of high-grade stenosis/occlusion of the proximal left SCA (or right brachiocephalic) *proximal to the origin of the VA*.

The exercise-induced increased arm perfusion demand effectively 'steals' blood from the ipsilateral patent VA (causing reverse flow in the VA). This results in hypoperfusion of the posterior cerebral circulation leading to vertebrobasilar symptoms (syncope, dizziness, nausea). Dynamic Duplex and angiogram will demonstrate reverse VA flow during limb exercise (which can also be asymptomatic). Treatment includes stenting of the SCA stenosis or carotid-SCA bypass (only necessary if symptomatic!).

Thromboembolism and acute ischaemia

An embolism may affect any of the upper limb vessels but usually occurs at or above the brachial bifurcation. Treatment decisions can be made on clinical grounds alone without further imaging and includes anticoagulation, catheter-directed thrombolysis/thrombectomy and open brachial embolectomy.

Brachial embolectomy

The brachial artery is exposed at the medial aspect of the upper arm (natural 'groove' between biceps and triceps). The accompanying bra-chial vein (often paired), basilic vein and median nerve (occasionally ulnar nerve) should be identified and preserved. The brachial artery can be dissected distally to expose the brachial bifurcation (origin of ulnar and radial arteries) at the lower edge of the antecubital fossa using a 'lazy S' incision (as it is crossing the joint). These vessels may then be embolectomised individually. If there has been a prolonged ischaemic time (>4–6 hours), then a forearm fasciotomy may be necessary.

Aberrant right SCA + Kommerall's diverticulum

An aberrant right SCA affects 0.5–1% of the population. It arises directly from the aortic arch, typically distal to the left SCA origin (in contrast to the normal origin as a branch from the brachiocephalic artery). As it travels towards the right upper limb, it may pass between oesophagus and spine or between oesophagus and trachea giving rise to SCA stenosis with or without tracheal stenosis (stridor) or oesophageal compression (dysphagia lusoria).

The aberrant SCA is also prone to aneurysmal degeneration (i.e. Kommerall's diverticulum), which may thrombose (right upper limb ischaemia), embolise (ischaemia or stroke) or rupture with free haemorrhage (very high mortality). Treatment is necessary for symptomatic disease or aneurysmal change and includes ligation with reconstruction (graft from aortic arch to SCA or transposition of right common carotid artery to SCA).

Upper limb venous disease
Upper limb DVT (5–10% of venous thrombosis)

Upper limb DVTs are less common compared with lower limb (2 in 100,000 persons per year) and may be *primary* or *secondary*.

Primary causes
- *Idiopathic venous thrombosis.* Although by definition no cause is identified, all patients should be investigated for secondary causes, especially malignancy and other hypercoagulable disorders.
- *Effort thrombosis (Paget-Schroetter syndrome).* This is axillary-subclavian vein thrombosis following vigorous arm activity (e.g. swimming, weight lifting) and accounts for 2% of upper limb DVT.
- *Venous thoracic outlet syndrome (V-TOS).* This overlaps with 'effort thrombosis' but in patients in whom TOS has been diagnosed with impingement on the subclavian vein (SCV) (see Chapter 45).

Secondary causes
There are numerous secondary causes of upper limb DVT including instrumentation (e.g. central venous catheterisation, cardiac pacemaker insertion, IVDU, Hickman lines, peripherally inserted central catheter [PICC] lines), malignancy and other hypercoagulable disease states (see Chapters 50–52).

Presentation
- A 'tightness' or 'heaviness' in the hand and arm.
- Oedema and warm cyanosis of the upper limb.
- Dilated superficial veins (as venous hypertension progresses).
- Less likely to embolise and cause PE.
- If PE occurs (36% of upper limb DVTs), it is often smaller and less lethal than lower limb.

45 Thoracic outlet syndrome

Figure 45.1 Anatomy and boundaries of the thoracic outlet.

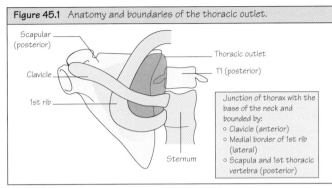

Scapular (posterior)
Clavicle
1st rib
Thoracic outlet
T1 (posterior)
Sternum

Junction of thorax with the base of the neck and bounded by:
○ Clavicle (anterior)
○ Medial border of 1st rib (lateral)
○ Scapula and 1st thoracic vertebra (posterior)

Figure 45.2 Anatomy of the thoracic outlet (left side).

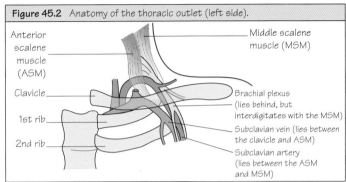

Anterior scalene muscle (ASM)
Clavicle
1st rib
2nd rib
Middle scalene muscle (MSM)
Brachial plexus (lies behind, but interdigitates with the MSM)
Subclavian vein (lies between the clavicle and ASM)
Subclavian artery (lies between the ASM and MSM)

Figure 45.3 Anatomical spaces for compression at the thoracic outlet.

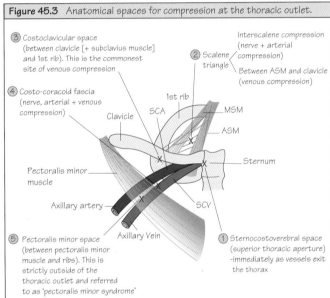

③ Costoclavicular space (between clavicle [+ subclavius muscle] and 1st rib). This is the commonest site of venous compression

④ Costo-coracoid fascia (nerve, arterial + venous compression)

Pectoralis minor muscle

Axillary artery

⑤ Pectoralis minor space (between pectoralis minor muscle and ribs). This is strictly outside of the thoracic outlet and referred to as 'pectoralis minor syndrome'

② Scalene triangle
Interscalene compression (nerve + arterial compression)
Between ASM and clavicle (venous compression)

1st rib
Clavicle
SCA
MSM
ASM
Sternum
SCV
Axillary Vein

① Sternocostovertebral space (superior thoracic aperture) –immediately as vessels exit the thorax

Figure 45.4 Anatomy of the scalene triangle.

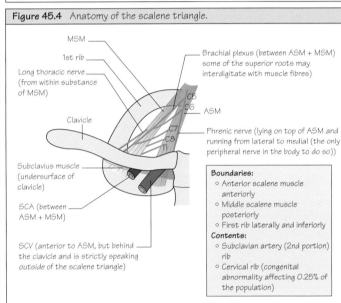

MSM
1st rib
Long thoracic nerve (from within substance of MSM)
Clavicle
Subclavius muscle (undersurface of clavicle)
SCA (between ASM + MSM)
SCV (anterior to ASM, but behind the clavicle and is strictly speaking outside of the scalene triangle)

Brachial plexus (between ASM + MSM) some of the superior roots may interdigitate with muscle fibres)
C5
C6
ASM
C7
C8
T1
Phrenic nerve (lying on top of ASM and running from lateral to medial (the only peripheral nerve in the body to do so))

Boundaries:
○ Anterior scalene muscle anteriorly
○ Middle scalene muscle posteriorly
○ First rib laterally and inferiorly
Contents:
○ Subclavian artery (2nd portion) rib
○ Cervical rib (congenital abnormality affecting 0.25% of the population)

Figure 45.5 Costoclavicular space: (as viewed from below (transaxillary view)).

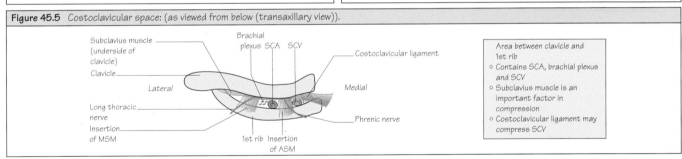

Subclavius muscle (underside of clavicle)
Clavicle
Lateral
Long thoracic nerve
Insertion of MSM
Brachial plexus SCA SCV
Costoclavicular ligament
Medial
Phrenic nerve
1st rib Insertion of ASM

Area between clavicle and 1st rib
○ Contains SCA, brachial plexus and SCV
○ Subclavius muscle is an important factor in compression
○ Costoclavicular ligament may compress SCV

Clinical manoeuvres in the diagnosis of TOS

Figure 45.6 (a and b) Hyperabduction manoeuvre. The examiner palpates the radial pulse with the arms at rest by the sides. There is disappearance of the pulse as the arm is abducted to 90° (or higher).

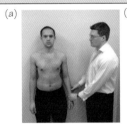
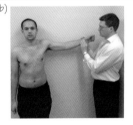

(a) (b)

Figure 45.7 (a and b) Roo's Test (also known as EAST (Elevated Arm Stress Test)). The arms are held in the "I surrender" position and the fists repetitively opened and closed for up to three minutes. This is a good test for N-TOS if pain and paraesthesia are reproduced.

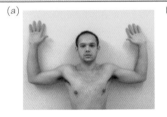
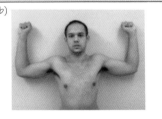

(a) (b)

Thoracic outlet syndrome (TOS) is a neurovascular compression at the level of the thoracic outlet.

Aetiology

There are numerous causes including abnormal angulation of first rib, congenital cervical rib, scalene muscle hypertrophy, abnormality at the level of the scalene tubercle (congenital or acquired) and post-trauma (e.g. malunion of clavicle fracture). It has a female preponderance (3:1) The causes and sites of compression are shown in Figures 45.3–45.5.

Classification

Neurogenic (N-TOS) – 95%.
Venous (V-TOS) – 3%.
Arterial (A-TOS) – 2%.

Anatomical spaces for compression

- Sternocostovertebral space/superior thoracic aperture (immediately as vessels exit the thorax).
- Scalene triangle.
  - Interscalene (arterial and nerve compression).
  - Between the anterior scalene muscle and clavicle (venous compression).
- Costoclavicular space (between the clavicle (with subclavius muscle) and 1st rib). This is the commonest site of venous compression.
- Costo-coracoid fascia (nerve, arterial and venous compression).
- Pectoralis minor space (between pectoralis minor muscle and ribs). This is actually outside the thoracic outlet and leads to 'pectoralis minor syndrome'.

Causes of compression

Within the scalene triangle

- Hypertrophied scalene muscles with a narrowed space within the triangle and first rib
- Abnormal (possibly congenital) fibrous bands with the scalene muscles (usually MSM)
- Anomalous first rib (e.g. vertically placed)
- Cervical rib (congenital abnormality) which has variable amounts of bone, cartilage and fibrous material

Beyond the scalene triangle

- Fracture callus (e.g. healed clavicle fracture).
- Narrowed space between clavicle and first rib (just beyond the scalene triangle).
- Pectoralis minor syndrome.

Anatomy of the thoracic outlet

Junction of thorax with the base of neck bounded by:
- Clavical (anterior).
- Medial border of first rib (lateral).
- Scapula and 1st thoracic vertebra (posterior).

Within the thoracic outlet is the scalenus anterior muscle, with the subclavian vein in front, the scalenus medius muscle (with the subclavian artery and brachial plexus between the two muscles).

Anatomy of scalene triangle

Boundaries

- Anterior scalene muscle anteriorly.
- Middle scalene muscle posteriorly.
- First rib laterally and inferior.

Contents

- Subclavian artery (2nd portion).
- Brachial plexus.

Cervical rib (congenital abnormality affecting 0.25% of the population)

Other important points

- The phrenic nerve traverses from lateral to medial (only peripheral nerve in the body to do so) on top of the ASM within its fascia.
- The SCV lies anterior to the ASM, but behind the clavicle (strictly speaking this is outside the scalene triangle).

Clinical examination

Look for signs of upper limb ischaemia (chronic and acute).
Looks for signs of upper limb DVT.
Full upper limb neurological examination (sensory and motor).
Look for evidence of upper limb muscle wasting.

Clinical (provocative) manoeuvres

Because of the anatomical abnormality, symptoms are precipitated by any action that further narrows the costo-clavicular angle.

Hyperabduction manoeuvre: Disappearance of the radial pulse as the straight arm is hyperabducted (compression by pectoralis muscle).

Roo's test: Repeated fist clenching with both arms held in the '*I surrender' position* (shoulders abducted to 90° + elbows flexed at 90°. There will be reproduction of symptoms (paraesthesia) if positive.

Adson's test: With arms loosely held by the sides, the patient inhales deeply and turns their head towards the affected side. It is positive if the pulse disappears (narrowing of the interscalene triangle). If positive on inhalation alone, then suspect a cervical rib!

Costoclavicular compression manoeuvre: Disappearance of the radial pulse as the shoulders are actively forced into an 'exaggerated military position' (backwards and downwards) leading to compression between the clavicle and first rib.

Investigations

There is no one absolute diagnostic test (especially N-TOS).
CXR (abnormal first rib or cervical rib (often poorly calcified). The presence of a cervical rib makes either N-TOS or A-TOS likely.
Dynamic Duplex scan (at rest and during provocation) to look for evidence of vessel obstruction, although this can be a normal finding.
Dynamic CTA/MRA to look at the anatomical space, and for signs of vessel compression and a cervical rib.
Nerve conduction studies for neuropathy (late sign).

Figure 45.8 Adson's Test. The radial pulse is palpated with arms in a relaxed position by the patient's side. The patient is asked to take in a deep breath and hold and then to turn the head to look towards the affected side. There may be a disappearance of the radial pulse during this manoeuvre. Some authorities also advocate turning the face away from the affected side in an attempt to alter the mechanical dynamics within the scalene triangle and compress the vessel.

(a)   (b)

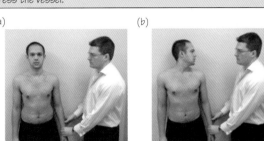

Figure 45.9 Costoclavicular Compression Manoeuvre. The patient stands in an 'exaggerated military position' with the arms by the sides, chin up and the shoulders forced backwards and downwards thereby reducing the space between the clavicle and first rib.

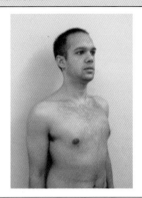

Figure 45.10 (a) Cheat X-ray demonstrating right-sided cervical rib. (b) Same rib magnified on CXR (1, first rib, 2, second rib, C, clavical).

(a)

(b)

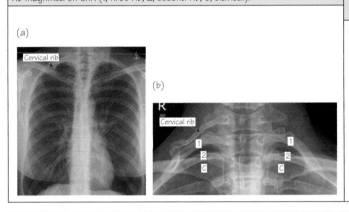

Figure 45.11 (a and b) CT angicgram for A-TOS displaying intimal injury with thrombus in the subclavian artery. (a) cross section image, (b) coronal image.

(a)   (b)

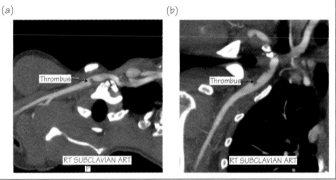

Figure 45.12 Surgical exposure of the thoracic outlet. (a) Displays the surface anatomical markings for exposure. (b) Demonstrates open exposure. The right phrenic nerve (traversing from lateral to medial) and anterior to the scaleous anterior. The contents of the scalene triangle with the scaleous medius posterior (which should also be divided at its insertion and excised).

(a)   (b)

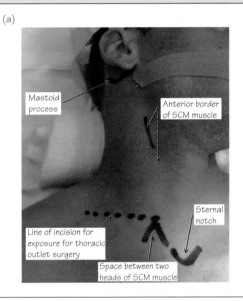

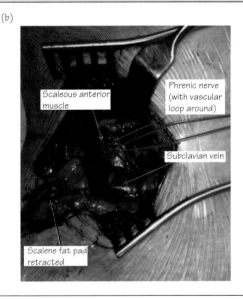

Abbreviations: ASM, anterior scalene muscle; A-TOS, arterial-TOS; MSM, middle scalene muscle; N-TOS, neurogenic-TOS; SCA, subclavian artery; SCM, sternocleidomastoid; SCV, subclavian vein; TOS, thoracic outlet syndrome; V-TOS, venous-TOS

Neurogenic TOS (N-TOS)

Typically there is compression of the lower brachial plexus roots ($C8/T1 \rightarrow$ *ulnar nerve*) where the cords converge within the scalene triangle and may be in association with a cervical rib or anomalous first rib. Predisposing factors include previous injury and repetitive strain conditions.

Presentation. Neck pain with radiation and paraesthesia in ulnar nerve distribution that is often effort-related but may occur at rest and may mimic carpal tunnel syndrome. May present with Raynaud's syndrome. Small muscle wasting in the hand is a late sign. Provocative manoeuvres are useful in the diagnosis.

Treatment. Usually conservative (>95%) with physiotherapy, postural exercises, occupational management and analgesia. Surgery is rarely indicated.

Venous TOS (V-TOS)

SCV compression at the level of the thoracic outlet, classically caused by narrowing at the costoclavicular space (by the costoclavicular ligament or the subclavius muscle) causing SCV stenosis ± thrombosis. Rarely thrombophilia presents as SCV thrombosis. It often starts with effort-related activity, especially with repetitive overhead shoulder movement (e.g. weight lifting, swimming, martial arts) affecting the right more frequently.

Presentation. Upper limb DVT (15% chance of PE) with swelling, suffusion, pain with dilated superficial veins. Rarely venous ischaemia (think malignancy!).

Treatment. Rest, limb elevation, compression, anticoagulation (≥3 months) and thrombolysis (best results <10days). Early surgical decompression post-thrombolysis is recommended (high recurrence rates [>50%]). Venous patch repair may be necessary (stenosis).

Arterial TOS (A-TOS)

This is typically associated with a cervical rib, congenital band or anomalous first rib causing compression occurring within the scalene triangle. Complications include SCA stenosis, thrombosis, embolisation and post-stenotic dilatation (aneurysmal change) with or without mural thrombus.

Presentation. Effort-related arm pain and fatigue (arm claudication), acute upper limb (thrombosis/distal embolisation) or secondary Raynaud's. Examination may reveal pulselessness (especially with Adson's test) and/or signs of distal embolisation (digital ischaemia). There may be a bruit on auscultation (SCA aneurysm).

Treatment. Restoration of perfusion (if acute limb) includes catheter-directed thrombolysis ± brachial embolectomy. Surgical decompression is usually recommended, especially if complications have occurred. SCA aneurysm should be resected and repaired (direct anastomosis or interposition graft, or ligation and bypass). The pectoralis minor muscle may be resected (to treat pectoralis minor syndrome) or a claviculectomy performed (compression from fracture malunion).

Surgical decompression of TOS

Decompression may be performed, either *transaxillary* or *transthoracic*.

Decompression aims to create space within the thoracic outlet with preservation of the phrenic nerve, brachial plexus and vessels:

- Cervical rib resection (if present).
- First rib resection.
- Anterior + middle scalenectomy.

A transaxillary approach is most suitable for pure N-TOS decompression, in the *absence* of a cervical rib. It is associated with less post-operative pain and a more cosmetically pleasing scar (under the axilla). It also allows for a future transthoracic approach if necessary. However, both the cervical rib excision and magnitude of scalenectomy is limited with this approach.

46 Vasculitis I: Overview

Table 46.1 Table of principal vasculitis conditions and the principal vessel size affected.

Aorta and branches	Large and medium sized vessels	Medium sized vessels only	Small vessels only	Microvascular occlusion
Takayasu's	Buerger's	Polyarteritis nodosa	Wegener's granulomatosis	Connective tissue disorders
Buerger's	Giant cell arteritis	Wegener's granulomatosis	Connective tissue disorders	Rheumatoid vasculitis
Giant cell arteritis	Polyarteritis nodosa		Rheumatoid vasculitis	Cutaneous vasculitis

Table 46.2 Serum autoantibody test and its associated vasculitis condition.

Autoantibody test	Associated disease
Anti-nuclear antibody (ANA) (indirect)	SLE, Sjogren's, rheumatoid arthritis, scleroderma
Extractable antinuclear antibody (ENA)	
Anti-Ro (anti-SSA antibody)	Sjogren's syndrome, SLE
Anti-La (anti-SSB antibodies)	Sjogren's syndrome
P-ANCA (antineutrophil cytoplasmic)	Polyarteritis nodosa
C-ANCA (antineutrophil cytoplasmic)	Wegener's granulomatosis
Rheumatoid factor (extracellular)	Rheumatoid arthritis, Takayasu's
Antiphospholipid (multiple locations)	Antiphospholipid syndrome, SLE
Anticardiolipin (anti-mitochondrial)	Antiphospholipid syndrome, SLE, Bechet's
Others	
Cryoglobulins and gold agglutinins	SLE, rheumatoid arthritis, mycoplasma pneumonia, blood dysrasias, hyperviscosity syndromes (including nephrotic syndrome) and hepatitis C
Complement levels	Low in urticarial vasculitis and lupus

Figure 46.1 Algorithm for the work-up and investigation of suspected vasculitis.

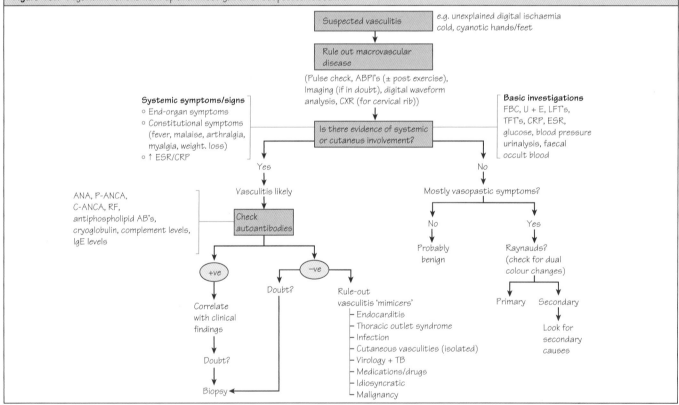

Abbreviations: ABPI's, ankle-brachial pressure index; CRP, C-reactive protein; CXR, chest X-ray; ESR, erythrocyte sedimentation rate; FBC, full blood count LFT's, liver function tests; SLE, systemic lupus erythematosus; TB, tuberculosis; TFT's, thyroid function tests; U+E, urea and electrolytes

Vascular and Endovascular Surgery at a Glance, First Edition. Morgan McMonagle and Matthew Stephenson.

Vasculitis is a spectrum of disorders characterised by acute and chronic inflammatory changes in the vessel wall.

While the management of vasculitis is rarely surgical, many patients may present to a vascular service for an opinion on managing the ischaemic component. There are numerous disorders, most of whose aetiology is unknown. Long-term complications may include vessel fibrosis, stenosis and occlusion (often microvascular occlusion) with tissue ischaemia ± end-organ injury.

Broad classification

The condition may be confined to the *skin* (*cutaneous vasculitis*) or may be *systemic*. Systemic vasculitis is characterised by:
- Constitutional symptoms (malaise, fever, weight loss)
- End-organ symptoms
- ↑ ESR/CRP.

In addition there is further classification according to the size and therefore type (elastic versus muscular) of vessel predominantly affected (see Figure 46.1).
- Large vessel vasculitis.
- Medium vessel vasculitis.
- Small vessel vasculitis.

Clinical picture and examination

- Symptoms and signs of peripheral ischaemia including cold hands and feet, discolouration and cyanosis of digits, tissue loss (ulceration) and gangrene.
- Nail-fold infarcts and splinter haemorrhages are common.
- Clinical signs of infection (malaise, etc.) or pyrexia of unknown origin (PUO) are common.
- Cutaneous vasculitis is common.
- Rarely there is aneurysmal degeneration of vessel.
- Signs of systemic involvement and end-organ injury (renal, GIT, respiratory, liver and eye).
- A full vascular examination to identify macrovascular disease should be performed to distinguish from microvascular ischaemia.
- TOS should be excluded (see Chapter 45).

Investigations

Basic serology. Full blood count (FBC) (anaemia, thrombocytopaenia), *urea and electrolytes (U&E)* and *creatinine* (renal injury), *LFTs* (liver dysfunction) and *thyroid function tests* (hypothyroidism). *Inflammatory markers* (CRP, ESR, serum osmolality) reflect disease severity and treatment response.

Autoantibodies. There are over 100 autoantibodies described in association with a multitude of disease processes. Figure 46.2 summarises the principal antibodies associated with vasculitis that may present to a vascular service. These tests are often difficult to interpret and referral to a rheumatologist is useful.

Diagnostic imaging

- *CXR* to look for a cervical rib or chronic pulmonary changes and fibrosis (e.g. Wegener's granulomatosis, rheumatoid disease).
- *Duplex U/S* to look for macrovascular occlusions and/or aneurysmal degeneration (e.g. Bechet's). A *'Halo' sign* may be seen in temporal arteritis.
- *Angiography* if macrovascular suspected as well as specific vascular 'patterns' seen in certain vasculitides (e.g. Polyarteritis, Buerger's).

Histopathology

A skin or vessel biopsy may be performed and stained for microscopy (specific histological changes) or direct immunofluorescence (on fresh frozen tissue) for difficult cases. However, many of the vasculitides display *non-specific inflammatory changes* affecting vessels and the diagnosis depends more on the clinical pattern as well as other investigations.

Other investigations

- ABPI measurement for macrovascular ischaemia.
- Digital pressure studies for small vessel ischaemia.
- Nail fold capillaroscopy (see Chapter 48).
- Infection screen (if malaise/systemic upset/PUO).
- Virology (e.g. hepatitis B a/w PAN).
- Echocardiogram (e.g. infective endocarditis)
- Urinalysis (dipstick and a 24-hour urinary protein collection)
- Faecal occult blood (associated with PAN).
- Targeted investigations for malignancy (if indicated).

Management

In mild cases, no treatment may be necessary other than observation, especially with cutaneous small vessel vasculitis (CSVV). With medium to larger vessel involvement, where there is an increased risk of end-organ damage, active treatment may be needed.

General management

- Cessation of smoking (for all vasculitis) but especially Buerger's.
- Keep warm/avoiding cold and wet conditions to relieve symptoms.
- Rest and elevation of the affected limb with simple analgesia and non-steroidal anti-inflammatory medications.

Treatment of the malperfusion

- BMT as per treatment of atherosclerotic disease with antiplatelet agents (often dual agents).
- Anticoagulation (warfarin) for more severe occlusive disease.
- Vasodilators to improve blood flow in small vessels and collaterals. Iloprost (prostacyclin analogue) has both antiplatelet and vasodilatory properties and is administered by i.v. infusion (5 days). The infusion can be titrated to side effects (flushing, headache, nausea and hypotension).
- Angioplasty/stenting for macrovascular disease (if short segment stenosis); occasionally surgery is required in difficult cases, but often there isn't a healthy distal target vessel (e.g. in Takayasu's).
- Amputation is necessary for gangrene.

Treatment of the inflammatory and systemic component

Therapeutic response to treatment can be graded by an improvement in clinical symptoms as well as falling inflammatory markers and/or angiographic appearances.

Mild attacks: Rest and elevation, non-steroidal anti-inflammatories, low-dose prednisolone and antihistamine (if urticarial component).

Moderate attacks: Increase steroid dose, colchicine, dapsone.

Severe attacks: Chronic steroids, azathioprine, mycophenolate, cyclophosphamide, methotrexate, IV immunoglobulin, rituximab.

Vasculitis II: Specific conditions

Figure 47.1 Severe vasculitis of lower limb with advance skin changes, cyanosis and ischaemic skin and digits.

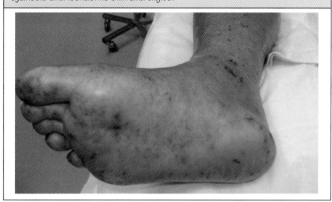

Figure 47.2 Advanced Buerger's disease (thromboangiitis obliterans) affecting the upper limb with ulceration of ring finger on right hand and evidence of previous distal digital amputation on the left (index and middle fingers). Note the brown staining on the left hand consistent with continuing cigarette smoking despite advanced disease.

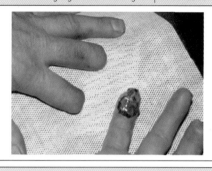

Figure 47.3 Diagrammatic representation of the spectrum of affected vessels in vasculitis.

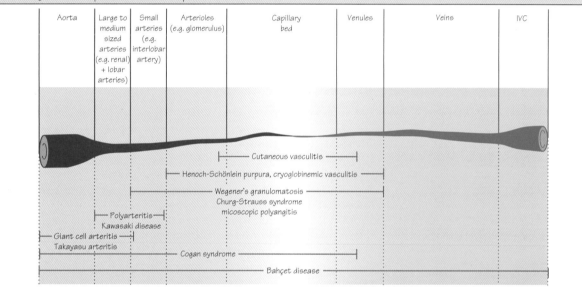

Figure 47.4 DSA angiogram demonstrating Buerger's disease of the upper limb with occlusion of multiple vessels (including ulnar artery) and numerous 'cork-screw' collaterals.

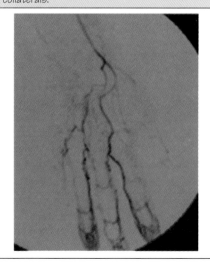

Figure 47.5 DSA angiogram of aortic arch branches with Takayasu's arteritis demonstrating numerous fibrotic stenosis of the extracranial carotid and vertebral vessels.

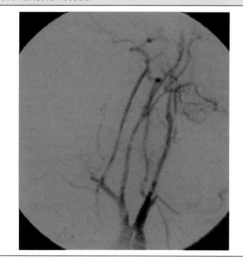

Vascular and Endovascular Surgery at a Glance, First Edition. Morgan McMonagle and Matthew Stephenson.

108 © 2014 John Wiley & Sons, Ltd. Published 2014 by John Wiley & Sons, Ltd. Companion website: www.ataglanceseries.com/vascular

Takayasu's arteritis

Clinical features. Prevalent in South-East Asia in young adults (female preponderance 8:1) and affecting aorta and its branches (elastic arteries). *Two phases* of disease described: *acute systemic phase* (prepulseless) and *chronic obliterative phase* (pulseless).

Prepulseless phase: Non-specific systemic upset (fever, malaise, myalgia, arthralgia, headache, weight loss) with vessel tenderness.

Pulseless phase: Obliteration of vessel (nodular thickening, stenosis, fibrosis). Late aneurysmal degeneration may also occur. *Pulmonary artery* is involved in 50% of cases. Hypertension is common (renal artery stenosis).

Diagnosis. Clinical pattern of disease (large vessel involvement with angiographic changes). Histology shows inflammation of all *three vessel wall layers* progressing to *chronic granulomatous formation, intimal nodular thickening* and *medial-adventitial fibrosis ('skip' pattern)*. Fifteen per cent are rheumatoid factor positive. ANA usually negative.

Treatment. Anti-inflammatory agents and steroids, escalating to more potent immunosuppressant therapy as required. Surgical treatment of occlusive or aneurysmal disease (if indicated) is considered only when the acute inflammatory component is in remission and the target vessel is free of active inflammation.

Giant cell arteritis (temporal arteritis)

Clinical features. Disease of middle-aged and elderly patients (female preponderance 5:1) being more common in smokers and those with established atherosclerosis. It affects the small and medium-sized arteries (especially the cranial branches of the aorta [external carotid artery]).

There may be non-specific systemic involvement (general malaise, fatigue, pyrexia [PUO]) with headache and scalp tenderness (temporal or occipital artery inflammation). Sudden, irreversible blindness (ophthalmic/posterior ciliary artery occlusion) is the most serious complication in untreated patients. This may be preceded by amaurosis fugax. Jaw claudication occurs in 50% (maxillary and facial artery inflammation).

Diagnosis. Largely clinical pattern supported by a high ESR (>100 mm min^{-1}). Duplex may demonstrate characteristic 'halo' sign around affected temporal artery. The gold standard is a histological diagnosis (granulomatous arteritis) via open (temporal artery) biopsy but lesions occur in a 'skip' pattern (risks false negative result).

Treatment. Steroids are the mainstay of treatment escalating to other more potent anti-inflammatories and immunosuppressants as indicated. When clinically suspected, treatment should be empirically started (and before biopsy results) because of the high risk of blindness.

Buerger's disease

Clinical features. Also known as *'thromboangiitis obliterans'* and largely a disease of young male smokers. It is a *non-atherosclerotic thrombotic occlusive vasculitis* affecting medium and smaller sized vessels in both the upper (25%) and lower limbs (>95%), especially tibial vessels. The presenting complaint is usually foot (not calf) claudication with absent pedal pulses (but preserved femoral and popliteal pulses). It may progress to rest pain and tissue loss. It has a strong association with both Raynaud's phenomenon and superficial migratory thrombophlebitis.

Diagnosis. Largely clinical pattern of disease in a young male smoker with characteristic angiographic pattern (abruptly occluded tibial vessels with multitudes of tortuous *'cork-screw' collaterals*). The remaining proximal vessels are relatively free of atherosclerosis. Histology consists of *hypercellular thrombus* in affected vessels.

Treatment. Cessation of smoking, BMT and exercise will effectively treat most patients. Vasodilators and sympathectomy may aid in symptom control. Surgical bypass is usually not possible because of small distal target vessels.

Polyarteritis nodosa (PAN)

Clinical features. This is a disease of middle age with a male preponderance (2:1) and affecting small and medium sized arteries. There are two recognised subtypes: *cutaneous (c-PAN)* and *microscopic (MPA)* (microscopic polyangiitis). There is a strong association with hepatitis B infection.

c-PAN. Affects 20–50% of patients and lesions include palpable purpura, livedo reticularis, ulceration and digital infarcts.

MPA. Forty per cent of patients will also have c-PAN. Systemic manifestations include non-specific symptoms (malaise, weight loss, pyrexia). End-organ involvement (*systemic necrotizing vasculitis*) includes *renal* (70%) (hypertension, proteinuria and progressive renal failure, necrotizing glomerulonephritis), *pulmonary* (pulmonary haemorrhage), *gastrointestinal* (abdominal pain, nausea, vomiting and rarely haemorrhage, infarction and perforation), *mononeuritis multiplex* (inflammation of vasa vasora) and, rarely, retina and testes. *Aneurysmal degeneration* (saccular or fusiform) may also occur.

Diagnosis. Largely clinical pattern supported by high p-ANCA levels. Angiography displays arterial stenosis +/− aneurysmal changes. The gold standard is skin biopsy showing *fibrinoid necrosis* of the vessel wall, *microaneurysms, thrombosis* and *tissue infarction*.

Treatment. Steroids escalating to more potent immunomodulators (cyclophosphamide, methotrexate, azathioprine) as required.

Wegener's granulomatosis

Clinical features. Affects the medium and small vessels. *Triad* of *respiratory* tract (upper and lower), *renal* and *cutaneous* (palpable purpura and nodules) disease. May progress to a necrotising vasculitis with ulceration and gangrene.

Diagnosis. Clinical pattern of disease supported by raised c-ANCA. The gold standard is with histopathology.

Treatment. Anti-inflammatories, steroids and immunosuppressants.

Behçet's disease

Clinical features. This is a multisystem recurrent systemic vasculitis affecting small vessels, most prevalent in Asian and Middle Eastern communities. *Triad* of recurrent (≥3 per annum) *oral and genital ulceration, chronic iridocyclitis* and *vasculitis* (30%). The vasculitis affects venous system (90%) with DVT and superficial thrombophlebitis and Budd-Chiari. Arterial involvement is rare but can lead to obliterative endarteritis +/− aneurysmal degeneration.

Diagnosis. Largely clinical pattern with venous involvement. Arteriography may show occlusion and aneurysmal formation.

Treatment. Steroids escalating to more potent cytotoxic agents as required. Arterial disease and venous thrombosis treated as standard.

Table 48.1 Causes of secondary Raynaud's syndrome.

Connective tissue	Medication	Occupational	Vascular	Other
Systemic sclerosis (scleroderma) CREST syndrome Rheumatoid arthritis Systemic lupus erythematosis Sjogren's syndrome Dermatomyositis/polymyositis	β-blockers Cyclosporine Ergotamine Cytotoxics Sulfasalazine	HAVS Vinyl chloride exposure Cold work environment (e.g. refridgeration)	Atherosclerosis Buerger's disease Thoracic outlet syndrome Microemboli Vasculitis (e.g. Wegener's, PAN)	Malignancy Tobacco smoke Firearm users Reflex sympathetic dystrophy Cryoglobinaemia Coagulopathy Hyperviscosity syndrome Hypothyroidism

Figure 48.1 Raynauld's disease of the hands. The fingers are cold with bi- or triphasic colour changes on exposure.

Figure 48.2 Frostbite. (a) Cold cyanotic toes progressing to (b) well-demarcated gangrene at tip of hallux which eventually went on to heal and auto-amputate leaving healthy underlying tissue (c).

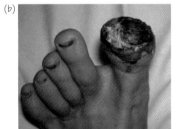

(a) (b) (c)

Figure 48.3 Algorithm for the clinical investigation of patient with suspected Raynaud's.

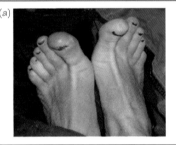

Suspected Raynaud's

Full history + clinical examination
- Attacks related to cold exposure/emotion
- Symmetrical symptoms and signs
- Normal nail fold capillaroscopy*
- Anything to suspect secondary Raynaud's?
- ESR levels + ANA

Normal findings → Primary Raynaud's

Abnormal findings → Rule-out macrovascular disease + thoracic outlet syndrome → Look for other secondary causes → ± Digital pressures → Normal / Abnormal → See chapter 46 + 47

*Normal nail fold capillaroscopy is required for a diagnosis of primary Raynaud's

Figure 48.4 Digital waveforms (as measured by digital plethsmography).

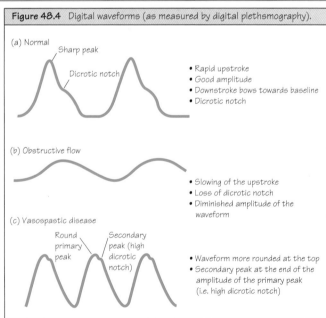

(a) Normal
Sharp peak
Dicrotic notch
- Rapid upstroke
- Good amplitude
- Downstroke bows towards baseline
- Dicrotic notch

(b) Obstructive flow
- Slowing of the upstroke
- Loss of dicrotic notch
- Diminished amplitude of the waveform

(c) Vasospastic disease
Round primary peak
Secondary peak (high dicrotic notch)
- Waveform more rounded at the top
- Secondary peak at the end of the amplitude of the primary peak (i.e. high dicrotic notch)

Abbreviations: CREST, calcinosis, Raynaud's oesophageal dysmotility, sclerodactyly, telangectasia; HAVS, hand-arm vibration syndrome; PAN, polyarteritis nodosa

Vascular and Endovascular Surgery at a Glance, First Edition. Morgan McMonagle and Matthew Stephenson.

Vasospastic disorders

A vasospastic disorder (primary or secondary) is any condition causing intense spasm in the arterial system resulting in ischaemia and pain.

Raynaud's syndrome and disease

Raynaud's is a <u>cold-induced</u> vasospastic disorder affecting the hands and feet.

It may be classified as either *primary* (Raynaud's disease) or *secondary* (Raynaud's syndrome). Raynaud's phenomenon is often used as a blanket term for any Raynaud's-type peripheral vasospasm.

Primary Raynaud's (Raynaud's disease)

This is an idiopathic vasospastic disorder, affecting about 10% of the population with a female preponderance (10:1). It occurs in isolation (i.e. without any other disease condition).

Secondary Raynaud's (Raynaud's syndrome)

This is a cold-induced, vasospastic disorder that occurs in association with other (usually systemic) conditions (e.g. connective tissue disorder) or with a triggering factor, other than cold (e.g. medication, occupational, etc).

Clinical features

The ischaemia induced by the intense vasospasm leads to cold, painful extremities, especially affecting the digits. Typically during a 'vasospastic attack', the digits will pass through a variety of clinically diagnostic, well-demarcated colour changes (*phases*):
- **White** (intense vasospasm with digital ischaemia and pain).
- **Blue** (as the levels of deoxygenated blood increase in the digits).
- **Red** (painful reactive hyperaemia (vasodilation) ± paraesthesia).

Although the symptoms and signs of Raynaud's cover a spectrum, the diagnostic clinical phases should be either *biphasic* or *triphasic* (i.e. the digital clinical features should go through at least two if not three of the colour phases). It affects both the fingers (most commonly) and toes, but may also affect other aspects of the extremities (nipples, tip of the nose, ear lobes and, rarely, the tongue. The affected digits may be symmetrical or asymmetrical. Rarely, it may progress to digital ulceration and gangrene.

Investigations

The diagnosis is largely a clinical one, although in severe cases an underlying secondary cause (including vasculitis) should be sought and all patients should have a CXR to look for a cervical rib.

Haematological Investigations

Standard blood investigations for Raynaud's include ESR, plasma viscosity, rheumatoid antibody, antinuclear antibody and cryoglobulins. Other investigations should be aimed at ruling out other secondary causes.

Digital systolic pressure measurement

This is taken before and after local cooling at 15°C of the digit. A pressure drop of >30 mmHg is considered significant, but no definitive gold standard exists. It should be carried out 2–3 hours after an attack and only after complete resolution of symptoms.

Nail-fold capillaroscopy

Examine the nails using an ophthalmoscope at high power. Normally, vessels are not visible in the nail-folds, but in certain connective tissue diseases (CTDs) abnormally large blood vessels are seen. A combination of abnormal nail-fold vessels and an abnormal immunological test has a >90% positive predictive value for CTD.

Management
General

- Differentiate between primary and secondary Raynaud's and treat the underlying condition if present (e.g. TOS, hypothyroidism, etc.).
- Avoid the underlying trigger (e.g. occupational, medication, smoking, environmental).
- As the condition is cold-induced, then avoidance of cold and keeping warm is recommended (e.g. wearing heated gloves, avoiding cold environments, wrapping up warm).

Medical

- Vasodilators to improve blood flow to the tissues (e.g. calcium channel blockers [e.g. nifedepine], pentoxifylline, naftidrofuryl, sildenafil, inositol nicotinate and moxisylate [thymoxamine]).

Nifedepine is a good first-line agent although side effects include headache, light-headedness, flushing, ankle swelling and reflex tachycardia (caution with ischaemic heart disease). In severe cases, intravenous prostaglandin (iloprost) may be necessary.

Surgical

- Sympathectomy removes the autonomic vasospastic element of the sympathetic nervous system and can be performed for both the upper limbs and lower limbs (cervical and lumbar respectively).
- A digital arterial sympathectomy can also be performed for individual fingers (stripping the autonomically rich adventitia from digital arteries).
- Surgical management of a specific underlying condition (e.g. TOS, amputation, bypass).

Cold injury and frostbite

Cold injury may lead to tissue freezing, microvascular occlusion, ischaemia and gangrene, and is divided into three phases.

Phase 1: (Frostnip) affects skin only with pain, numbness and redness of the extremity and is fully reversible.

Phase 2: Skin blistering, which may ulcerate. In general this is reversible over time, but can result in cold-sensitivity with neuralgia, pain, paraesthesia and ↓ sensation.

Phase 3: Irreversible, often full-thickness tissue damage, hardening of the tissue, nerve damage and necrosis.

Treatment consists of tetanus prophylaxis and rapid rewarming of the extremity in warm water (38–40°C), elevation, analgesia (opiates), and allowing the surrounding area to demarcate before a decision on surgical debridement or digital amputation can be made. An escharotomy may be required (if circumferential).

Figure 49.1 Diagrammatic representation sympathetic outflow from spinal cord to supply the upper limbs and its relay within the autonomic ganglia and chain.

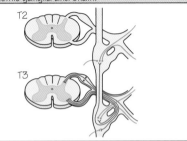

Figure 49.2 Iontophoresis of palmar hyperhidrosis.

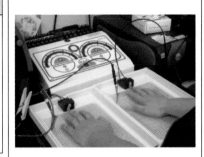

Figure 49.3 Illustration of thorascopic sympathectomy. usually only two ports are required (one for camera and one for instrument insertion).

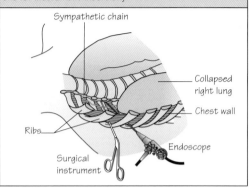

Figure 49.4 Diagrammatic illustration of sympathetic outflow to eye and heart (above T2). These tracts should be preserved to avoid Horner's syndrome and bradycardia.

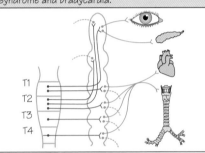

Figure 49.5 (a) Illustration of sympathectomy chain (with ganglia) along the spinal vertebrae and the extra-anatomical bypass autonomic tracts ('Nerve of Kuntz') which may explain failure of sympathectomy. (b) The correct segment of sympathetic chain should be divided and resected to prevent recurrence and avoid side effects (Horner's and bradycardia).

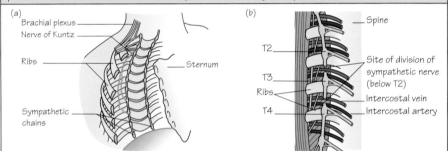

Table 49.1 Social consequences of untreated palmar hyperhidrosis (Adapted from British Journal of Dermatol. 2002;147:1218–1226).

Social complications of palmar hyperhidrosis	
Low confidence	71.8%
Feelings of unhappiness/depression	48.7%
Changes in leisure activities	44.6%
Frustrated with daily activities	30.4%
Miss social engagements	25%
Decrease in time spent at leisure activities	19.3%

Horner's syndrome
Miosis
Ptosis
Anhidrosis
Enophthalmus (may not occur in humans)

Figure 49.6 Diagrammatic Illustration of sympathetic outflow from spinal cord to supply the upper limbs and the points for division during sympathectomy to treat palmar hyperhidrosis.

Do not divide chain above T2 ganglion, as this will result in a Horner's syndrome

Spinal cord (T2–T6)
segment T2–T6 supply upper limbs; after exiting the dorsal nerve root and entering the sympathetic chain via the white ramus communicans, fibres travel upwards in the sympathetic chain; before joining brachial plexus (C1–T1). The brachial plexus consists of spinal nerves onto which autonomic nerve fibres have 'hitch-hiked' along to gain access to the upper limbs.

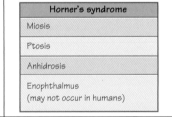

Vascular and Endovascular Surgery at a Glance, First Edition. Morgan McMonagle and Matthew Stephenson.
© 2014 John Wiley & Sons, Ltd. Published 2014 by John Wiley & Sons, Ltd. Companion website: www.ataglanceseries.com/vascular

Primary hyperhidrosis is the excessive, localised, uncontrollable production of sweat with no discernable cause.

It affects 0.5–1% of the general population with an equal male to female preponderance. Although no true diagnostic definition exists, the condition has been objectively diagnosed gravimetrically as a measured axillary sweat production >50 mg/min.

However, if sweating is excessive to the point of having a negative lifestyle effect, then it may be considered problematic to the point of necessitating further treatment (see Table 49.1).

Pathophysiology
- Eccrine sweat glands innervated by sympathetic nervous system (SNS).
- Uniquely has acetylcholine as neurotransmitter.
- Spinal cord segments T2–T6 supply the sympathetic innervation to the upper limbs and passe cephalad to join the brachial plexus.
- All postganglionic sympathetic fibres to entire upper limb except axillae run via brachial plexus (C5–T1).
- An aberrant (anatomical variant) thoracic origin of the sympathetic supply to the upper limbs may also exist is referred to as the *Nerve of Kuntz* (variable intrathoracic ramus arising caudal to the normal sympathetic outflow offering an alternative pathway to the upper limbs) This may explain failure or recurrence post-surgical treatment).

Clinical features
- Avoid stress triggers and certain foods (e.g. spices, alcohol).
- Palms, axillae, soles of feet and, rarely, the entire body.
- Patients complain of the social and psychosocial consequences including dripping hands, slippery handgrip, dripping into computer keyboards, embarrassment, offensive odour, wet clothing and depression, as well as the side effects of treatment.

Management
- Medical.
- Surgical (severe cases where medical management has failed).

Medical management
This includes the use of various topical agents applied to the affected skin, botulinum toxin, systemic treatment and iontophoresis.

Topical agents
Numerous agents have been tried with variable success including aluminium compounds, anticholinergics, potassium permanganate, tannic acid solutions, boric acid, resorcinol, formaldehyde, glutaraldehyde.

Aluminium hexahydrate 20%
Applied directly to the skin (axillary disease only), this acts by causing sweat to thicken into clumps, thereby blocking sweat ducts and preventing further sweat release. Side effects include skin irritation, rashes, stinging sensation, pruritus and damage to clothing.

Anticholinergics
These include oxybutynin, benztropine, glycopyrrolate. Side effects include dry mouth, blurred vision, mydriasis, retention and constipation.

Botulinum toxin A (BTX-A)
This is a highly toxic *neurotoxin* from the bacterium Clostridium botulinum that is injected intradermally. It inhibits the release of acetylcholine (ACh) from nerve fibres at the axonal-gland synapse (muscarinic receptor-stimulated). Side effects include; bleeding, bruising, flu-like symptoms, dry eyes and compensatory sweating.

Other therapeutic uses of botulinum toxin include achalasia, muscle spasm, torticollis, blepharospasm, neurogenic bladder, anal fissure, migraine, vocal cord dysfunction and cosmetic wrinkles.

Iontophoresis
Affected body parts (palmar or plantar) are immersed in an electrochemical solution as a low-intensity electrical current (15–20 mA) is passed ($\uparrow$ as tolerated [painful paraesthesia]). Charged ions are electrically driven into the skin, thereby temporarily disrupting sweat gland function. A course is typically ~20 mins per session, twice weekly for 7–8 sessions, and improvements are typically seen after 4 sessions. Maintenance sessions are used as needed when sweating recurs. Side effects include pain, skin cracking, blistering and erythema. Contraindications include: pregnancy, cardiac arrhythmias and the presence of a cardiac pacemaker.

Surgical management
Excision of affected skin
This involves the direct excision of skin with the removal of subcutaneous tissue-containing sweat glands, but leaves scarring. The *Skoog procedure* involves suction currettage of the sub-cutaneous axillary tissue (incl. sweat glands) via a 1–2 cm incision under local anaesthesia.

Sympathectomy
Surgical interruption (*open* or *thoracoscopic*) of the sympathetic chain at the level of T2 removes the autonomic innervation to the palmar sweat glands (but not always axillary). It is an invasive procedure usually reserved for palmar hyperhidrosis and Raynaud's.

Thoracoscopic sympathectomy
After intubation with a double lumen endotracheal (ET) tube, CO_2 is insufflated to deflate the lung and visualise the sympathetic chain via a thoracoscopic port inserted through the third intercostal space. The sympathetic chain runs along the posterior thoracic wall overlying the heads of the ribs. The head of the second rib is identified (most prominent rib) and corresponds to the T2 ganglion. The sympathetic chain is divided below, thereby interrupting the sympathetic supply running cranially (upper limb supply) on the respective side.

Open sympathectomy
Largely superseded because of the less invasive thoracoscopic approach but includes Telford's (supraclavicular), Atkin's (transaxillary) and Cloward's (dorsal midline) approaches.

Complications of sympathectomy
The treating physician needs to weigh up the risks of such an invasive procedure against the condition in a young population.
- *General.* Pneumothorax, phrenic nerve injury (diaphragmatic paralysis), vagus nerve injury, pleural effusion, haemorrhage, haemothorax, chylothorax and empyaema.
- *Compensatory sweating.* Affects up to 60% where hyperhidrosis occurs at a previously unaffected region. Gustatory (related to eating) sweating occurs in up to 10% (similar to Frey's syndrome).
- *Horner's syndrome.* This is due to division of the sympathetic chain <u>above</u> the level of the T2 ganglion, thereby interrupting the cervical sympathetic supply eye leading to:
  1 *Miosis* (pupillary constriction).
  2 *Ptosis* (drooping eye lid).
  3 *Anhidrosis* (periorbital dryness due to $\downarrow$ sweating).
  4 *Enophthalmus* ('sunken eye' described in animal models and may not occur in humans).

Figure 50.1 Pathophysiology of thrombosis: Virchow's triad.

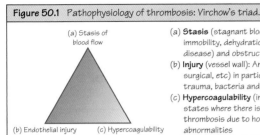

(a) Stasis of blood flow
(b) Endothelial injury
(c) Hypercoagulability

(a) **Stasis** (stagnant blood flow): Venous stasis from immobility, dehydration, turbulence (cardiac valve disease) and obstruction to vessel outflow
(b) **Injury** (vessel wall): Any vessel wall injury (traumatic, surgical, etc) in particular the endothelium including; trauma, bacteria and hypertension
(c) **Hypercoagulability** (intrinsic): Hypercoagulable states where there is a tendency towards inherent thrombosis due to host-related coagulation abnormalities

Secondary hypercoagulability

General causes: major surgery, medications (esp. oestrogens (OCP, HRT, tamoxifen, etc), sepsis, immobility, hyperviscosity (e.g. dehydration, nephrotic syndrome, congestive cardiac failure, HONK), pregnancy, etc. (see chapter 51).
Specific causes: HITS, antiphopholipid syndrome, hyperhomocysteinemia and paroxysmal nocturnal haemoglobinuria.

Table 50.1 Investigations for hypercoagulopathy and its associated condition.

Investigation	Hypercoagulopathy
Primary	
Antithrombin antigen and activity	Antithrombin deficiency
Prothrombin 20210A genetic analysis	Hyperprothrombinaemia
APC resistance test	Factor V Leiden deficiency
Factor V Leiden genetics	Factor V Leiden deficiency
Protein C antigen and activity	Protein S and C deficiency
Protein S antigen	Protein S and C deficiency
Factor VIII levels	Factor VIII elevation
Functional plasminogen	
Secondary	
Antiphospholipid/anticariolipin	Antiphospholipid syndrome
Homocysteine level	Hyperhomocysteinaemia
Cryoglobulins and cold agglutions	

Figure 50.2 Coagulation and how it interacts with the theory of Virchow's triad.

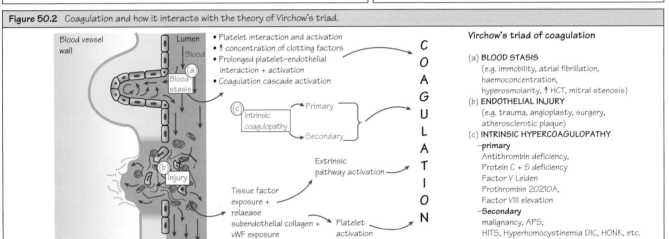

Blood vessel wall / Lumen / Blood

(a) Blood stasis
(b) Injury
(c) Intrinsic coagulopathy — Primary / Secondary

- Platelet interaction and activation
- ↑ concentration of clotting factors
- Prolonged platelet–endothelial interaction + activation
- Coagulation cascade activation

Extrinsic pathway activation

Tissue factor exposure + relaease subendothelial collagen + vWF exposure

Platelet activation

COAGULATION

Virchow's triad of coagulation

(a) BLOOD STASIS
(e.g. immobility, atrial fibrillation, haemoconcentration, hyperosmolarity, ↑HCT, mitral stenosis)
(b) ENDOTHELIAL INJURY
(e.g. trauma, angioplasty, surgery, atherosclerotic plaque)
(c) INTRINSIC HYPERCOAGULOPATHY
–primary
Antithrombin deficiency, Protein C + S deficiency Factor V Leiden Prothrombin 20210A, Factor VIII elevation
–Secondary
malignancy, APS, HITS, Hyperhomocystinemia DIC, HONK, etc.

Figure 50.3 Diagrammatic illustration of the points along the coagulation cascade that the primary coagulopathies affect (a) intrinsic and (b) extrinsic pathways.

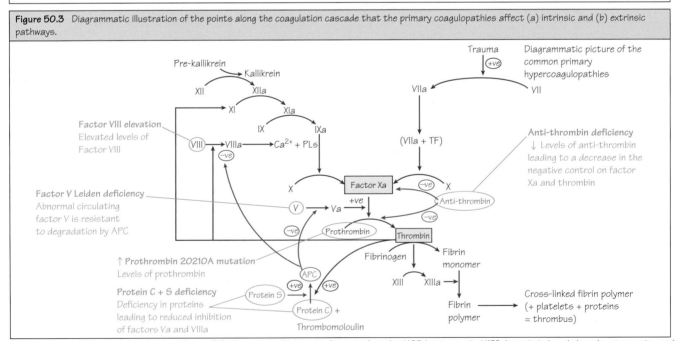

Diagrammatic picture of the common primary hypercoagulopathies

Factor VIII elevation
Elevated levels of Factor VIII

Factor V Leiden deficiency
Abnormal circulating factor V is resistant to degradation by APC

↑ Prothrombin 20210A mutation
Levels of prothrombin

Protein C + S deficiency
Deficiency in proteins leading to reduced inhibition of factors Va and VIIIa

Anti-thrombin deficiency
↓ Levels of anti-thrombin leading to a decrease in the negative control on factor Xa and thrombin

Abbreviations: APS, antiphospholipid syndrome; DIC, disseminated intravascular coagulopathy; HCT, haematocrit; HITS, heparin induced thrombocytopaenia syndrome; HONK, hyperosmolar non-ketotic coma; PLs, phospholipids

Vascular and Endovascular Surgery at a Glance, First Edition. Morgan McMonagle and Matthew Stephenson.

114 © 2014 John Wiley & Sons, Ltd. Published 2014 by John Wiley & Sons, Ltd. Companion website: www.ataglanceseries.com/vascular

Pathophysiology of thrombosis

This is broadly explained with Virchow's Triad: *Stasis* of blood flow, *Injury* (tissue factor exposure) and *Hypercoagulopathy*.

Hypercogulopathy

A hypercoagulopathy is an inherent and intrinsic increased tendency towards thrombosis.

It affects both venous (most common) and arterial systems and is classified as either *primary* or *secondary*.

Investigations

Coagulation and haematology including prothrombin time, APTT, international normalised ratio (INR), FBC (platelets), platelet aggregation, tests for malignancy (if indicated).

D-dimer assay. D-dimers are breakdown products of cross-linked fibrin and represent a very sensitive marker of thrombosis–fibrinolysis with a high negative predictive value. Therefore a normal test (in conjunction with a negative U/S if indicated) effectively excludes a venous thrombotic event with very high certainty. However, it is also very non-specific, rising in many other disease states (e.g. post-operative, malignancy, sepsis).

Thrombophilia screen. This is a test for primary hypercoagulopathy when an inherited or familial thrombophilia is suspected. It is useful to consult with a haematologist because not all patients require testing, but in general the following groups of patients warrant screening: *young* (<40 years), *familial history*, *recurrent thrombosis* (with no identifiable cause) and *'unusual'* venous thrombosis (e.g. mesenteric, cerebral).

Primary hypercoagulability

This includes the inherited thrombophilias and the risk of thrombosis is much greater when there is more than one abnormality or cause co-existing (e.g. two inherited disorders, inherited disorder + secondary risk factor [e.g. oral contraceptive pill, pregnancy, malignancy]). Most of the thrombophilias result in DVT, but multiple venous and arterial thromboses may occur. Therapy typically consists of long-term anticoagulation.

Deficiency in inhibitory enzymes of coagulation

- Antithrombin deficiency.
- Protein C and Protein S deficiency.

Increased function of procoagulation factors

- Factor V Leiden deficiency.
- Prothrombin 20210A.
- Factor VIII elevation.

Antithrombin (AT) deficiency

Mechanism. Deficiency in antithrombin (synthesised in liver), which normally inactivates thrombin and other factors (especially X and Xa).

Genetics. Rare autosomal dominant (homozygous or heterozygous) condition affecting 0.5% of population. Homozygous sufferers die in the neonatal period.

Clinical. Heterozygous form is divided into *type 1* (reduced levels of normal AT) or *type 2* (abnormal AT synthesis). The type 1 form is more aggressive (usually die in neonatal period). Type 2 sufferers have a ×10 increased risk of venous thrombosis.

Protein C and Protein S deficiency

Mechanism. Deficiency in the *vitamin-K dependent* (inhibited by warfarin) serine proteins produced by the liver, endothelial cells and megakaryocytes. Protein C is converted (by thrombin) to activated Protein C (APC) on the endothelial surface which (in conjunction with Protein S) acts as a cofactor (*Protein C/S complex*) inhibiting factors Va and VIIIa.

Genetics. Autosomal inheritance (*homozygous* or *heterozygous*). The heterozygous form has prevalence of 0.1–0.5% of population. Protein S deficiency affects about 1% of the general population.

Clinical. Homozygous form (Protein C deficiency) causes *purpura fulminans neonatalis* (neonatal death from disseminated intravascular coagulation [DIC] and organ infarction). In the heterozygous form, 50% will present by age 40 years with thrombosis (usually venous). *Warfarin-induced skin necrosis* is a specific condition occurring in Protein C or S deficiency resulting in skin necrosis (microthrombosis around adipose tissue) early after starting warfarin therapy, due to the inhibition of Protein C/S synthesis before the other vitamin-K dependent factors (II, VII, IX, X) have been inhibited, hence temporarily worsening the coagulopathy.

Factor V Leiden deficiency

Autosomal dominant condition also known as '*activated Protein C resistance (APR)*' because the abnormal circulating factor V cannot be degraded by APC. It is the most common genetically inherited thrombophilia (5% of population) but rare in African Americans.

Prothrombin 20210A mutation

This is increased levels of circulating prothrombin (precursor to thrombin) affecting about 1% of the general population.

Secondary hypercoagulability
Malignancy

Trousseau's syndrome (hypercoagulability in association with malignancy) was originally described with pancreatic cancer, but can occur with any malignancy. It is thought to result from '*tissue-factor like factor*' secreted by tumour cells or via direct platelet activation (haematological malignancies + myeloproliferative disorders).

Primary antiphospholipid syndrome (APS)

This is the persistent presence of antiphospholipid antibodies in plasma (anticardiolipin antibody and lupus anticoagulant) characterised by *venous and arterial thrombosis* (70:30 ratio respectively), *recurrent spontaneous abortion* (first and second trimester), *thrombocytopaenia* and *neurological disorders*.

Heparin-induced thrombocytopenia (HIT)

This is thrombocytopaenia (↓ platelets) but with a paradoxical increased tendency for thrombosis of which there are two types. *Type 1* begins early after heparin initiation (probably non-immune phenomenon) as a result of heparin binding directly to the platelet membrane. Platelets fall $<150 \times 10^9$/L and recover spontaneously. *Type 2* typically presents a week after heparin (earlier if repeat exposure) as an immune reaction. Platelets typically fall below 50×10^9/L and heparin resistance is displayed (APTT levels). Thromboembolic complications are more common. Treatment involves cessation of heparin (± instituting different anticoagulation).

Hyperhomocystinaemia

This is a disorder of methionine metabolism carrying a higher risk of venous thromboembolism.

Figure 51.1 Diagrammatic illustration of DVT: thrombus within the lumen of the vein with inflammation, occlusion and valve destruction.

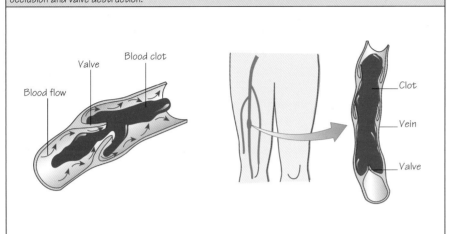

Figure 51.2 Anti-thrombotic compression stockings (below-knee).

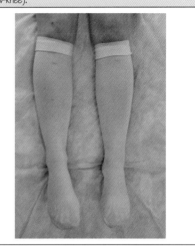

Figure 51.3 Full length sequential compression device (SCD).

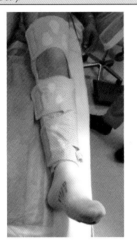

Figure 51.4 Measurement of calf circumference in the clinical examination for DVT. (a) The tibial tuberosity is identified and marked. (b) The skin on the anterior tibia is marked 10cm below the tibial tuberosity. (c) Using a measuring tape the circumference is measured (normal=35cm) on both sides. A difference of ≥2cm is considered significant (but not diagnostic).

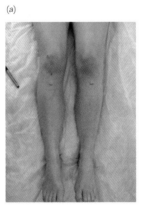
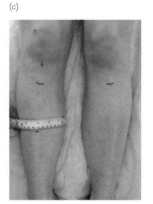

Figure 51.5 (a) normal appearance of CFA and CFV respectively, on ultrasound, without compression (b) demonstrating total compression of CVF by the external U/S probe (ie: negative for DVT).

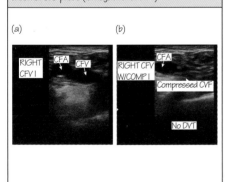

Figure 51.6 U/S demonstrating junction of CFV with LSV at the SFJ. There is a DVT present in the CFV as demonstrated by the inability to compress (W/comp) the CFV with the U/S probe.

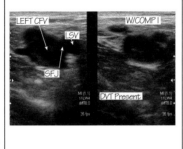

Figure 51.7 SFJ on U/S demonstrating thrombus within the LSV from acute thrombophlebitis and extending into deep venous system (CFV) via the SFJ. There is a risk of further extension and development of an above knee DVT. Treatment includes ligation of the SFJ.

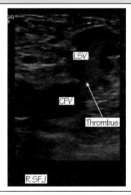

Abbreviations: CFA, common femoral artery; CFV, common femoral vein; DVT, deep vein thrombosis; IVC, inferior vena cava; LSV, long saphenous vein; PE, pulmonary embolism; SFJ, sapheno femoral junction; W/COMP, with compression

Vascular and Endovascular Surgery at a Glance, First Edition. Morgan McMonagle and Matthew Stephenson.

Figure 51.8 DVT in left iliac and SFV system secondary to May-Thurner syndrome (external compression of left common iliac vein by overlying right common iliac artery). A Trellis™ device is inserted and the thrombus cleared to re-establish flow followed by venous stenting to treat compression.

Multiple collateral venous tributeries

Femur

Lower SFV with occlusion from DVT above

IVC

Thrombus

Trellis catheter within common iliac vein

Left common iliac venous system with multiple 'shadows' consistent with thrombus (DVT)

Stent within left CIV to treat external compression secondary to May-Thurner syndrome

Good venous flow in iliac system after trellis procedure

Post trellis

Improved venous flow in SFV post-Trellis (compare with first images). Still residual thrombus (shadows)). but obstruction sucessfully cleared

Figure 51.9 Anatomical sites where a deep venous thrombosis may arise.

Site of DVT: 1. In calf sinuses, 2. Below knee tibial vessels, 3. Popliteal vein, 4. Superficial femoral vein-common femoral vein, 5. Iliac venous system, 6. IVC (below liver or renals), 7. IVC (above liver) with high risk of Budd-Chiari syndrome (hepatic venous outflow obstruction) ± acute liver failure, 8. Forearm, 9. Brachial vein (basilic vein will behave similar), 10. Axillary vein, 11. subclavian vein, 12. SVC (risk of SVC obstruction).

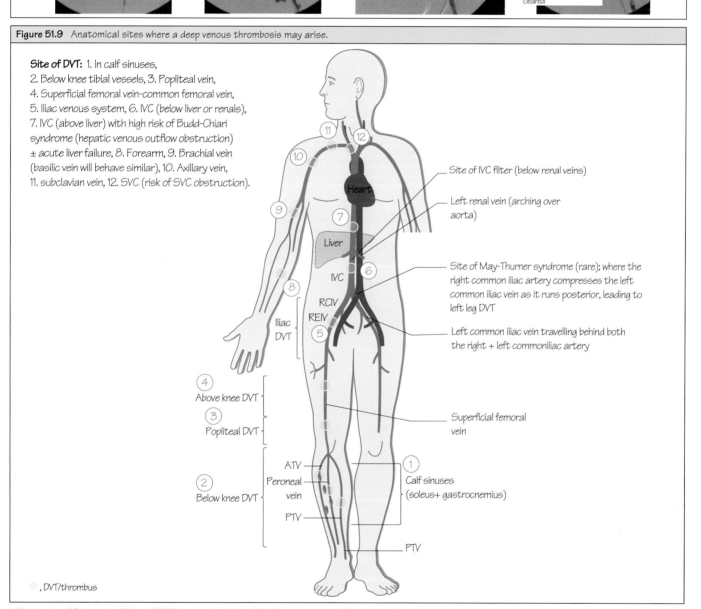

Site of IVC filter (below renal veins)

Left renal vein (arching over aorta)

Site of May-Thurner syndrome (rare); where the right common iliac artery compresses the left common iliac vein as it runs posterior, leading to left leg DVT

Left common iliac vein travelling behind both the right + left commoniliac artery

Superficial femoral vein

Heart

Liver

IVC

RCIV

REIV

Iliac DVT

Above knee DVT

Popliteal DVT

Below knee DVT

ATV

Peroneal vein

PTV

Calf sinuses (soleus+ gastrocnemius)

PTV

, DVT/thrombus

Abbreviations: ATV, anterior tibial vein; DVT, deep vein thrombosis; IVC, inferior vena cava; PTV, posterior tibial vein; RCIV, right common iliac vein; REIV, right external iliac vein; PTV, posterior tibial vein; SVC, superior vena cava

Deep venous thrombosis (DVT) is a thrombosis within the deep venous system.

It most commonly affects the lower limb but may also include the iliac veins, IVC, SVC and upper limb veins.

Incidence

This is variable depending on the population but is estimated to occur in 10–30% of hospital patients and as high as 80% in critical illness and major trauma. They are more common in the left leg (longer pelvic course running behind *both* the right and left common iliac arteries).

Risk factors, complications and management of DVT

Risk factors

- Major surgery (esp. lower limb and pelvic surgery)
- Major trauma
- Immobility
- Dehydration
- Prothrombotic medications (e.g. OCP)
- Hyperosmolarity (e.g. HONC, nephrotic syndrome)
- Coagulopathies (congenital and acquired)
- Malignancy
- Venous obstruction (e.g. external obstruction from a pelvic tumour, gravid uterus, May-Thurner syndrome)
- Pregnancy (gravid uterus and prothombotic state)

Complications

- Pulmonary embolism (PE)+/− sudden death
- Recurrent thrombosis
- Post-thrombotic syndrome. (Venous valvular incompetence with chronic reflux, venous hypertension and ulceration)
- Pulmonary hypertension
- Venous ischaemia (rare)
- Budd-Chiari syndrome (hepatic venous outflow obstruction)

Management

Prophylaxis

- General management
  - Treat underlying cause mobilise, hydrate
- Mechanical prophylaxis
  - SCDs (sequential compression devices)
  - Compression hosiery
- Chemical prophylaxis (prophylactic dose)
  - Heparin (unfractionated)
  - LMWH (fractionated heparin)

Treatment

- Anti-coagulation (therapeutic dose)
- Catheter-directed thrombolysis
- Percutaneous mechanical thrombectomy
- Open surgical thrombectomy

Lower limb DVT

The majority develop in the BK segment including soleal sinuses, tibial veins and BK-popliteal vein. Fragmentation and embolisation is less common compared with an AK-DVT (AK-popliteal, SFV, CFV and iliac veins). An AK-DVT has a much higher incidence of PE and sudden death, but without treatment BK DVTs may propagate proximally.

Table 51.1 Prevalence of DVT in high-risk, in-hospital population of patients.

Patient Group	Prevalence of DVT (%)
General Medical	10–20
General Surgery	15–40
Major Gynaecological Surgery	15–40
Post-stroke	20–50
Hip / knee / pelvic surgery	40–60
Major Trauma	40–80
Critical Care Patients	10–80

Symptoms and signs

- Asymptomatic (often picked up incidentally).
- Hot, tender, swollen and tender calf (or thigh if proximal).
- Dilated superficial veins (collateral drainage).
- Enlarged calf diameter in comparison to contralateral limb, measured at a fixed point (10 cm below the tibial tuberosity).
- *Homan's sign*. Calf tenderness with passive flexion–extension of the ankle joint (do not perform because of the risk [albeit small] of embolisation!).

Investigations

- *Venous Duplex*. This is the first investigation of choice and a good screening tool, but is very user-dependent. Venous thrombus may be visualised and is non-compressible (except if very fresh).
- *Contrast venography* is an invasive test performed by injecting contrast via a cannula in a dorsal foot vein and using fluoroscopy to visualise filling defects within the deep venous system.

DVT prophylaxis

General measures

This includes treatment of the underlying condition (e.g. removal of obstructing tumour) and identified risk factors if possible (e.g. early mobilisation, good hydration, cessation of risk-associated medications [e.g. OCP]).

Mechanical prophylaxis

- *Compression stockings*. These augment flow in the deep venous system by squeezing empty the superficial veins into the deep system thus increasing volume in the deep veins and preventing stasis. They also exert a gradually decreasing pressure gradient from the ankle (20 mmHg) upwards. Compression stockings should be specifically measured and are contraindicated if ABPI < 0.7.
- *Sequential compression devices (SCDs)*. These are pneumatic devices worn on the lower limbs that imitate the calf muscle pump by intermittently inflating and deflating. They are particularly useful during surgery or if compression stockings are contraindicated. They have similar prophylactic benefits to compression hosiery and the two may be used in combination.

Chemical prophylaxis

A smaller (prophylactic) dose of anticoagulant is given as a once-daily s.c. injection. The two commonly used agents are *heparin* and *LMWH* (superior) and they are both well absorbed through the skin. Although chemical is superior to mechanical prophylaxis, best practice is to use both in combination. Side effects include bleeding (usually minor at injection site) and, rarely, HIT syndrome (see Chapter 50).

Treatment of DVT

Anti-coagulation

Anticoagulation does not lyse thrombus, but helps to stabilise it (~7days) and prevent propagation (proximally or into the venules). Heparin or LMWH are prescribed as a weight-dependent dose. Heparin is administered i.v. as a bolus followed by infusion and the APTT must be monitored closely (therapeutic level is APTT 2–2.5 times normal). LMWH is preferred because it can be given s.c. and has a more predictable dose-response effect (APTT monitoring is not required), but, rarely, LMWH-resistance occurs (monitor anti-Xa levels). The incidence of HITS is much lower with LMWH.

If DVT is clinically suspected, then treatment should start empirically even in the absence of confirmatory tests. If DVT is confirmed, then treatment should be continued for 3–6 months usually with an oral anticoagulation (e.g. warfarin) to reduce the incidence of further thrombosis and complications (e.g. post-thrombotic syndrome).

Catheter-directed thrombolysis

This is usually reserved for more extensive proximal DVTs. Thrombolytic agent (e.g. tPA) is delivered via an intravenous catheter placed directly at the site of thrombosis. Up to 30% will get complete resolution if treatment is started within 10 days but it may be attempted up to 4 weeks. The risk of systemic absorption is low ($T_{1/2}$ 20–30 minutes) but contraindications are similar to systemic thrombolysis including active bleeding, recent surgery, recent stroke, history of intracranial haemorrhage, diabetic retinopathy and pregnancy.

Percutaneous mechanical thrombectomy (PMT)

This is also usually reserved for more extensive thrombosis. A variety of devices are commercially available (e.g. Trellis device) that mechanically break up the thrombus followed by aspiration.

Open surgical thrombectomy

This is largely a historical operation, but is occasionally undertaken (e.g. during TOS decompression with subclavian venous repair). There is a high rate of re-thrombosis and post-thrombotic syndrome.

Superficial thrombophlebitis

This is acute thrombosis of the *superficial venous system* presenting as an intense inflammatory reaction (pain, swelling and erythema). Risk factors include repeated trauma (e.g. cannulation) and venous incompetence. Treatment includes analgesia, elevation and compression. Anticoagulation is usually not required (controversial).

Over time the vein may become fibrotic and obliterate or develop incompetence with reflux. Occasionally the thrombus may extend to the deep system (e.g. at the saphenofemoral junction [SFJ]) with risk of DVT (ligation of the junction can be performed to prevent extension).

Figure 51.1 (a) Vena cava filter. This is placed within the IVC to trap emboli in patients with DVT and/or high risk of PE. (b) Filter seen in situ on plain X-ray. (c) Filter in situ in the infrarenal IVC seen during DSA venogram. Access for insertion may be via the femoral vein (this case) or via the internal jugular vein (retrograde insertion via the superior and inferior venae cavae and retrohepatic IVC to reach the infrarenal IVC).

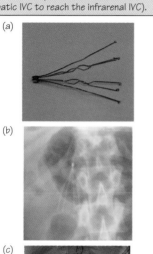

(a)

(b)

(c)

Filter in infra-renal IVC

Tip of venous catheter via femoral approach

Figure 52.2 Bilateral PE's on CT pulmonary angiogram seen in the RPA and LPA and extending into subsegmental branches on the left.

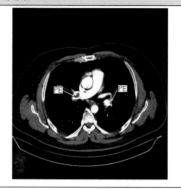

Figure 52.3 Venous phase CT scan demonstrating thrombus in the IVC up to the level of the RRV and LRV respectively which led to the PE's seen in image. Note the normal arrangement of the vessels with the LRV travelling in front of the aorta (<3% it is retro-aortic), with the SMA even more anterior as it exits off the aorta.

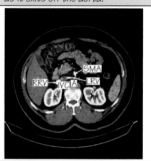

Figure 52.4 Left iliac venous thrombosis with extension into IVC. There is complete occlusion of the left iliac venous system.

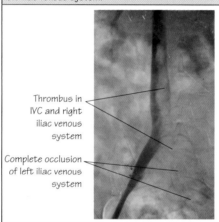

Thrombus in IVC and right iliac venous system

Complete occlusion of left iliac venous system

Figure 52.5 Early venous ischaemia of right foot. Note diffuse swelling and cyanosis with ischaemic skin on the forefoot.

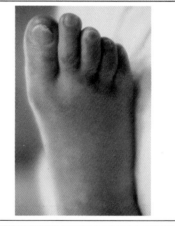

Figure 52.6 Complications of PE.

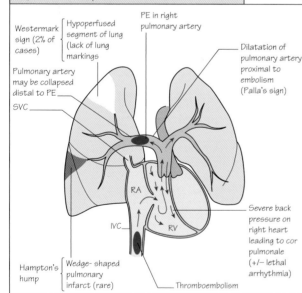

Westermark sign (2% of cases)

Hypoperfused segment of lung (lack of lung markings)

PE in right pulmonary artery

Dilatation of pulmonary artery proximal to embolism (Palla's sign)

Pulmonary artery may be collapsed distal to PE

SVC

RA

IVC

RV

Severe back pressure on right heart leading to cor pulmonale (+/– lethal arrhythmia)

Hampton's hump

Wedge-shaped pulmonary infarct (rare)

Thromboembolism

Figure 52.7 Complications of DVT.

Acute/chronal liver failure

Pleural effusion

Pulmonary infarct

Pulmonary embolism

Sudden death

Cor pulmonale and right heart failure

Hypoxia and respiratory failure

Arrhythmias

Hypotension

Budd-Chiari (very rare)

DVT

Recurrent thrombosis

Lower limb venous ishhaemia (rare)

Venous infarction

Phlegmasia alba dolens

Phlegmasia caerulea dolens

Post-thrombotic syndrome and lower limb venous hypertension

Venous ulceration

Chronic limb pain

Varicose veins

Lipodermatosclerosis and venous eczema

Abbreviations: A, aorta; CT, computed tomography; DVT, deep venous thrombosis; IVC, inferior vena cava; LMWH, low molecular weight heparin; LPA, left pulmonary artery; LRV, left renal vein; PE, pulmonary embolism; RA, right atrium; RPA, right pulmonary artery; RRV, right renal vein; RV, right ventricle; SCD'S, sequential compression devices; SMA, superior mesenteric artery

Vascular and Endovascular Surgery at a Glance, First Edition. Morgan McMonagle and Matthew Stephenson.

120 © 2014 John Wiley & Sons, Ltd. Published 2014 by John Wiley & Sons, Ltd. Companion website: www.ataglanceseries.com/vascular

Pulmonary embolism

Symptomatic venous thromboembolism occurs in 0.1–0.2% of adults each year with 33% presenting with PE, which carries a significant mortality (12–48%) depending on the *size* of the PE and the underlying *health status* of the patient. About 75% are first events with the remaining 25% recurrent presentations.

Complications of PE

- Acute hypoxia (ventilation/perfusion [V/Q] mismatch).
- Acute cor pulmonale (right heart failure from respiratory cause).
- Hypotension and sudden death.
- Rarely, pulmonary infarction (usually critically ill).

Symptoms

- Asymptomatic (silent). These are picked up incidentally.
- Dyspnoea (>90%) and cough.
- Chest pain (may be pleuritic or non-pleuritic).

Signs

- Hypoxia (SaO_2 < 95%, PaO_2 < 80%), tachypnoea and tachycardia (absent in up to 50%) and haemoptysis.
- Diaphoresis (sweating) and fever (usually low grade).
- Hypotension (often pre-terminal) and cardiac arrest (2%). Occasionally a PE may lead to a pulmonary wedge infarct after which patients often remain critically ill.
- DVT (<25% will have a symptomatic DVT).

Investigations

- **CXR.** (Low yield), but signs include dilated pulmonary vein with absent lung markings (Westermarks sign [2%]). Also aids in ruling out other causes of chest pain and hypoxia (e.g. pneumonia).
- **ECG.** (Low yield). Often normal, but may rule out other causes of chest pain. ECG changes in PE include sinus tachycardia (most common), right heart strain (right axis deviation, high voltage R-waves in right heart leads, peaked p-waves) and, very rarely, $S_IQ_{III}T_{III}$ (S-wave [lead I], Q-wave and T-wave inversion [lead III]).
- **Arterial blood gas (ABG).** An abnormal PaO_2 has a sensitivity of ~90% and specificity of ~15%.
- **D-dimer assay.** Highly sensitive (by ELISA) for PE and DVT with a low specificity (numerous conditions cause this). *A negative result effectively rules out a thrombotic event!*
- **V/Q scan.** Images the mismatch between ventilated and perfused lung corresponding to the obstructing PE. However, other disease processes may give rise to a false positive result (e.g. atelectasis, pneumonia). Results are reported as a *probability* of PE (*low, intermediate, high*) and must be correlated with a similar qualitative *clinical* scale. If the clinical picture is considered either intermediate or high probability, then a normal V/Q scan result effectively excludes a PE and a high probability V/Q result effectively confirms the diagnosis. But, 50% of patients with a low clinical suspicion but a high V/Q probability will have a PE!
- **Pulmonary phase CT scan.** Very accurate diagnostic modality. Injected contrast is scanned during the thoracic 'pulmonary phase' and thrombus visualised within the pulmonary vasculature. It is highly sensitive for large, central PEs, but less so for small, subsegmental ones because the accuracy is affected by the timing of the contrast bolus and any movement artefact.

- **Pulmonary angiography.** Historically this was the gold standard test involving direct catheterisation of the pulmonary artery and injection of contrast. It is an invasive procedure (1% mortality) and has now been superseded by CT scanning.

Management of PE

- Oxygenation and resuscitation. Maintain O_2 sats > 95%.
- Analgesia, and rule out other causes of chest pain (especially cardiac).
- Anticoagulation. As per DVT and should be started empirically pending investigations. Once diagnosed, patients will require warfarin (3–6 months or longer if recurrent).
- Catheter-directed thrombolysis may be considered if haemodynamic compromise present. Surgical (open) thrombectomy (Trendelenburg's operation) is now of historical interest only!
- Consider *IVC filter*. This is a small cage-like device placed within the infra-renal IVC in patients with an occurrence of PE despite anticoagulation or in whom it is contraindicated (e.g. trauma). Complications include haemorrhage, IVC perforation, failure to deploy, IVC obstruction, failure to retrieve. Ideally the filters should be removed within 2–6 weeks to avoid complications (thrombosis, IVC perforation, failure to retrieve).

Post-thrombotic syndrome

This is a late complication due to valvular destruction and residual venous obstruction leading to *ambulatory venous hypertension*. Patients develop symptoms and signs of venous hypertension as described and are at risk of venous ulceration (see Chapters 53–55).

Venous occlusion and ischaemia

Total iliofemoral outflow occlusion can threaten limb viability. The majority of patients have an underlying coagulopathy (malignancy!) with onset usually in the sixth decade with associated high mortalities (>20%). Two broad varieties are described.

- **Phlegmasia alba dolens (PAD)**: 'White' leg syndrome presents as a swollen, painful white limb due to deep venous obstruction. The venules and capillaries are unaffected.
- **Phlegmasia caerulea dolens (PCD)**: 'Blue' limb syndrome occurs when the thrombus propagates to involve the venules and capillaries and is a vascular emergency. The leg is intensely painful, cyanotic and swollen. As the venous pressure rises (up to fivefold), capillary and eventually arterial ischaemia develop (hydrostatic back-pressure). Up to 50% will progress to this stage (usually starting distally before progressing more proximally).

Management

- Fluid resuscitation. The fluid sequestration can lead to haemodynamic collapse in this sick elderly population.
- Treat the underlying cause (note: think malignancy!).
- Compression and limb elevation to reduce the hydrostatic pressure.
- Once symptoms begin to improve, the patient should be ambulated to improve venous flow.
- Analgesia including opiates may be required.
- Anticoagulation is the mainstay of treatment with unfractionated heparin or LMWH followed by warfarin.

For extensive thrombosis, catheter-directed thrombolysis and/or thrombectomy should be considered (see Chapter 51).

53 Varicose veins and venous hypertension

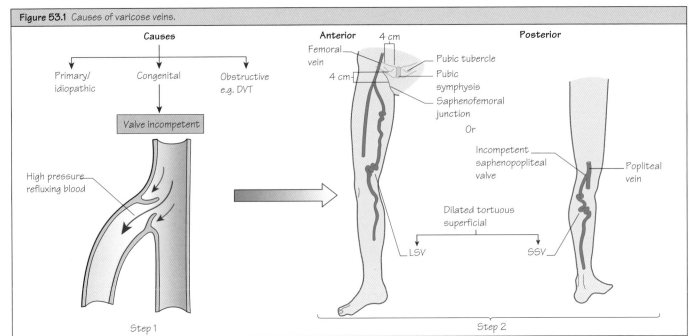

Figure 53.1 Causes of varicose veins.

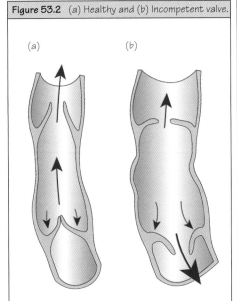

Figure 53.2 (a) Healthy and (b) Incompetent valve.

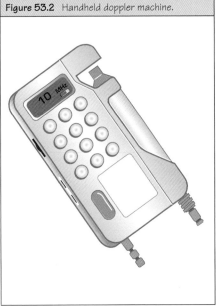

Figure 53.2 Handheld doppler machine.

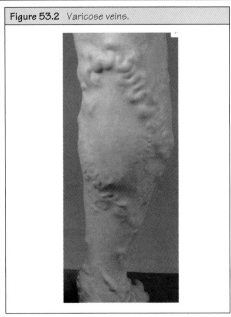

Figure 53.2 Varicose veins.

Abbreviations: DVT, deep vein thrombosis; LSV, long saphenous vein; SSV, short saphenous vein

Vascular and Endovascular Surgery at a Glance, First Edition. Morgan McMonagle and Matthew Stephenson.

122 © 2014 John Wiley & Sons, Ltd. Published 2014 by John Wiley & Sons, Ltd. Companion website: www.ataglanceseries.com/vascular

Definition

Varicose veins (VVs) are **dilated**, **tortuous**, **superficial** veins. By far, the legs are the most common site.

Epidemiology

They are extremely common, affecting approximately 30–40% of the population to some degree. They affect men and women roughly equally although women are more likely to present to their doctor.

Aetiology

There are two superficial systems of veins that drain from the foot into the deep leg veins at two key points: the **saphenofemoral junction** (SFJ) and the **saphenopopliteal junction** (SPJ) (see Chapter 2). The deep veins are under high pressure – imagine a column of blood all the way from the heart to your foot. The superficial veins, however, are normally **low pressure** veins and are protected from this high pressure system by veins at these junctions. Varicose veins develop because these **valves become incompetent** so blood **refluxes** back into them.

Consequently they become dilated and because they're fixed at certain points along their length they become tortuous. The causes are:

1 **Primary/idiopathic** (the most common): An inherent weakness in the valve that is most likely genetic.
2 Obstructive:
  • DVT.
  • Pregnancy.
  • Other pelvic mass.
3 **Congenital** anomaly, such as in Klippel-Trenauney syndrome.

As a consequence of this high pressure, the microcirculation in the skin around the ankle (where the pressure is highest) can't cope and can't return blood northwards as normal. Blood begins to seep out of the veins into the skin, the leg can swell and finally the skin can break down and cause a venous ulcer. All these signs are known as signs of chronic venous insufficiency; some you look for, some you feel for. The importance of looking for them is that they warn you of imminent skin breakdown, or ulceration.

Presentation
Symptoms
• Pressure.
• Aching.
• Pain (may indicate thrombophlebitis).
• Itching.
• Occasionally bleeding.
• Cosmetic dissatisfaction.

Signs
• Pitting oedema.
• Venous eczema.
• Lipodermatosclerosis.
• Haemosiderin deposition (pigmentation).
• Venous ulceration.

Investigations

Varicose veins and the signs of chronic venous insufficiency can be diagnosed clinically. However, to treat them you need to know two further things that aren't always immediately obvious:

1 Which valve is defective, the SFJ or the SPJ?
2 Are the deep veins working well or is there (a) an occlusion or (b) reflux? Both of these tend to be the result of a DVT in the past. This is important to know, because significant deep venous problems preclude VV surgery.

There are only two investigative modalities in common use for VVs.

Handheld Doppler

This is usually sufficient to determine whether the valves at the SFJ or SPJ, or both, are defective (see Chapter 14 for full details on how to use it).

Duplex

This clearly shows the site(s) of valvular incompetence and in addition shows whether the deep veins are obstructed or refluxing. This is also very helpful in recurrent varicose veins where the anatomy can be different from expected.

Classification

The clinical and Duplex findings help to classify your patient's VVs: the internationally accepted CEAP Classification. This has become very important in healthcare systems like the one in the UK where treatments need to be rationed and only the most severe VVs are treated.

Clinical classification
• C0: No visible or palpable signs of venous disease.
• C1: Telangiectasia or reticular veins.
• C2: Varicose veins.
• C3: Oedema.
• C4a: Pigmentation.
• C4b: Lipodermatosclerosis.
• C5: Healed venous ulcer.
• C6: Active venous ulcer.

aEtiological classification
• Ec: Congenital.
• Ep: Primary.
• Es: Secondary (post-thrombotic).
• En: No venous cause found.

Anatomical classification
• As: Superficial veins.
• Ap: Perforator veins.
• Ad: Deep veins.
• An: No venous location identified.

Pathological classification
• Pr: Reflux.
• Po: Obstruction.
• Pr,o: Reflux and obstruction.
• Pn: No venous pathophysiology identified.

Figure 54.1 Conservative measures.

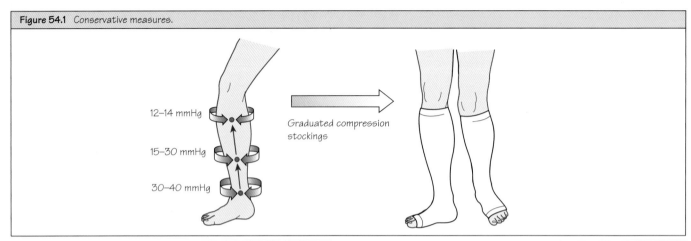

12–14 mmHg

15–30 mmHg

30–40 mmHg

Graduated compression stockings

Figure 54.2 Endovenous ablation.

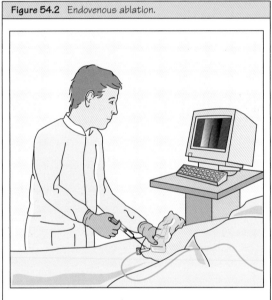

Figure 54.3 Superficial veins of the leg.

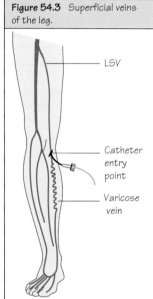

LSV

Catheter entry point

Varicose vein

Figure 54.4 Vein ablation (a) Catheter in vein (b) Vein is heated (c) Vein closes as catheter is withdrawn.

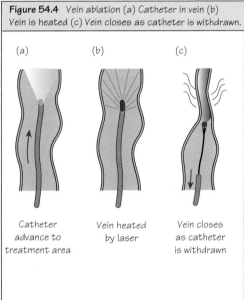

(a) Catheter advance to treatment area

(b) Vein heated by laser

(c) Vein closes as catheter is withdrawn

Figure 54.5 Open surgery.

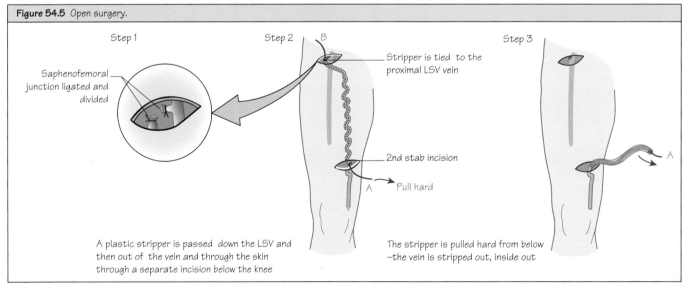

Step 1

Saphenofemoral junction ligated and divided

A plastic stripper is passed down the LSV and then out of the vein and through the skin through a separate incision below the knee

Step 2

B

Stripper is tied to the proximal LSV vein

2nd stab incision

A Pull hard

Step 3

A

The stripper is pulled hard from below —the vein is stripped out, inside out

Abbreviation: LSV, long saphenous vein; GSV, long saphenous vein

Vascular and Endovascular Surgery at a Glance, First Edition. Morgan McMonagle and Matthew Stephenson.

124 © 2014 John Wiley & Sons, Ltd. Published 2014 by John Wiley & Sons, Ltd. Companion website: www.ataglanceseries.com/vascular

The treatment of VVs is largely conservative, mainly consisting of patient reassurance in uncomplicated VVs without signs of venous insufficiency. In mild venous insufficiency, compression stockings usually suffice but in significant venous insufficiency, surgery is usually indicated (as well as stockings postoperatively). Surgery for VVs has been revolutionised in the last decade or so.

Treatment
Conservative
The principles of conservative management are first to reduce the duration of high pressure. So, first, advise the patient to:
• avoid standing for too long (stops gravity from creating a hydrostatic column of blood)
• put their feet up when resting.
Second, fight pressure with pressure, which means compression stockings:
• Patients with VVs without ulceration can wear Class II (25–35 mmHg) BK graduated compression stockings. They are graduated from high pressure distally to lower pressure proximally
• When ulceration has developed, patients should have four-layer compression bandaging, which usually results in healing in approximately 6 weeks.

Surgical
Some patients seek surgery for their veins just because they don't like their appearance or because they're uncomfortable, but, at the other end of the spectrum, some have severe venous ulceration. In the latter case, the venous ulceration should ideally be treated first using the compression described earlier; once it has healed, the patient should be considered for surgery.

There are two options: traditional **open** surgery or the newer **endovenous** treatment.

Open surgery
There are two operations, one for SFJ incompetence and one for SPJ incompetence, but the principles are the same: to surgically disconnect the problematic superficial vein from the deep vein so that reflux can no longer occur. The only significant difference is that the LSV should not only be disconnected but should also be stripped out from its junction with the femoral vein to just below the knee. This is because, in addition to the SFJ and SPJ, there are in fact other points along the length of the LSV where it drains into the thigh; these can also become incompetent. The short vein isn't usually stripped because first this isn't such a problem with the SSV but also because there are some nerves (especially common peroneal and sural) that run very close with it, and could be inadvertently injured.

Endovenous surgery
This newer technique is rapidly becoming the standard procedure for VVs. The advantages are that it can be performed under LA and doesn't require a surgical wound.

The varicose vein is cannulated and a catheter is passed up inside the vein to just distal to either the SFJ or SPJ under Duplex guidance. The vein is then ablated from inside using one of the following (there are pros and cons to each but they all aim to achieve occlusion of the LSV from within the vein):
• *Radiofrequency*, or
• *Laser*, or
• *Sclerotherapy*.
Whether you use the traditional open surgery or endovenous surgery, these only deal with the main trunk varicose veins (the LSV or the SSV). In reality, other superficial veins draining into these trunk veins do also become varicose (hence why varicose veins don't always appear to be in the expected distributions of the long or short saphenous veins). These may need to be dealt with separately by multiple tiny stab avulsions under LA and pulling the veins out individually.

Prognosis
The vast majority of patients with varicose veins never develop ulceration or even get signs of chronic venous insufficiency. These patients learn to live alongside their veins lifelong. However, when venous ulceration develops, this is a major cause of morbidity and is a considerable burden on the health service. Ulceration is usually reversible with compression; however, recurrence is high if compression is removed.

Figure 55.1 Anatomy of an ulcer.

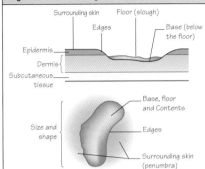

The following should be described when examining an ulcer to identify the dominant underlying pathology as well as the presence or absence of established infection:

a Site (e.g. on a pressure area: heel, gaiter area, etc)
b Size of the ulcer (centimetres)
c Shape of the ulcer (e.g. round, 'punched-out', serpiginous, regular, irregular, deep, shallow)
d Floor of the ulcer (this is the visible floor and is a description of the contents lying there e.g. slough)
e Base of the ulcer (if visible. This is under the floor and may contain granulation tissue, subcutaneous tissue, muscle, tendon, bone, etc)
f Edges of the ulcer (regular or irregular and whether it is 'raised and rolling' in appearance: clinical sign of malignant change)
g Discharge from the ulcer and its odour
h Surrounding skin (the skin in the 'penumbra' around the ulcer. This includes presence/absence of cellulitis, tracking pus, oedema, dry tissue, lipodermatosclerosis as well as how well-perfused looking it is)
i Any other clinical signs of the potential aetiology (e.g. sensation, presence of varicose veins, etc)
j Comment on whether the ulcer is improving or deteriorating and whether there is established infection or not

Figure 55.2 Venous hypertension with haemosiderin deposition (brown pigmentation) and venous ulceration at the gaiter area. Note the lipodermatosclerotic-looking features ('inverted champagne-bottle').

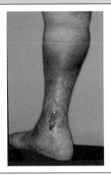

Figure 55.3 Lower limb displaying skin changes associated with venous hypertension including haemosiderin deposition (brown pigment) with surrounding dry pruritic venous eczema with early venous ulceration at the centre (initiated by minor trauma). This patient was successfully treated by compression bandaging followed by varicose vein surgery.

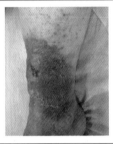

Figure 55.4 Deep 'punched-out' ulceration over heel (pressure area) in a neuropathic diabetic foot. Note surrounding skin is healthy and well-perfused looking.

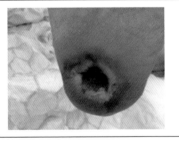

Figure 55.5 Necrotic (dry) venous ulceration at right gaiter area with surrounding erythema.

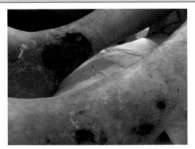

Figure 55.6 Dry gangrenous ulceration of tip of second toe secondary to ischaemia in a diabetic patient.

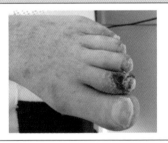

Table 55.1 Differentiation between arterial, venous and neuropathic ulceration on clinical grounds.

Examination	Neuropathic ulcer	Venous ulcer	Arterial ulcer
Pulses	Present	Present (difficult to palpate if oedematous)	Absent
Skin perfusion	Normal and warm	Normal and warm	Cool, prolonged capillary refill time
ABPI	Normal	Normal	Reduced (usually <0.5)
Ulcer location	Pressure areas	Medial malleolus (gaiter area)	Pressure and friction areas
Ulcer margin	Small and round ('punched-out')	Large and irregular	Small and round ('punched-out')
Ulcer contents	Clean granulating wound	Yellow wet appearance	Black necrotic tissue (dry or wet)
Ulcer drainage	Small	Moderate to large	Small
Skin	Healthy	Signs of venous hypertension	Pale, thin, ischaemic, friable
Pruritus	No	Yes	No
Oedema	Minimal	Moderate to severe	Minimal
Pain	Insensate	Painful	Minimal pain in ulcer, but there may be rest pain in the limb

Abbreviation: ABPI, ankle-brachial pressure index

Vascular and Endovascular Surgery at a Glance, First Edition. Morgan McMonagle and Matthew Stephenson.

Ulceration is an established defect in an epithelial surface.

Aetiology
- Neuropathic (most common).
- Venous.
- Arterial.
- Mixed (10%) (e.g. neuropathic–arterial, venous–arterial, etc).

Neuropathic ulceration
Pathophysiology
Chronically reduced sensation leaves the limb vulnerable to injury that may go undetected, thereby leading to ulceration at pressure areas (heel, ankle, metatarsal heads). There may be associated chronic joint destruction and malformation (e.g. Charcot's joint).

Aetiology
- Diabetes mellitus (by far the most common!).
- Ischaemic neuropathy (e.g. post-acute limb).
- Alcoholic neuropathy.
- Vitamin B12 deficiency.
- Certain medications (amiodarone, isoniazid, cytotoxic agents).
- Rare causes include chronic renal failure, hypothyroidism, tabes dorsalis, leprosy, porphyria, amyloidosis, progressive sensory neuropathy, Charcot-Marie-Tooth disease.

Clinical
Decreased or absent sensation in the foot ± decreased vibration sense and joint position sense (if posterior spinal columns affected). If there is no arterial element, perfusion (+pulses) will be normal or even increased because of vasodilatation (associated infection or autonomic neuropathy [both common in diabetes!]).

Venous ulceration
Pathophysiology
Chronic venous hypertension leads to tissue oedema with venous + capillary congestion and relative tissue hypoxia. The skin is vulnerable to minor trauma or spontaneous breakdown with poor healing ability. Ulceration is large and irregular because the surrounding ischaemic tissue area (penumbra) is large.

Aetiology of venous hypertension (VHT)
- Deep venous reflux with calf-pump failure (ambulatory VHT).
- DVT (usually proximal and obstruction).
- Venous trauma (ligation of proximal vein).
- Congenital absence of deep veins (e.g. Klippel-Trenaunay syndrome [KTS]).

Clinical
The legs are oedematous, moist and malodorous, and ulceration classically occurs just above the medial malleolus (gaiter area), where the skin is most vulnerable (may be bimallelolar and circumferential). Gangrene is usually absent (base of the ulcer may be necrotic) and the foot is warm with normal pulses (difficult to palpate because of oedema) if arterial disease is absent. The stigmata of venous disease will be present (varicose veins, venous eczema, haemosiderin deposition, lipodermatosclerosis and atrophie blanche).

Arterial ulceration
Pathophysiology
Arterial ulceration results directly from poor arterial supply leading to direct tissue hypoxia affecting all the tissues in the ischaemic zone. The decreased perfusion also renders these more prone to infection with poorer healing ability.

Aetiology
- PVD.
- Diabetes mellitus (macro- and micro-vascular occlusion).
- Arterial trauma.
- Arterial embolism.
- Ionising radiation and vasculitis.

Clinical
Ulcers develop over points of friction and weight bearing (heel, first and fifth metatarsal–phalangeal joints, Achilles tendon, and between the toes). There will be clinical signs of PVD and ABPIs (caution in diabetes!) will be critically low (<0.4) (see Chapter 34–36).

Mixed ulceration
Many ulcers have a mixed aetiology (e.g. arterial–venous, arterial–neuropathic [e.g. diabetes]), although one is usually dominant. In addition, established infection will contribute to ulcer deterioration.

Investigations
Investigations are tailored at diagnosing the underlying aetiology:
- ABPIs and Duplex U/S (arterial and venous).
- Nerve conduction studies (if suspected neuropathy).
- Angiogram (as required for arterial disease).
- Wound swab for culture (if ulcer infected).
- Biopsy of ulcer edge (for non-healing or suspicion of malignancy).

Management
Management includes:
- treating the underlying cause
- relieving pressure on the tissues
- treating any infection.

Treating the underlying cause
- *Neuropathic.* Generally irreversible (except hypothyroidism) but good control of diabetes may reduce recurrent infection.
- *Arterial.* Correction of poor tissue perfusion as per Chapter 36. In general a pedal pressure >50 mmHg is required for healing (although higher pressures are typically required).
- *Venous.* Management is aimed at reducing swelling and VHT as per Chapter 53–54 including elevation and compression (if ABPI > 0.7). Of the four grades of compression, the highest grade tolerated may be used although most will heal with two-layered compression, which can be escalated as required. Compliance and time are often the biggest challenges.

Relief of friction/pressure
- Both neuropathic and ischaemic feet should have low-pressure footwear fitted and regular podiatry checks.

Treatment of infection
- This includes regular dressing changes to de-slough the wound ± sharp debridement and wound wash-out (e.g. hydrogen peroxide).
- Antibiotics are indicated (empirically) if there is marked deterioration or failure to heal despite treatment, or if there is spreading infection/septicaemia. A wound swab should be taken for culture and sensitivities (see Chapter 56).

Hyperbaric therapy
May have a role in stubborn non-healing wounds when there is reversible hypoxia (e.g. difficult venous, neuropathic, radiation-induced ulcers or poor healing of skin grafts).

56 General wound care

Figure 56.1 Diagrammatic illustration of skin cross-section with accompanying typical infections affecting individual layers.

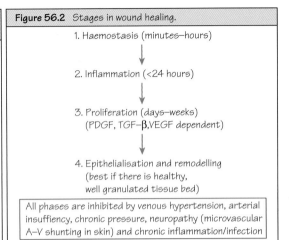

	Infection site	Aetiologic organism
Epidermis	Impetigo	*S. aureus, strep. pyogenes*
Hair follicle	Erysipelas	*Strep. pyogenes*
Dermis	Folliculitis	*S. aureus*
	Cellulitis	*Strep. pyogenes* (common) *S. aureus* (uncommon) *H. influenzae* (rare) Others
Subcutaneous fat	Necrotising fasciitis	*Strep. pyogenes* or mixed bowel flora
Fascia and muscle		

Figure 56.2 Stages in wound healing.

1. Haemostasis (minutes–hours)

   ↓

2. Inflammation (<24 hours)

   ↓

3. Proliferation (days–weeks) (PDGF, TGF–β,VEGF dependent)

   ↓

4. Epithelialisation and remodelling (best if there is healthy, well granulated tissue bed)

All phases are inhibited by venous hypertension, arterial insuffiency, chronic pressure, neuropathy (microvascular A–V shunting in skin) and chronic inflammation/infection

Figure 56.3 Negative-pressure wound therapy (vac therapy).

Applied to amputated hallux post reperfusion. The sponge dressing (black) is applied to the wound bed and an air-tight (similar to 'cling wrap') is applied over this. The vacuum device is then applied over this after making a small incision in the air-tight seal and negative pressure (vacuum) is applied to the wound via a portable machine. Note the third toe has also been amputated (overlying dressing).

- Applies controlled suction to wound after filling wound with specialised foam
- Continuous or intermittent negative pressure (vacuum) may be applied
- Removes excess exudate
- Stimulates angiogenesis + wound healing

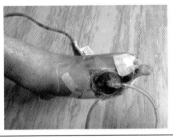

Figure 56.4 Same wound (Fig.56.3) two weeks later with healthy granulation tissue and surrounding skin. There is some infected fibrinous material in the wound (yellowish) which required sharp debridement to hasten healing and the vac-dressing was reapplied.

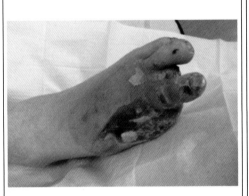

Figure 56.5 Healing ulceration at base of 5th toe (post-amputation) in a neuropathic foot. Note healthy, well-perfused surrounding skin.

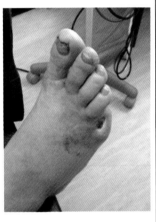

Figure 56.6 Wound dressing characteristics.

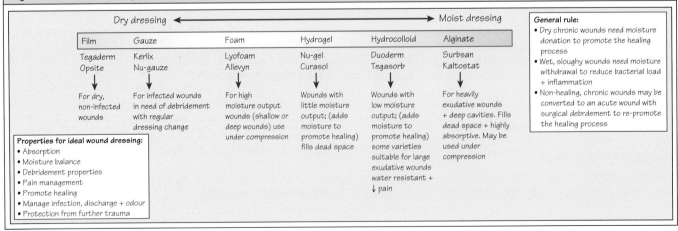

Dry dressing ←——————————→ Moist dressing

Film	Gauze	Foam	Hydrogel	Hydrocolloid	Alginate
Tegaderm Opsite	Kerlix Nu-gauze	Lyofoam Allevyn	Nu-gel Curasol	Duoderm Tegasorb	Surbsan Kaltostat
For dry, non-infected wounds	For infected wounds in need of debridement with regular dressing change	For high moisture output wounds (shallow or deep wounds) use under compression	Wounds with little moisture output; (adds moisture to promote healing) fills dead space	Wounds with low moisture output; (adds moisture to promote healing) some varieties suitable for large exudative wounds water resistant + ↓ pain	For heavily exudative wounds + deep cavities. Fills dead space + highly absorptive. May be used under compression

Properties for ideal wound dressing:
- Absorption
- Moisture balance
- Debridement properties
- Pain management
- Promote healing
- Manage infection, discharge + odour
- Protection from further trauma

General rule:
- Dry chronic wounds need moisture donation to promote the healing process
- Wet, sloughy wounds need moisture withdrawal to reduce bacterial load + inflammation
- Non-healing, chronic wounds may be converted to an acute wound with surgical debrdement to re-promote the healing process

Abbreviations: PDGF, platelet derived growth factor; TGF-β, transforming growth factor beta; VEGF, vascular endothelial growth factor

Vascular and Endovascular Surgery at a Glance, First Edition. Morgan McMonagle and Matthew Stephenson.

Important wound concepts

• All chronic wounds are contaminated with bacteria.
• Wound healing occurs in the presence of bacteria.
• Certain bacteria appear to aid wound healing.
• It is not the presence of bacteria, but their interaction with the host tissue, that determines their influence on wound healing.
• The flora in an open wound will change over time.

Although all open wounds will have bacteria present, they may not need treatment unless infection becomes established. Infection of an ulcer should be strongly considered in any wound that fails to heal or deteriorates despite adequate care.

Definitions

Wound contamination

This is the presence of non-replicating organisms in a wound. All chronic wounds are contaminated (usually indigenous bacteria or from the environment), but the majority of contaminating organisms are unable to replicate in a wound (e.g. from soil).

Wound colonisation

This is the presence of replicating organisms inhabiting a wound in the absence of injury to the host. Most of these are from the normal skin flora (e.g. staph epidermidis, other coagulase negative organisms, corynebacterium sp).

Wound infection

This is the presence of replicating organisms within a wound causing injury to the host (e.g. Staph. Aureus, haemolytic strep [S. Pyogenes, S. Agalactiae], E. Coli, Proteus, klebsiella, anaerobes, pseudomonas, acinetobacter).

Evolving microbiology of a wound

The microbiology of a wound will change over time!

Early acute wound

The primary bacteria are normal skin flora (Staph. Aureus, β-haemolytic strep).

After about 4 weeks

Facultative anaerobic Gram-negative organisms will generally colonise the wound (e.g. proteus, E coli, klebsiella). If the wound deteriorates and deepens, then anaerobes predominate (often polymicrobial [>4 species]).

Chronic wound

This is essentially a wound that has failed to heal or has deteriorated and generally contains more anaerobes than aerobes, including *gram negative rods* often from *exogenous sources* such as baths, toilets, wash rooms (e.g. pseudomonas, acinetobacter). Enterococcus and candida are also commonly isolated but treatment is only indicated if they occur in isolation or are present in high concentrations (>10^6 colony-forming units [CFUs] per gram of tissue). As wounds become deeper and more complex, they can involve underlying structures (muscle, ligaments and bone). This may lead to osteomyelitis (S aureus, coliforms and anaerobes).

Transition from colonisation to infection

A continuum exists from simple colonisation to infection, but infection of a chronic wound should be considered in any wound that fails to heal or deteriorates. There are many contributing factors including *organism factors* and *host factors* (*systemic* and *local*).

• *Organism factors.* The *number of organisms* present and *virulence* of the organisms (versus host resistance). Some organisms need high concentrations to produce injury (e.g. candida, enterococcus) while others display synergistic injury in combination (e.g. Group B strep and Staph. Aureus). Pseudomonas is not very invasive (unless the host is compromised), but there may be marked deterioration of the wound due to its endotoxins and exotoxins (the wound becomes moist with foul-smelling green slough).

• *Systemic host factors.* Poorly controlled glucose, ischaemia, venous hypertension, oedema, malnutrition, chronic illness, alcohol abuse, smoking, corticosteroid use and immunosuppression.

• *Local (wound) host factors.* Necrotic tissue, deep wounds, chronic wounds, location of the wound (extremities, perineum), prior surgery and radiation.

Host resistance (both local and systemic) is the single most important determinant in wound healing

Clinical features of an infected deteriorating wound

• Increased swelling and exudate (wet looking!)
• Increased pain and erythema (angry looking!).
• Increased local temperature (± cellulitis and ascending infection).
• Change in appearance of granulation tissue (friable and bleeding).

Cellulitis and erysipelas are quite common in an acute infection of a chronic wound, but always consider *strep. pyogenes* (may lead to toxic shock and necrotising fasciitis) as well as *clostridium tetani*.

Management of an infected wound

• Treat the underlying cause and manage systemic complications (systemic sepsis, acute kidney injury, acute respiratory distress syndrome [ARDS], etc.).
• Ensure tetanus vaccination is up to date.
• Debulking the wound (chemical and mechanical [surgical debridement or regular dressing with desloughing agents]).
• Antimicrobials (empirical versus specific).

If infection is to be treated, then the gold standard microbiology sample is a tissue biopsy from the leading wound edge. If there is >10^6 CFU/gm tissue, then sepsis is more likely. A swab may suffice in the absence of a biopsy, but growth often takes 3–5 days and may be affected by current antibiotic treatment. In the presence of sepsis, empirical antimicrobial treatment should be started.

Organisms that should be treated regardless

Certain organisms should always be considered pathogenic and treated regardless of interaction with the host tissue. These include Beta-haemolytic strep, mycobacteria sp, bacillus anthracis, yersinia pestis, corynebacterium diphtheria, erysipelothrix rhusiopathiae, leptospira sp, treponema sp, brucella sp, clostridium sp, varicella virus (VZV), herpes simplex virus (HSV), dimorphic fungi, leishmaniasis.

Figure 57.1 Signs.

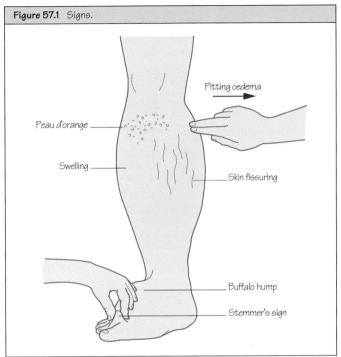

- Pitting oedema
- Peau d'orange
- Swelling
- Skin fissuring
- Buffalo hump
- Stemmer's sign

Figure 57.2 Causes.

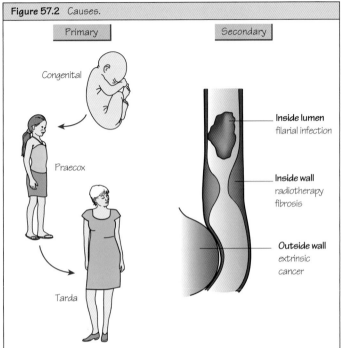

Primary

- Congenital
- Praecox
- Tarda

Secondary

- **Inside lumen** filarial infection
- **Inside wall** radiotherapy fibrosis
- **Outside wall** extrinsic cancer

Figure 57.3 Management.

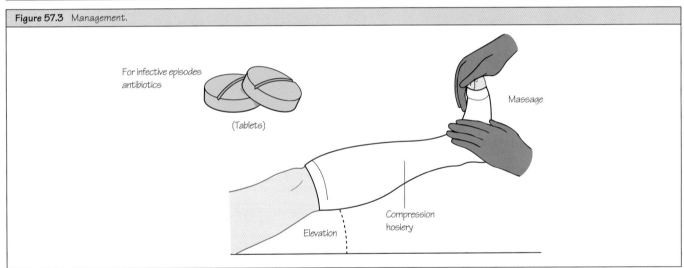

- For infective episodes antibiotics
- (Tablets)
- Massage
- Compression hosiery
- Elevation

Vascular and Endovascular Surgery at a Glance, First Edition. Morgan McMonagle and Matthew Stephenson.

Definition

Progressive swelling of a limb due to failure of the lymphatic system to drain fluid distally to proximally. The lymphatic system drains excess fluid from the interstitium back to the venous circulation. Lymphoedema occurs when this system fails. It can be a debilitating condition for which there is no cure, only palliative treatment. The most common lymphoedema problem in the Western world is due to cancer or its treatment (radiotherapy); the most common cause worldwide is filarial infection (elephantiasis).

Causes
Primary

These all share some similarities with the common themes being aplasia, hypoplasia or even hyperplasia of lymphatic vessels.
• **Congenital** (from or soon after birth). Sometimes this is inherited as an autosomal dominant condition.
• **Lymphodema praecox** (before age 35), most common primary form. Especially in women. Often follows seemingly trivial ankle trauma – for instance, during adolescence, from which the leg swelling never improves.
• **Lymphoedema tarda**, after age 35.

Secondary

Occlusion of proximal lymphatic vessels or lymph nodes by a specific process. Like all obstructive processes, these can be loosely remembered in the following way:
• **Outside the lumen**: e.g. pelvic tumours.
• **Inside the lumen**: e.g. filarial infection.
• **Inside the wall**: e.g. radiotherapy.

Presentation
History

• Slowly progressive limb swelling – distal to proximal.
• Unable to fit footwear.
• Worse by end of day.
• Heavy and uncomfortable.

Examination

• Swollen limb.
• Primary usually bilateral.
• Secondary usually unilateral.
• Thickened skin.
• *Peau d'orange* appearance.

• Initially pitting oedema, later non-pitting.
• Hyperkeratosis and fissuring of skin.
• 'Buffalo hump' on dorsum of skin.
• Reduced skin elasticity (Stemmer's sign is the inability to pinch the skin of the dorsum of the second toe).

Investigations

The main purpose of investigating clinically suspected lymphoedema is to rule out other causes, or in rare cases where lymphoedema surgery is considered. There are three most common methods:
• **Duplex U/S:** Principally to exclude chronic venous insufficiency.
• **Lymphangioscintigraphy:** Radiolabelled isotopes are injected into the web spaces in the foot and a gamma-camera takes pictures of the leg to watch the flow of the isotopes.
• **CT:** Especially if considering a pelvic malignancy, for example.

Treatment
Non-surgical

• Explanation and patient education.
• Elevation when possible (e.g. raise the foot end of the bed).
• Meticulous skin and nail hygiene (to prevent infection).
• Exercise (encourages muscle pump action and lymphatic contractility).
• Lose weight.
• Manual lymphatic drainage (essentially massage of fluid back up the limb).
• Graduated elastic compression (up to 60 mmHg).
• Antibiotics for superficial skin infections.
• For filarial infection – diethylcarbamazine.
• Note: diuretics have no long-term value.

Surgical

Very rarely used because of high morbidity and high failure rates.
   Bypass operations. Very rarely performed, in only a few centres. High failure rates, and technically very demanding requiring microvascular anastomoses. Consists of using autologous lymphatic vessels, muscle, or even omentum to bridge defective lymphatic channels.
   Debulking operations. Very high morbidity. Reserved for the most severe cases and largely obsolete.
• **Homan's operation:** Excision of a large section of skin and subcutaneous tissues with primary closure.
• **Charles operation:** Excision of all skin and subcutaneous tissue down to deep fascia with subsequent skin grafting.

58 The diabetic foot

Table 58.1 Wagner's classification of diabetic foot lesions.

Grade 0	High risk foot with no ulceration or a pre-ulcerative lesion
Grade 1	Superficial ulcer (no deeper than skin) with no infection
Grade 2	Deeper ulcer penetrating to tendon or muscle, but no bone involvement. There may be cellulitis but no abscess formation
Grade 3	Deep ulcer with abscess or involvement (osteomyelitis)
Grade 4	Localised gangrene (toes, heel)
Grade 5	Extensive gangrene involving whole foot

Figure 58.1 Diabetic foot with flat base and prominent metatarsal heads. There is in-drawing of the toes ('hammer-toes'/ 'claw-toes') and chronically deformed joints at mid-foot and ankle (osterarthropathy) all leading to weight maldistribution and high propensity for injury and ulceration. There is a deep neuropathic ulcer on the heel.

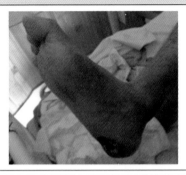

Figure 58.2 Diabetic dermopathy: dark brown non-blanching skin spots.

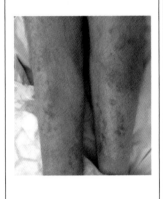

Figure 58.3 Severe destruction secondary to infected diabetic foot. Wide debridement was performed followed by BKA.

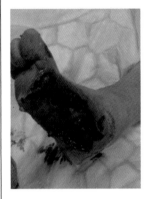

Figure 58.4 Severe diabetic foot gangrene and infection. There has been wide debridement of the skin and tissue on the sole of the foot to manage acute infection with septicaemia.

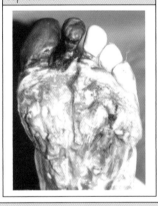

Figure 58.5 Severe destruction and infection in a mixed ischaemia-neuropathic diabetic foot. Note the 'claw-like' toes and flat sole of foot. There has been an amputation of the 4th and 5th toe complex but with further 'die-back' of tissue from a combination of ischaemia and infection.

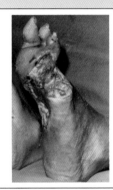

Figure 58.6 Clinical features of advanced diabetic foot.

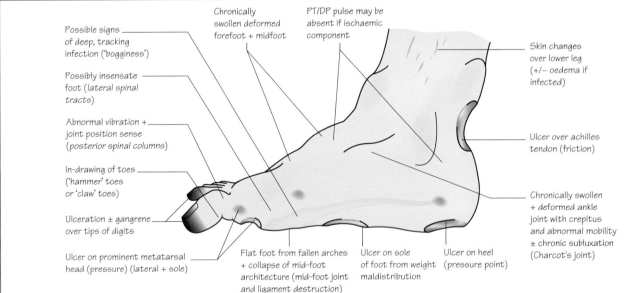

Possible signs of deep, tracking infection ('bogginess')

Possibly insensate foot (lateral spinal tracts)

Abnormal vibration + joint position sense (posterior spinal columns)

In-drawing of toes ('hammer' toes or 'claw' toes)

Ulceration ± gangrene over tips of digits

Ulcer on prominent metatarsal head (pressure) (lateral + sole)

Chronically swollen deformed forefoot + midfoot

PT/DP pulse may be absent if ischaemic component

Skin changes over lower leg (+/− oedema if infected)

Ulcer over achilles tendon (friction)

Chronically swollen + deformed ankle joint with crepitus and abnormal mobility ± chronic subluxation (Charcot's joint)

Flat foot from fallen arches + collapse of mid-foot architecture (mid-foot joint and ligament destruction)

Ulcer on sole of foot from weight maldistribution

Ulcer on heel (pressure point)

Abbreviations: BKA, below knee; DP, dorsal pedis; PT, posterior tibial

Vascular and Endovascular Surgery at a Glance, First Edition. Morgan McMonagle and Matthew Stephenson.

132 © 2014 John Wiley & Sons, Ltd. Published 2014 by John Wiley & Sons, Ltd. Companion website: www.ataglanceseries.com/vascular

The diabetic foot represents a special problem for vascular surgeons and is truly a condition requiring a multidisciplinary team approach, including diabetology, ophthalmology, nephrology, podiatry, tissue viability and diabetic nurse specialists.

Aetiology
- Neuropathy.
- Vasculopathy:
  - Macrovascular disease.
  - Microvascular disease.
- Infection.

Neuropathy
Most common aetiology in both diabetic foot and diabetic ulceration.

Pathophysiology. Diabetic neuropathy is complex. Often there is loss of the posterior spinal columns resulting in decreased joint position and vibration sense. Eventually there is a loss of the lateral spinal tracts leading to decreased sensation loss for pain and temperature, leaving the foot vulnerable to even trivial injury. In addition, microvascular disease affecting the peripheral nerves (including mononeuritis multiplex) leads to further loss of sensation and protective reflexes. Autonomic neuropathy, although leading to vasodilatation in the feet, also gives rise to microvascular shunting within cutaneous tissue, which is also thought to contribute to skin vulnerability, leading to ulceration and poor healing ability.

Clinical features
- Ulceration over pressure areas (heads of the metatarsal–phalangeal joints (especially first and fifth), lateral aspects of the sole and heel of the foot (often initiated by minor injury or chronic pressure/friction).
- Chronic friction also leads to callus formation over pressure areas.

Vasculopathy
Pathophysiology. Both *macrovascular* and *microvascular* disease contribute to ischaemia in diabetic foot. Macrovascular disease refers to PVD, which is common in diabetes especially if patients are also smokers. The atherosclerosis is often diffuse and multilevel throughout the lower limb, particularly affecting the profunda (hence poorer ability to collateralise), and vessels are often smaller and heavily calcified (especially tibial vessels). Unreconstructable disease is more common compared with non-diabetic patients with PVD).

Microvascular angiopathy is non-atherosclerotic disease affecting the vessels (skin, skeletal muscle, retina and kidney). It results in hyperglycaemia-related thickening of the basement membranes in the arterioles and capillaries leading to impaired oxygen diffusion. This microangiopathy contributes to the development of retinopathy, nephropathy and neuropathy seen in diabetes.

Clinical features
- Ischaemic ulceration and gangrene over friction and pressure points.
- Infection is more common in diabetes, especially if there is a diabetic foot with ulceration. Infection and pus often track proximal through the foot, aggressively spreading to joint, bone and tendon if not promptly treated (open drainage and antibiotics).
- Check the glycosylated HbA1c (long-term glucose control).
- Diabetic nephropathy (monitor urea and creatinine).
- Glycosuria and microalbuminuria (check with dipstick).

- Diabetic retinopathy (regular ophthalmology review).
- Skin pathology (ulceration [neuropathic/arterial]), diabetic dermopathy, necrobiosis lipodica diabeticorum, erythema nodosum).

Charcot's joint
Chronic, progressive, degenerative arthropathy as a result of a loss of sensory innervation of the affected joint and its ligaments.

Pathophysiology
- Peripheral neuropathy eventually affecting the joints (*neuropathic arthropathy*), in particular of the foot and ankle.
- Neuropathic arthropathy with loss of protective joint and tendon sensory reflexes allows repetitive minor trauma and chronic pressure maldistribution to go undetected (cycle of injury and poor healing). Eventually the joints (ankle and metatarsal–phalangeal joints) are painlessly destroyed.
- Results in gross joint deformity, osteoarthropathy and new bone formation (callosities).
- Motor neuropathy leads to wasting of the small muscles in the foot with loss of protective arch architecture (transverse and longitudinal arches) and in-drawing of toes ('hammer' or 'claw' toes).
- Eventually there is a chronic change and malformation of the foot with weight maldistribution, thereby adding to the cycle of injury.
- Autonomic neuropathy reduces sweating and opens up microscopic arteriovenous shunts within the skin with increased vulnerability.

Clinical features of a Charcot's foot
- Sensory neuropathy (stocking distribution):
  - Pin-prick and light touch.
  - Loss of temperature sensation.
- Posterior column changes:
  - Loss of proprioception and vibration sense.
- There may be impaired deep tendon reflexes.
- Warm, swollen and tender foot (infection or neuropathic vasodilatation).
- Grossly deformed, chronically swollen ankle joint with decreased or abnormal mobility (including hypermobility) and joint instability.
- Other swollen and deformed joints include first metatarsal and tarsal, tarsometatarsal, metatarsophalangeal joints.
- Gross osteoarthrosis with new bone formation (enlarged deformed joints).
- Loss of the normal architecture of the foot including fallen arches (collapse of the mid-foot from destruction of tarsal–metatarsal joints) leading to 'flat foot' with in-drawn 'claw-like' toes.
- Joint crepitus (chronic inflammation and tendonitis).
- Abnormal redistribution of the normal pressure areas of the foot leading to vulnerability to injury.
- Ulceration may be present (painless if neuropathic) and often plantar.

Causes of Charcot's joint
- Diabetes mellitus (>98%):
  - Typically affects the tarsal, tarsometatarsal and metatarsophalangeal joints.
- Other rare causes: tabes dorsalis (knee, hip, ankle, lumbar and lower dorsal vertebrae), syringomyelia (elbow, shoulder and cervical vertebrae), myelomeningocoele (ankle, tarsus), leprosy and various hereditary neuropathies (Charcot-Marie-Tooth disease, neurofibromatosis, congenital insensitivity to pain [e.g. Riley-Day syndrome]).

Figure 59.1 Complications of central venous lines.

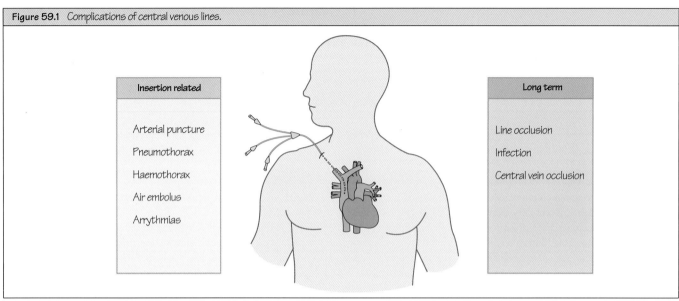

Insertion related	Long term
Arterial puncture	Line occlusion
Pneumothorax	Infection
Haemothorax	Central vein occlusion
Air embolus	
Arrythmias	

Figure 59.2 Types of arteriovenous fistulae and grafts.

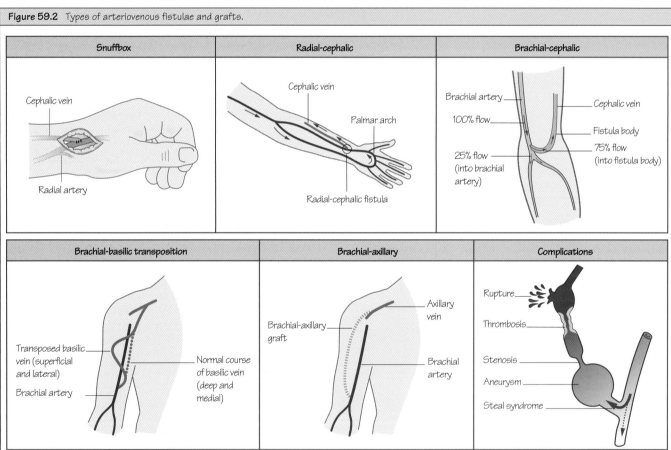

Snuffbox
- Cephalic vein
- Radial artery

Radial-cephalic
- Cephalic vein
- Palmar arch
- Radial-cephalic fistula

Brachial-cephalic
- Brachial artery
- 100% flow
- 25% flow (into brachial artery)
- Cephalic vein
- Fistula body
- 75% flow (into fistula body)

Brachial-basilic transposition
- Transposed basilic vein (superficial and lateral)
- Brachial artery
- Normal course of basilic vein (deep and medial)

Brachial-axillary
- Brachial-axillary graft
- Axillary vein
- Brachial artery

Complications
- Rupture
- Thrombosis
- Stenosis
- Aneurysm
- Steal syndrome

Vascular and Endovascular Surgery at a Glance, First Edition. Morgan McMonagle and Matthew Stephenson.

Haemodialysis patients need vessels that can be regularly cannulated and have large volumes of blood drained out of them (without collapsing) and large volumes of blood replaced back into them (without bursting). Unfortunately only central veins exist naturally that can perform these functions and perhaps the simplest way to haemodialyse a patient would be through a central line, which can be tunnelled under the skin (to reduce infection risk) into the internal jugular vein with its tip in the SVC. However, these occlude over time, they can become infected and they are thrombogenic, which can result in central vein occlusion. They are good as a short-term solution only.

That's where the surgically created AVF comes in. By joining an artery to a superficial vein, high-pressure blood is redirected up the vein back to the heart. Over time, this expands the vein, which becomes thick walled ('arterialises') and eventually, on average, a litre of blood may pass though the fistula every minute (this is very variable on the fistula and the patient but you would aim for >600 ml/min).

Principles of fistula creation

Because patients may be on haemodialysis for many years, they may need several over time because they may thrombose.

1 *Start distally and work proximally.* If a distal fistula fails, you can still try the next level up; however, the converse is not true (see 'Hierarchy of haemodialysis access').

2 For this reason, end-stage renal failure patients should only ever have their most distal veins (e.g. the back of the hand) used for taking blood or cannulae: this *preserves the main veins for fistula use.*

3 *Autogeneous vein is better than graft*: higher patency and lower infection risk. Reserve graft for when there is no peripheral vein left.

4 *Plan early:* if a patient is developing end-stage renal failure, the fistula should be created many weeks before anticipated dialysis because they take time to mature. Otherwise you have to use a central line.

Hierarchy of haemodialysis access

- *Snuffbox*: dorsal branch of the radial artery and the cephalic vein.
- *Radial-cephalic*: radial artery to cephalic vein at the wrist.
- *Brachial-cephalic*: brachial artery to cephalic vein (the most common overall) at the cubital fossa.
- *Brachial-basilic*: brachial artery to basilic vein (more complicated than the cephalic because the vein is deep and so requires full mobilisation to a superficial position to be needled) at the cubital fossa.
- *Brachial-axillary* graft: when arm vein options are exhausted. Brachial artery in the cubital fossa to axillary vein.
- More complex ('tertiary') procedures, such as:
  - Popliteal artery to femoral vein using LSV.
  - Axillo-femoral.
  - Axillo-axillary, etc.

Complications of central lines

- Insertion-related:
  - Arterial puncture.
  - Pneumothorax.
  - Haemothorax.
  - Air embolus.
  - Arrythmias.
- Long term:
  - Occlusion.
  - Infection.
  - Central vein occlusion.

Complications of fistulae

- Stenosis.
- Occlusion (thrombosis).
- Haemorrhage.
- Steal syndrome – fistulae lower peripheral resistance so arterial blood may be diverted away from the hand (i.e. 'stealing' it). This can result in a pale cool hand, which may become painful or at worse develop critical ischaemia. If severe, these fistulae need revision.
- Ischaemic monomelic neuropathy – like an extreme form of steal syndrome that develops within hours of surgery and requires immediate revision of the fistula to prevent irreversible loss of hand function.
- Aneurysmal degeneration.
- Cardiac failure – with very high flow fistulae.
- Venous hypertension – especially when there is a central venous stenosis.

Planning which fistula to make

- **Clinical examination**: to assess for a suitable superficial vein and nearby artery with a good pulse. This is considered sufficient by many surgeons.
- **Duplex examination**: increasingly becoming the norm as an adjunct to clinical examination. Can accurately assess venous patency, which helps guide which vein to use.

Managing fistulae

- Many units will keep their fistulae under surveillance with regular clinical examination and Duplex U/S.
- Reduced flows on Duplex suggest stenosis and fistulography are indicated.
- Significant stenoses should be treated during fistulography with balloon angioplasties and occasionally a stent. Alternatively, open surgery with a patch.
- Large aneurysms with thin threatened overlying skin should be treated by ligation or repair.

Figure 60.1 Mesenteric vascular anatomy.

Median arcuate ligament of diaphragm
Splenic artery
Celiac axis
Gastro-duodenal collaterals
SMA
IMA
Mesenteric collaterals
Hypogastric artery (internal iliac artery)
Sigmoidal arteries

Mesenteric Arterial Supply
- **Coeliac artery** This supplies the foregut and liver (25% hepatic blood flow, but 75% of oxygen supply is via the hepatic artery)
- **SMA** This supplies the mid-gut from duodenum to about the mid-transverse colon where it overlaps with the IMA
- **IMA** This supplies the hind gut from the splenic flexure down

Mesenteric venous supply
- **Portal vein** This supplies 75% of hepatic blood flow, but 25% of hepatic oxygen and is the confluence of SMV and splenic vein. All GI venous drainage goes via the portal system and to the liver
- **SMV** This joins splenic vein to become portal vein
- **IMV** This joins splenic vein along its course

Collaterals
- Arc of Riolan
- Marginal artery of Drummond
- Internal iliac arteries

Diagrammatic outline of mesenteric vascular supply + collaterals

Principal vessel	Collateral supply
Coeliac artery	Superior + Inferior pancreaticoduodenal arteries
SMA	Arc of Riolan (meandering mesenteric artery)
IMA	Internal iliac arteries

Table 60.1 Aetiology of arterial mesenteric ischaemia.

Chronic	Acute
• Atherosclerosis (>90%)	• Thromboembolism (e.g. cardiac, aneurysm)
• Dissection flap (static or dynamic)	• In situ thrombosis of atherosclerotic plaque
• Fibromuscular dysplasia	• Dissection flap (static or dynamic)
• Intimal flap (e.g. post-trauma)	• Iatrogenic injury during intervention
• Radiation endarteritis	• Extrinsic compression (unusual)
• Extrinsic compression (e.g. median arcuate ligament syndrome)	• Vasospasm (e.g. ergot poisoning, cocaine, vasopressors)
• Arteritis	• EVAR stenting (covering vessel origin)

Figure 60.2 Grossly ischaemic small bowel with gangrenous patches.

Figure 60.3 Colour flow Doppler of mesenteric arteries showing critical coeliac stenosis but normal SMA.

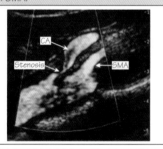

CA
Stenosis
SMA

Figure 60.4 Cross-section contrast-enhanced CT scan demonstrating dissection of aorta with extension of dissection flap into the coeliac artery. The coeliac artery is supplied by both the false (F) and true (T) lumens of the dissected aorta.

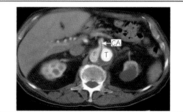

CA
F
T

Figure 60.6 (a) Angiocatheter (AP view) at origin of CA demonstrating outline of CA and its branches with tight stenosis at origin. (b) Catheter-directed angiogram (lateral view) of aorta and mesenteric vessels demonstrating tight stenosis at coeliac artery origin. Note pig-tailed catheter within aortic lumen.

(a)

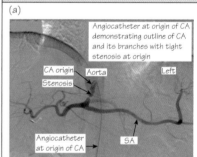

Angiocatheter at origin of CA demonstrating outline of CA and its branches with tight stenosis at origin
CA origin
Aorta
Left
Stenosis
Angiocatheter at origin of CA
SA

(b)

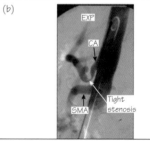

EXP
CA
SMA
Tight stenosis

Figure 60.5 CT reconstruction image of successful venous bypass from aorta + coeliac origin (hood patch-plasty of coeliac artery origin stenosis) to mid-SMA, thereby treating stenosis of both mesenteric vessels. (b) Aorta-to-SMA bypass for chronic SMA occlusion.

(a)

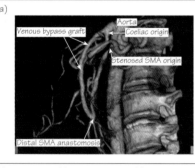

Aorta
Venous bypass graft
Coeliac origin
Stenosed SMA origin
Distal SMA anastomosis

(b)

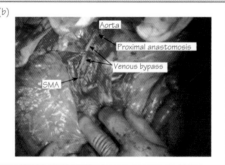

Aorta
Proximal anastomosis
Venous bypass
SMA

Abbreviations: CA, coeliac artery; CT, computed tomography; GI, gastrointestinal; IMA, inferior mesenteric artery; IMV, inferior mesenteric vein; SMA, superior mesenteric artery; SMV, superior mesenteric vein

Vascular and Endovascular Surgery at a Glance, First Edition. Morgan McMonagle and Matthew Stephenson.

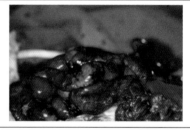

Classification

- Arterial ischaemia (80%).
- Venous ischaemia (15%).
- Non-occlusive mesenteric ischaemia (5%).

Mesenteric arterial ischaemia

Severe occlusive disease of at least two of the three mesenteric vessels, resulting in a reduction in blood flow to the gut.

Presentation

- Chronic.
- Acute.
- Acute-on-chronic.

Chronic mesenteric ischaemia (CMI)

This is caused by mesenteric artery stenosis (usually at the vessel origin) leading to a chronic or intermittent decrease in mesenteric perfusion. Theoretically, two vessels need to be involved for symptoms to develop (controversial).

Clinical features

Patients often complain of post-prandial abdominal pain (due to gut malperfusion during digestion) referred to as *mesenteric angina*. In addition, they may practise f*ood avoidance* (due to pain) with *weight loss* (malabsorption and food avoidance), but can compensate by eating smaller meals more frequently ('*small meal syndrome*'). Malabsorption may lead to *diarrhoea* and *steatorrhoea* with a risk of vitamin deficiency (especially fat-soluble [A, D, E, K]). Other non-specific features include anorexia, nausea and vomiting.

Investigations and diagnosis

- Duplex U/S. Velocity changes may be visualised during the respiratory cycle (dynamic study).
- Angiography. CTA, MRA or catheter-directed. Mesenteric angiography is the gold standard but it is invasive and best reserved for patients undergoing endovascular treatment.

Treatment

- *Endovascular:* This is the first-line treatment and includes angioplasty and stenting of the stenosis. Usually only one vessel requires treatment (preferably the SMA). Risks include acute thrombosis or dissection leading to acute ischaemia.
- *Surgery:* Perfusion may be re-established by widening the stenosis (e.g. patch angioplasty) or bypass grafting. In-flow may be *antegrade* (e.g. direct from healthy mesenteric artery or aorta) or *retrograde* (e.g. iliac artery). Distal anastomosis may be to a healthy mesenteric artery or one of its branches (e.g. hepatic). The SMA can also be anastomosed directly (transposition) to another vessel for in-flow (e.g. hepatic artery, aorta).

Median arcuate ligament (MAL) syndrome

This is an unusual condition where the MAL (conjoint right and left crus of diaphragm as it arches over the aorta) pinches and obstructs the coeliac artery during inspiration leading to intermittent abdominal pain. Weight loss and food avoidance is not usually a feature. Treatment is by dividing the ligament (open or laparoscopically).

Acute mesenteric ischaemia (AMI)

This is a surgical emergency caused by the sudden and complete occlusion of a mesenteric vessel (or distal branches). The small bowel can withstand only about 60 minutes of total ischaemia before irreversible infarction occurs. Overall, AMI is associated with a high mortality (>80%) or severe long-term disability (if the patient survives), including *short-bowel syndrome* [<200 cm of viable gut remaining].

Clinical features

Patients present with non-specific central abdominal pain (variable intensity) often with vomiting (perhaps faeculent) and diarrhoea (perhaps bloody). There are often few clinical signs with the abdomen remaining soft until very late when bowel infarction or perforation has occurred leading to peritonitis. *The abdominal pain is often described as 'out of proportion' to the clinical findings.* Systemic sepsis with haemodynamic collapse (late presentation) may occur.

Investigations and diagnosis

A high index of suspicion is necessary because of the non-specific clinical signs and lack of any one reliable test!
- Raised inflammatory markers (white cell count [WCC], CRP, ESR), but these are non-specific and unreliable.
- Raised lactate with acidaemia is sensitive for ischaemic tissue but it is a non-specific finding that may occur in many septic conditions. In addition, by the time lactate has risen significantly, the ischaemia may be irreversible.
- CT angiogram may visualise the occluded vessel segment and ischaemic segment of bowel.
- Mesenteric angiogram is the gold standard test that may demonstrate occluded vessels. However, it cannot visualise affected bowel effectively. In addition, a filling defect may not be appreciated in a distal branch. The narrow ischaemic window and high mortality make this an impractical test for diagnosis.

Management

- Manage the haemodynamic instability with fluid resuscitation, inotropic support and broad spectrum antibiotics (bowel flora).
- Anticoagulation may limit the thrombosis but offers little acutely because of the narrow ischaemic window and high mortality.
- Laparotomy with resection of gangrenous or perforated bowel and restoration of perfusion (embolectomy with direct closure or patch angioplasty/bypass as necessary).
- If bowel viability is in doubt, warm packs should be applied while perfusion is restored. If viability is still uncertain, then perform a re-look laparotomy after demarcation (12–24 hours).
- Endovascular options include catheter-directed thrombolysis or suction embolectomy (±angioplasty/stenting of any stenosis). However, this carries high risks because of the narrow ischaemic window and, regardless of success, it should be followed by an exploratory laparotomy to inspect the bowel.
- The acidosis may worsen after reperfusion due to the 'washout' period and all patients should be monitored in a critical care environment as inotropic support is frequently required.
- If there is total bowel necrosis (non-survivable), then the abdomen should be closed and the patient palliated.

Figure 61.1 DSA angiogram of IMA outlining the marginal artery as it supplies the left side of the colon and its anastomosis with the middle colic artery branch of the SMA.

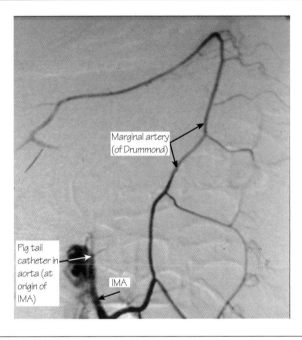

Marginal artery (of Drummond)

Pig tail catheter in aorta (at origin of IMA)

IMA

Abbreviations: DSA, digital subtraction angiogram; IMA, inferior mesenteric artery; SMA, superior mesenteric artery

Vascular and Endovascular Surgery at a Glance, First Edition. Morgan McMonagle and Matthew Stephenson.

138 © 2014 John Wiley & Sons, Ltd. Published 2014 by John Wiley & Sons, Ltd. Companion website: www.ataglanceseries.com/vascular

Colonic ischaemia

Colonic ischaemia typically affects areas supplied within the IMA perfusion territory, typically occurring at 'watershed' areas of large bowel, where there is 'overlap' or a physiological anastomosis between the IMA branches and the most distal branches of another blood supply (e.g. SMA).

Watershed areas of bowel

- Splenic flexure (IMA and SMA overlap).
- Sigmoid colon (IMA and pudendal artery overlap).
- Caecum (ileocolic and ileal artery overlap).

Clinical presentation

- Transient reversible ischaemic colitis.
- Chronic ischaemic colitis.
  - ± stricture formation.
- Acute total ischaemia (of a segment).
  - Necrosis.
  - Perforation.
- Fulminant total necrosis (high mortality).

Aetiology

- Atherosclerosis (>95%).
- Ligation of IMA (e.g. AAA repair).
- Intimal flap/dissection.
- Trauma (e.g. iatrogenic).

Investigations

- Contrast-enhanced CT.
- Colonoscopy.
- Barium enema.

CT scanning may demonstrate occluded vessel and malperfused, thickened bowel with/without perforation. Colonoscopy has a low sensitivity (unless there is full-thickness ischaemia of the bowel or a stricture is present) because often the mucosa is spared. Barium enema may visualise a stricture but should be avoided in acute presentation because of the high risk of perforation.

Management

- If peritonitis/sepsis present, then patients should be fluid resuscitated and broad spectrum antibiotics started.
- Indications for surgery and bowel resection include acute total ischaemia, perforation, gangrene or stricture (sigmoid colectomy/left hemi-colectomy).
- Non-resected bowel left behind must have an adequate blood supply, especially if re-anastomosed.
- If blood supply is in doubt (or in an acute presentation), then an end colostomy should be fashioned.
- Occasionally a sub-total colectomy with end ileostomy will be required if there is fulminant total necrosis.
- The rectum is usually spared because of its pudendal artery supply.

Mesenteric venous thrombosis (MVT)

This covers a spectrum of mesenteric venous disease from non-occlusive thrombosis to complete and extensive thrombosis of the portal venous system. *Pathophysiology*. Venous thrombosis leads to capillary and arterial congestion and hypoxia. Loss of arterial pulsation is a very late sign.

Classification

- *Primary* (<25%). No identifiable underlying cause.
- *Secondary* (>75%). Intrinsic thrombophilia (especially malignancy).

Secondary MVT

Numerous causes including malignancy (the most common), liver cirrhosis, intra-abdominal sepsis (e.g. appendicitis, diverticulitis), thrombophilia (primary or secondary) or external compression (tumour mass).

Presentation

- Asymptomatic.
- Non-specific abdominal pain, nausea, vomiting and distension.
- Septicaemia with or without peritonitis (gangrene/perforation).
- Variceal bleeding (from increased venous pressure).

Investigations

- Contrast-enhanced CT abdomen (portal-venous phase).
- Venous Duplex (may visualise portal vein thrombus).

Management

- Fluid resuscitation, oxygenation and inotropic support (as required).
- Therapeutic anticoagulation is the mainstay of treatment.
- Treatment of the underlying aetiology (if appropriate).
- Successful thrombolysis has been reported but carries a high risk of bleeding and bowel perforation.
- Surgery is reserved for complications (e.g. necrosis, perforation), but is associated with a very high mortality and re-thrombosis rate. Often the whole small bowel is involved, being oedematous, haemorrhagic and cyanotic-looking without a clear demarcation (unlike arterial ischaemia) for resection (unless frankly necrotic).

Non-occlusive mesenteric ischaemia

- Generally a condition occurring in critically ill patients, often with advanced systemic disease. Mostly affects 'watershed' areas.
- Results from generalised low-flow systemic perfusion (e.g. severe congestive cardiac failure, shock, sepsis).
- Supportive inotropic agents may further aggravate the condition (especially if strongly vasoconstrictive [i.e. alpha-agonists]).
- Management includes treatment of the underlying cause, fluid resuscitation, oxygenation and restoration of effective cardiac output, and end-organ perfusion.
- Other therapies have included mesenteric catheter-directed injection of papaverine (vasodilator) or intravenous glucagon (selective splanchnic vasodilator).
- These patients are often already critically ill and mortality rates remain high regardless of treatment (>80%).

Figure 62.1 Diagrammatic representation of stenosis at the origin of the right renal artery. This may induce hypertension by stimulating increased renin output from the kidney in response to proximal tubule hypoperfusion. Paradoxically the contralateral (normal) kidney may be affected first as a direct result of hypertensive injury as the stenosis in the right renal artery protects the right renal parenchyma from the effects of chronic hypertension.

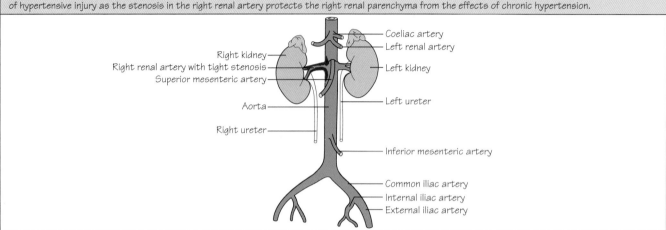

Figure 62.2 Pathophysiology of hypertension from RAS.

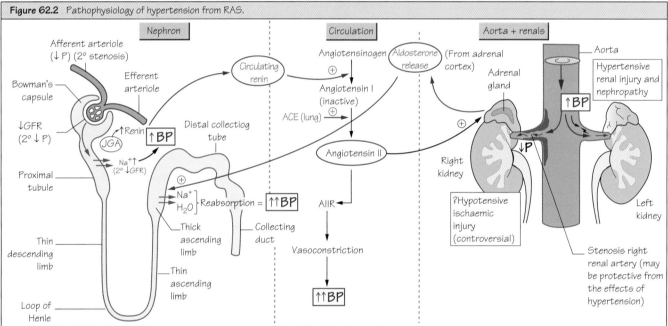

Figure 62.3 Algorithm for the investigation and management of RAS.

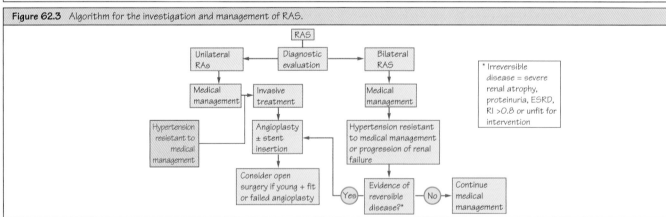

Abbreviations: ACE, angiotensin converting enzyme; AIIR, angiotensin II receptor; BP, blood pressure; GFR, glomerular filtration rate; JGA, juxtaglomerular apparatus; Na$^+$, sodium; P, pressure; RAS, renal artery stenosis

Vascular and Endovascular Surgery at a Glance, First Edition. Morgan McMonagle and Matthew Stephenson.

Renal artery stenosis (RAS) is a stenotic lesion affecting one or both renal arteries.

It affects 1–5% of the general population and may be unilateral or bilateral. Although there is no absolute consensus as to what constitutes significant RAS, a stenosis >70% (PSV > 200 cm/s or ratio ≥ 3.5) or a cross-lesion pressure gradient drop of 15–20 mmHg is a useful objective guide.

Aetiology
- Atherosclerosis (>85%).
- Fibromuscular dysplasia (10%).
- Intimal flap (e.g. dissection, iatrogenic trauma).
- Vasculitis.

Clinical presentation
- Majority are asymptomatic (silent) discovered incidentally.
- Hypertension (most common symptom), often in younger patients.
- Acute ('flash') pulmonary oedema (due to severe hypertension).
- Renal dysfunction (due to malperfusion [controversial] or hypertension-related renal injury).

Pathophysiology
Hypoperfusion of the nephron stimulates sodium re-absorption in the proximal tubule with renin release from the juxta-glomerular apparatus (JGA). Circulating renin cleaves angiotensinogen to form angiotensin I (inactive), which in turn is converted to angiotensin II (AII) by ACE in the lung. AII acts on the AII receptor directly causing vasoconstriction (↑ BP) and stimulates aldosterone-release (adrenal cortex) which leads to Na^+ and H_2O re-absorption in the distal tubule (↑ BP).

Ironically, the RAS-affected kidney may be protected from the hypertension by the stenosis, while the RAS-free contralateral kidney is exposed (leading to atrophy, scarring and eventually renal failure). The contribution of chronic post-RAS renal hypoperfusion towards ipsilateral renal insufficiency is unclear and controversial.

Complications of RAS
- **Hypertension.** This can lead to systemic effects including congestive cardiac failure, 'flash' (sudden) pulmonary oedema, chronic renal impairment, hypertensive retinopathy, stroke and MI.
- **Renal hypoperfusion.** Chronic hypoperfusion is a rare cause of renal failure. ACE inhibition (ACEi) or AII receptor blockers (ARBs) may worsen the renal failure because the affected kidney is more reliant on the renin–angiotensin system to maintain post-stenotic perfusion. But, controversially ACEi/ARBs have also been shown to slow the progression of renal disease!

Clinical examination
There may be evidence of hypertension-related end-organ damage (retinopathy, renal failure, cardiac failure, pulmonary oedema). An audible abdominal bruit is a non-specific finding of RAS.

Investigations
- Imaging (Duplex and angiography [CTA, MRA, catheter-directed]).
- Captopril stimulation test (indirect, non-invasive test measuring decrease in blood flow and glomerular filtration rate [GFR] after administration of ACEi).

Duplex assessment
There is high flow into low resistance capillary bed and therefore there is significant blood flow during diastole (waveforms more pulsatile proximally and dampen distally). *The normal renal systolic velocity is 100–150 cm/s. A significant stenosis is PSV > 180–200 cm/s or RAR ≥ 3.5. A PSV > 400 cm/s corresponds to a 90% stenosis.*

In addition, the RI measured in an interlobar artery reflects diastolic flow and is calculated as PSV-EDV/PSV (normal RI: 0.55–0.7). Diastolic flow reduction is reflected by an increased RI (may predict response to revascularisation).

Atherosclerosis
This is the most common cause of RAS (>95%) and the lesion occurs at or within 1 cm of the renal artery ostium (>90%) and is often bilateral. It is also often associated with aortic and mesenteric vessel plaque as well as systemic atherosclerosis (coronary and carotid).

Fibromuscular dysplasia (FMD)
This is a non-atherosclerotic, non-inflammatory disorder affecting medium-sized muscular arteries (e.g. mesenteric, carotid) usually in young patients (female preponderance). There are five different subtypes, typically affecting the middle and distal renal artery (or intrarenal branches). Radiological imaging is described as '*chain of lakes*' appearance because of multiple smooth, regular appearing lesions. Progression occurs in up to 1/3 of patients rarely to total occlusion (see also Chapter 64).

Management of RAS
Hypertension can be managed medically in most patients with revascularisation reserved for difficult cases (failure of medical management [at least 3 agents]), young patient, FMD (responds better than atherosclerosis) or if there has been an acute severe life-threatening complication (e.g. flash pulmonary oedema, CCF). Little evidence exists that revascularisation improves RAS-induced renal failure, but it is still used in difficult cases or young patients.

Medical management
- General management of atherosclerosis including BMT.
- Antihypertensive agents. Aim for *BP < 140/90 mmHg.* Lower BP targets (<130/80 mmHg) are preferable in diabetes or significant renal injury (proteinuria). ACEi or ARBs are still first-line agents!

Revascularisation
- Renal artery angioplasty and stenting.
- Surgical revascularisation (endarterectomy + patching, bypass).

Indications for revascularisation
- Recurrent flash pulmonary oedema.
- Hypertension resistant to medical management.
- High-grade bilateral RAS.
- ACE inhibition-related reduction in renal function.
- RAS in patients who require ACE inhibition or AII blockers for the treatment of other medical problems (e.g. CCF).
- Deteriorating renal function in bilateral disease (i.e. evidence of renal hypoperfusion contributing to the deteriorating renal function).

63 Congenital vascular malformations

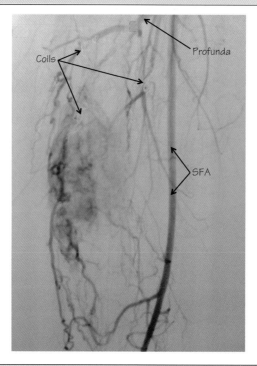

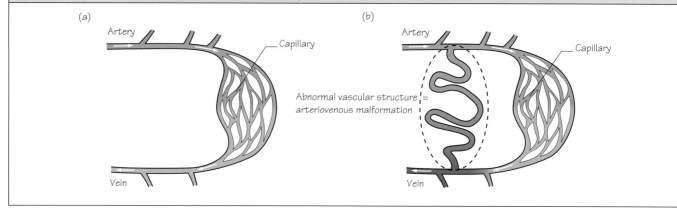

Vascular and Endovascular Surgery at a Glance, First Edition. Morgan McMonagle and Matthew Stephenson.

While congenital vascular malformations (CVM) are a considerable cause of morbidity in some patients, they have historically been poorly described and explained with considerable confusion among clinicians. Originally lesions were named according to the size of the lumen of the channels in the CVM, which gave rise to names such as: capillary haemangioma, strawberry haemangioma and cavernous haemangioma for blood-containing lesions, and lymphangiomas or cystic hygroma for lymphatic lesions. However, much has since been learnt about CVMs and, while these terms are still in common use, a more scientific approach is now considered more appropriate. The classification system currently in use is the Mulliken and Glowacki Classification, which divides all lesions simply into two types:

1 **Haemangiomas** (tumours).
2 **Congenital vascular malformations**.

Haemangiomas tend to appear after birth, often grow quite rapidly and then usually regress. In contrast, CVMs are present at birth and grow with the child as they grow. In order to prognosticate and guide treatment, it is important to distinguish between these two at an early stage, because they behave differently.

Haemangiomas

These are true, benign tumours of the endothelial cells. They often have a characteristic strawberry appearance when cutaneous. They can affect anywhere but particularly the head and neck. They may be warm and pulsatile. There are two main types: **infantile** and **congenital**. The much more common infantile one, as mentioned, appears after birth and regresses. The congenital ones are present at birth, like CVMs, but still usually regress. Rarely do they need any treatment because of this spontaneous regression over the first year of life.

Vascular malformations

In 1988, the Hamburg Classification was developed for CVMs. This divides them up using two criteria: (A) the predominant vascular defect, and (B) the embryological artery of origin. This latter point is important to grasp – they can be one of two types:

1 *Truncular:* Arise late in the embryological development from less primitive stem cell types. Much better prognosis.
2 *Extratruncular:* Arise during early embryological development and are therefore derived from earlier progenitor cells. These have a worse prognosis.

Therefore:

A: Anatomical type
• Predominantly arterial.
• Predominantly venous.
• Predominantly AV shunting.
• Predominantly lymphatic.
• Combined.

B: Embryological type
• Truncular.
• Extratruncular.

The other way of classifying CVMs is simply into slow flow or fast flow, based on Duplex characteristics. Overall the most common CVM is a venous malformation.

Investigations

Clinical examination is the mainstay of diagnosis supported by:
• *Duplex U/S:* Very good non-invasive modality that ascertains predominantly arterial or venous constitution by assessing slow or fast flow.
• *CT:* Excellent at establishing the anatomical configuration.
• *MRI:* Excellent at establishing the anatomical configuration without the radiation exposure.
• *Lymphoscintigraphy:* For predominantly lymphatic malformations.

Treatment

Often not necessary unless causing symptoms such as bleeding or high-output cardiac failure. The principal problem with any treatment is recurrence so usually treatment is conservative. Where necessary, in general, treatment is either:
• **Open surgery**: Aiming to ablate the CVM. Works better for truncular CVMs.
• **Endovascular therapy**: Using a range of treatments, these aim to ablate the vessels from within. Those in use include:
  • Coiling.
  • Glues.
  • Absolute ethanol.
  • Sclerosing agents such as polidocanol or sodium tetradecyl sulphate.

Combined CVMs

There are some eponymous CVMs that are of mixed type, are complex and tend to be managed conservatively because of poor outcomes with surgery and frequent recurrence. These are two classic examples:

Klippel-Trenauney syndrome

Classically identified clinically by the triad:
• Port wine stains.
• Varicose veins.
• Hypertrophy of affected limbs.

Pathologically there is involvement of mainly venous and lymphatic abnormalities. Treatment is generally conservative, however. Debulking surgery is occasionally tried with sclerotherapy for particularly troublesome varicosities or lymphatic cysts, along with limb compression and physical therapy.

Parkes-Weber syndrome

A fast-flowing CVM resulting in limb hypertrophy in the presence of a cutaneous capillary malformation.

Figure 64.1 Diagrammatic representation of the spectrum of disorders that may be classified as 'acute aortic syndrome' including penetrating aortic ulcer and intramural haematoma. Both these conditions may give rise to acute aortic dissection.

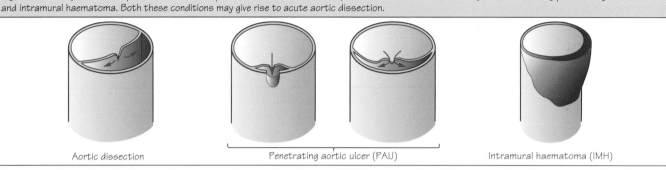

Aortic dissection   Penetrating aortic ulcer (PAU)   Intramural haematoma (IMH)

Figure 64.2 PA with cystic adventitial lesion in situ as seen during surgery (a) and after resection displaying the multiple cysts within the thickened adventitia (b).

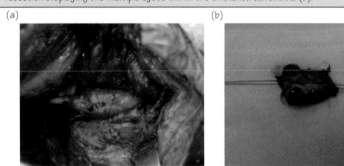

(a)   (b)

Figure 64.3 Normal anatomical relationship of popliteal fossa and its contents (right side).

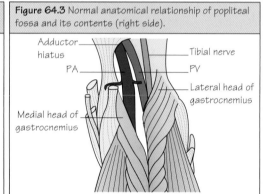

Adductor hiatus
PA
Medial head of gastrocnemius
Tibial nerve
PV
Lateral head of gastrocnemius

Figure 64.4 Popliteal entrapment types I–IV. Type I: PA passes medial to and under the medial head of gastrocnemius and PV remains in normal position. Type II: Medial head of gastrocnemius originates more lateral than normal and PA descend in a more straight-lined fashion around the medial border of the medial head. Type III: PA passes in a straight-lined fashion and through the body of the medial head of gastrocnemius. A slip of muscle originates more laterally which may compress the vessel. Type IV: PA passes deep to the popliteus muscle (or an associated band) in the absence of a gastrocnemius muscle abnormality. Type V is any of the types I–IV but both PA and PV are involved (10% of cases). Type VI is a 'functional' entrapment syndrome where the anatomical arrangements are normal. There may by hypertrophy of the otherwise normal gastrocnemius muscle.

Type I — Popliteal artery swings around medial head os gastrocnemius

Type II — Medial head of gastrocnemius originates from an abnormal position (more lateral) whilst popliteal artery descends relatively normally

Type III — Popliteal artery descends in a normal fashion, but then passes between an abnormally shaped medial head of gastrocnemius muscle (ie: separate slip of muscle passing laterally)

Type IV — Medial head of gastrocnemius (removed for illustrative purposes). Popliteal artery descends normally behind gastrocnemius muscle, but then goes deep to popliteus (or other band) causing compression. Lateral head of gastrocnemius (removed for illustrative purposes). Popliteus muscle

Figure 64.5 (a) HSK overlying aorta. (b) Renal artery is seen arising anterior from the aorta (arrow).

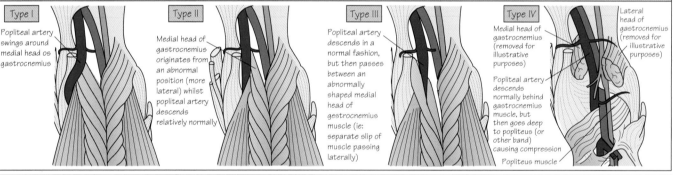

(a)   (b)

Abbreviations: A, aorta; HSK, horse shoe kidney; PA, popliteal artery; PV, popliteal vein

Acute aortic syndrome

Spectrum of degenerative aortic pathology (now thought to be a variant of acute aortic dissection pathology) leading to acute, painful conditions affecting the aorta (at any point). Patients often present with pain (back pain/interscapular pain). The syndrome includes *penetrating aortic ulcer* (PAU) and *intramural haematoma* (IMH), and may represent a prequel to acute aortic dissection (or aneurysm formation).

An IMH is a haematoma confined to the medial layer of the aorta (in the absence of communication between the haematoma in the false lumen and the true lumen or an identifiable aortic flap), whereas a PAU has breached the endothelium and internal elastic lamina to penetrate into the media with a risk of dissection or free rupture. An intramural haematoma may be due to spontaneous rupture of vasa vasora. A penetrating ulcer is restricted by the atherosclerotic process, thereby limiting the dissection of the vessel wall. They are both found more commonly in older patients with hypertension and typically affect the descending thoracic aorta. It is thought that an IMH is more likely to behave like a classic aortic dissection, whereas a PAU is more prone to aneurysmal degeneration (50%) and is less prone to dissection.

Fifty to eighty per cent of patients with asymptomatic IMH or PAU of the descending aorta (type B) will heal spontaneously and should be treated with medical therapy alone (as in aortic dissection) with CT scan surveillance, unless the aortic diameter exceeds 4 cm (best predictor of complications). Treatment may be with stenting (preferred) or open surgery. Ascending pathology should be treated surgically because of the higher risk of complications and true progression to either dissection of aneurysmal degeneration.

Arterial endofibrosis

Recurrent trauma or repetitive motion, typically in high-performing athletes (especially cyclists), affects the external iliac artery, giving rise to claudication on extreme exercise. Repetitive trauma leads to medial fibrosis and thickening of the tunica intima. May be treated conservatively by reducing exercise workload.

Buerger's disease (thromboangiitis obliterans)

Classically affects younger males and heavy smokers. Also prevalent among people of Middle Eastern and Asian origin. Numerous thrombotic occlusions of small and medium-sized arteries (i.e. BK). Vessels on angiogram are normal to a sudden point of occlusion with numerous, tortuous, cork-screw collaterals. Raynaud's phenomenon is also associated. Excellent prognosis with smoking cessation and exercise.

Carotid artery dissection

Usually spontaneous occurrence (although traumatic dissection is associated with head and neck trauma) that may be asymptomatic or symptomatic (unexplained neurological deficit such as stroke [>50%)], TIA, Horner's syndrome). There are three recognised subtypes: type I has vessel irregularity but no significant stenosis; type II has >70% stenosis or 50% dilatation; and type III has a characteristic 'flame-shaped' occlusion just above the bifurcation. Twenty-five per cent are bilateral. Treatment is with anticoagulation to reduce the risk of stroke, and most will heal within 3 and 6 months.

Carotid body tumour (CBT)

Typically benign tumour within the adventitial layer of the common carotid artery (typically at the bifurcation), derived from embryonic neural crest cells. They are often asymptomatic, but may present as a painless neck lump. Compressive symptoms may also occur (e.g. dysphagia, hoarseness, XII nerve palsy, Horner's syndrome). They are well encapsulated, thus allowing complete dissection from the carotid complex usually without the need for reconstruction. Five per cent are bilateral and 5% malignant (with either local or distant metastasis).

Cockett syndrome

See 'May-Thurner syndrome'.

Cystic adventitial disease

Cystic degeneration of the tunica adventitia of an artery, typically affecting the popliteal artery leading to stenosis, chronic ischaemia and/or acute thrombosis. Pathologically it consists of a true cyst (epithelial lined) within the adventitia, which may be in continuity with the synovium of the knee joint. On examination, pulses are present at rest, but disappear on knee flexion. Surgical resection with popliteal artery reconstruction is the management of choice. Angioplasty should be avoided because results are poor and associated with a high complication rate (acute thrombosis and distal embolisation of cystic material).

Ehlers-Danlos syndrome

Inherited connective tissue disorder (defect in type III collagen) of which there are 10 recognised subtypes (varying genotype and phenotype), but characterised by increased elasticity of the skin, joint hypermobility, thin skin and easy bruisability. Incidence is 1:150,000. Types I and IV are most likely to present to a vascular service in a young population. Type I (Gravis) may have varicose veins. Type IV (Sack-Barabas) may have aneurysmal degeneration (especially thoracic and abdominal aorta) or even spontaneous arterial rupture (and/or gravid uterine and intestinal rupture).

Fibromuscular dysplasia

Disease of unknown aetiology with fibrotic thickening and muscular hyperplasia affecting the tunic media of the vessel, more commonly affecting women. It usually affects the renal and carotid arteries but the external iliac artery may also be affected). Angiograms classically show a beaded appearance to the affected vessel ('chain of lakes').

There are five different histological subtypes (the most common is medial fibroplasia), but more usefully three radiological classifications: type I (80%) alternating segments of stenosis and dilatation of the vessel; type II (10–15%) unifocal or multifocal tubular stenosis (more intimal fibroplasia), which may be more prone to dissection and occlusion; and type III (5–10%) thinning of the vessel with saccular aneurysmal degeneration. Treatment of the stenosis is with angioplasty (±stenting), with surgery now reserved for failed angiointervention.

HIV-associated arterial disease

This is arterial disease (mostly large vessel disease) associated with chronic HIV infection. It is a spectrum of conditions including occlusive disease and aneurysmal degeneration (both true and false aneurysms). The condition is due to a large vessel vasculitis (leucocytoclastic vasculitis) and less commonly is associated with mycotic aneurysmal degeneration. Patients are generally young with multiple aneurysmal change both in usual and unusual sites (e.g. carotid). Graft infection rates have been recorded as high as 10–30% (which may be an overestimation with current anti-HIV treatments) with intravenous drug abuse associated with higher infection rates.

Horse-shoe shaped kidney

Congenital shaped kidney (affects 1:500 of the population) where both right and left kidneys are fused across the midline overlying the aorta. There is a wide variation in the amount of fusion, but typically there are numerous accessory renal arteries supplying each organ (and coming off the anterior aspect of the aorta instead of laterally) and/or duplicate draining ureters. Access to the aorta during dissection (e.g. AAA repair) is also hampered by the overlying structure with a high risk of bleeding and renal ischaemia from misidentified perfusing vessels. A retroperitoneal approach and Carrel patch may be necessary (akin to a type IV thoraco-abdominal aneurysm repair) where the entire organ along with the remaining abdominal organs are dissected from the left-hand side and mobilised medially to gain access to the aneurysm free of renal vessels. The isthmus may be divided if it contains little renal tissue and no substantial accessory artery.

Hypothenar hammer syndrome

Typically an occupational condition secondary to repetitive trauma where the dominant hand is used as a hammer (e.g. carpenters, mechanics). The position of the terminal ulnar artery at the hypothenar eminence leaves it vulnerable to chronic injury leading to aneurysmal degeneration or fibrosis, thrombosis and embolisation (often to digital arteries). Treatment is often supportive, although thrombolysis and vasodilatory agents may be used with acute ischaemia. Ulnar artery aneurysms should be resected to remove the source of embolisation.

Intramural haematoma

See 'Acute aortic syndrome'.

Klippel-Trenaunay syndrome (KTS)

Congenital condition consisting of a triad of venous malformations/varicose veins, capillary malformations (port-wine stains) and bone/soft tissue hypertrophy affecting the limb (>80% lower limb). The deep veins of the limb may be absent, hypoplastic or aneurysmal (typically affecting the SFV and popliteal veins) with or without venous hypertension. Caution is needed if embarking on surgery because of the high propensity for haemorrhage, and it is contraindicated in the absence of deep veins. There is also a higher propensity for thromboembolic disease.

Kommerall's diverticulum

This is an aneurysm of an aberrant right SCA. The aberrant origin of the right SCA typically arises directly from the descending aorta just distal to the origin of the left SCA and is prone to aneurysmal degeneration (i.e. the Kommerall's diverticulum) and acute thrombosis. It may also compress the oesophagus and/or trachea as it travels from the left chest to the right upper limb giving rise to dysphagia lusoria or stridor respectively.

LeRiche syndrome

Triad of intermittent claudication (typically affecting the buttocks), erectile dysfunction and absent femoral pulses secondary to aorto-iliac occlusion. Longstanding disease may also have lower limb muscle atrophy.

Marfan's syndrome

Genetic disorder in connective tissue (fibrillin-1) development leading to tall thin stature with long limbs and digits. Marfan's patients are prone to heart and aortic defects including aortic aneurysm formation (especially aortic root ± aortic regurgitation) and aortic dissection (types A and B).

May-Thurner syndrome

Venous outflow obstruction affecting the left lower limb due to compression of the left common iliac vein by the overlying right common iliac artery (often leading to venous thrombosis). It may be treated with venous thrombolysis and stent placement or with surgery (Palma-Dale procedure) where the LSV on the contralateral (normal) leg is dissected and tunnelled across the midline while leaving the proximal SFJ intact. The tunnelled LSV is anastomosed to the ipsilateral common femoral vein (CFV), thereby providing venous drainage for the affected limb.

Medial cystic disease

Disease of large vessels (e.g. aorta) with the development of cyst-like lesions within the tunica media with a higher incidence in certain connective tissue disorders.

Mid-aortic syndrome

Also known as 'abdominal coarctation'. Occurs primarily in children and young adults due to narrowing of the aorta (typically the visceral portion) with stenosis of the renal and visceral branches. Typically patients present with severe hypertension and lower limb hypoperfusion, and (uncommonly) renal failure may also occur. Treatment includes management of hypertension and surgical reconstruction of the diseased aortic segment. Renal artery stenting may aid in the management of the hypertension.

Moyamoya disease

Progressive occlusive disease affecting the intracerebral (supraclinoid) internal carotid artery and proximal middle and anterior cerebral arteries. The term means 'wavering puff of smoke', which describes the appearance on angiography in advanced disease. It tends to affect children and young adults presenting with cerebral ischaemia, stroke and intracerebral haemorrhages. There are six recognised stages in the disease development.

Nutcracker syndrome

See 'Renal vein entrapment syndrome'.

Pelvic congestion syndrome

Controversial syndrome consisting of pelvic and/or vulval varices leading to chronic pelvic pain and discomfort due to ovarian vein or internal iliac vein incompetence. Treatment includes endovenous coiling of the refluxing vessel, but the non-specific symptoms may persist even after successful ablation.

Penetrating aortic ulcer

See 'Acute aortic syndrome'.

Persistent sciatic artery

The sciatic artery is an embryonic vessel, a continuation of the internal iliac artery and the principal vascular supply to the developing lower limb. The popliteal and peroneal arteries are the normal remnants of this, which later join up with the femoral artery complex later in development.

A persistent sciatic artery is a congenital persistence of the embryonic sciatic artery (in part or total) and may be bilateral (22%) with proximal symptoms and ilio-femoral hypoplasia. The artery is prone to premature atherosclerosis, and aneurysmal degeneration with thrombosis and embolisation. Cowie's sign is characteristic (absent proximal pulses with present distal pulses).

Popliteal entrapment syndrome

Popliteal artery compression by the surrounding musculo-tendinous complex of the knee (abnormal anatomical arrangement) leading to claudication and paraesthesia during exercise. It is generally a condition of young, fit patients with symptoms associated with exercise. There are six variants of the condition described according to the anatomical relationship of the popliteal artery to the gastrocnemius muscle. The popliteal artery courses around or within an abnormal medial head of gastrocnemius (types I–III) or deep to popliteus muscle (type IV). Type V is any of the previous descriptions but with the popliteal vein also involved. Type VI is a 'functional' entrapment in the absence of an anatomical abnormality.

The compressed artery is prone to aneurysmal degeneration, fibrosis, occlusion, thrombosis and distal embolisation. Diagnosis is made by imaging with the patient at rest and then during plantar-flexion and dorsi-flexion in an attempt to induce arterial compression. Treatment is aimed at release of compression with reconstruction of the vessel if occlusion/aneurysmal degeneration has occurred. The condition is bilateral in two-thirds of patients.

Paget-Schroetter syndrome

Effort thrombosis (e.g. exercise) of the subclavian-axillary vein typically in association with external venous compression (thoracic outlet syndrome, often at the costo-clavicular space).

Radiation arterial disease

Radiation endarteritis may affect arteries of all sizes with the endothelial layer particularly susceptible to its effects leading to thickened intima ('heaped-up' endothelial cells), fibrosis, stenosis and eventually luminal occlusion ± distal embolisation. There is little propensity for collateral formation because of the effects of the radiation on surrounding tissues. These changes may occur from 6 months to 20 years post-radiation treatment.

Renal vein entrapment syndrome

Also known as 'Nutcracker syndrome', this is entrapment of the left renal vein between the abdominal aorta and superior mesenteric artery.

It may be asymptomatic or present with left flank pain, microscopic haematuria or with testicular pain and varicocoele (via distension of the left gonadal vein branch).

Replaced hepatic artery

The right or left hepatic arteries have an atypical or aberrant origin affecting 10–15% of the population and are more prone to injury during dissection if not recognised. Typically a replaced left hepatic artery will arise from the left gastric artery (as opposed to being a branch off the common hepatic artery off the coeliac axis) and travels in the gastrohepatic ligament. A replaced right hepatic artery typically arises from SMA (or occasionally coeliac axis). Although a normal common hepatic artery arises from the coeliac axis and branches into the left and right hepatic arteries, it may also be 'replaced', arising directly from the aorta or SMA (rare).

Subclavian steal syndrome

Exercise-induced reverse flow in the vertebral artery due to occlusion in an SCA (proximal to the origin of the VA). As the arm exercises, demand via the SCA cannot be adequately met, thereby 'stealing' blood from the ipsilateral vertebral artery. This may be asymptomatic and seen only on imaging (incidental finding), or it may be associated with posterior circulation symptoms (dizziness, syncope, nausea, vertigo).

Blood may also be 'stolen' from the ipsilateral internal thoracic artery, which, if this has been used for coronary artery bypass grafting, may lead to acute angina during arm use. Treatment is by stenting the SCA lesion (if possible) of bypass (e.g. carotid-SCA bypass, SCA transposition).

Superior mesenteric artery syndrome

Also known as 'Wilkies syndrome', this is compression of the third part of the duodenum between the aorta (posterior) and superior mesenteric artery (anterior), typically due to a short angle (<30°) and width (<10 mm) between SMA and aorta. Typical presentation includes severe epigastric pain, nausea and vomiting secondary to compression on the duodenum. Patients will develop electrolyte imbalance and weight loss. It may be due to a lack of retroperitoneal tissue.

Wilkies syndrome

See 'Superior mesenteric artery syndrome'.

Table 65.1 Approximate overall primary patency rates for angiointervention vs. bypass grafting for peripheral vascular disease from best published evidence.
* There is no demonstrable difference between in situ LSV and reversed LSV vein grafting (arm vein has demonstrably much poorer patency rates)
**Equivalence between Dacron and ePTFE grafting. Subintimal angioplasty not included (more useful for limb salvage). Best patency rates are for stenosis over total occlusion and for claudication over critical limb ischaemia.

	Aorto-iliac/femoral	Fem-AK pop	Fem-BK pop	Fem-distal	AX fem	Fem-fem, X-over
Angioplasty/stenting						
	70–95% 1yr 60–85% 3yr 55–80% 5yr	65–80% 1yr 50–70% 3yr 40–55% 5yr		55–60% 1yr 40–50% 3yr 30–40% 5yr	N/A	N/A
Bypass grafting						
*Vein	N/A	80–85% 1yr 70–75% 3yr 60–70% 5yr	80–85% 1yr 75–80% 3yr 65–70% 5yr	70–75% 1yr 60–65% 3yr 50–60% 5yr	N/A	N/A
**Synthetic	85–90% 5yr 70–85% 10yr	70–75% 1yr 50–60% 3yr 40–50% 5yr	60–70% 1yr 35–45% 3yr 30–40% 5yr	40–45% 1yr 25–30% 3yr 20–25% 5yr	50–70% 5yr	65–80% 5yr

Risk factors and best medical therapy

- The risk of PVD increases with age.
- Claudicants who smoke have 1.5–3 times the mortality of those who do not. Those who stop smoking will decrease this risk to that of non-smokers over 2–4 years.
- Nicotine replacement therapy doubles the success rate of smoking cessation at 1 year compared with placebo.
- Diabetes has a 2–4 fold increased risk of PVD with a 10–16 fold increase in the risk of limb amputation compared with non-diabetics.
- For every 1% increase in HbA1c levels, there is an almost 30% increased risk of the development of PVD.
- For every 10 mmHg decrease in systolic BP treatment, there is a 12% decreased risk in cardiovascular morbidity and 16% decrease in PVD-related morbidity.
- Even with a modest decrease in BP (10/5 decrease), there is a decrease in:
  - stroke mortality: 40%.
  - ischaemic heart disease (IHD): 16%.
  - all cardiovascular (CVS) mortality: 30%.
  - peripheral vascular events: 26%.
- A fasting cholesterol >7 mmol/L is associated with a doubling of the PVD risk.
- There is a reduction in CVS death or non-fatal MI by up to 50% in patients treated with statin therapy.

- Treatment with statin therapy has been shown to reduce fatal and non-fatal IHD and stroke events by 30–40%.
- The use of an antiplatelet agent reduces the risk of serious vascular events by almost 25%.
- β-blockade appears to reduce peri-operative MI in high-risk vascular patients undergoing major vascular surgery.

Abdominal aortic aneurysm

- Focal dilatation of an artery with a diameter increase ≥50% than its non-dilated segment (male ≥3 cm, female ≥2.5 cm).
- Affects 7–8% of men >65 years in the UK; 15–25% of males (6% females) with AAA display familial 'clustering'.
- Three to five times more common in the Caucasian population compared with Afro-Caribbean.
Indications for repair:
  - Symptomatic/rupture.
  - ≥5.5 cm (rupture risk > surgical mortality [5.8%]).
  - Aneurysm growth ≥0.5 cm in 6 months).
  - Saccular aneurysm.
- Five-year risk of rupture:
  - 5–5.9 cm: 25%.
  - 6–6.9 cm: 35%.
  - >7 cm: 75%.

- Seventy-five per cent are asymptomatic with 50% identifiable on physical examination alone.
- Eighty-five per cent are infrarenal.
- Seventy-five per cent of patients with ruptured AAA will die before reaching hospital.
- AAAs account for the sixteenth leading cause of death in the USA in males aged 65–85 years.
- Twenty-five per cent of AAA patients will have a concomitant iliac aneurysm.
- Five per cent of AAA patients will have an associated peripheral aneurysm and 2% will have a visceral aneurysm.

Repair of AAA
- Open surgery mortality: 5–6% (elective) versus 37–50% (emergency).
- Graft infection rate: 7% (without prophylactic antibiotics) and 1% (with prophylactic antibiotics).
- Long-term survival (post-repair):
  - 1 year: 85%.
  - 3 years: 70%.
  - 5 years: 60%.
- EVAR versus open repair mortality: 1.7% versus 4.7% respectively.
- Ten per cent of elective patients require cardiac revascularisation before AAA repair.
- Heparin reduces the peri-operative MI rate from 5.7% to 1.4%.

Peripheral aneurysms
- Eighty per cent are popliteal.
- Fifty per cent of popliteal aneurysms are bilateral.
- Popliteal aneurysms are prone to thrombosis/embolisation rather than rupture.
- Forty to fifty per cent of popliteal aneurysms will have an AAA.
- Consideration for repair of peripheral aneurysms:
  - 2–3 cm: popliteal.
  - 3–3.5 cm: femoral.
  - 4 cm: iliac.
- External iliac aneurysms are extremely rare.

Stroke
- Eighty per cent are thromboembolic (20% haemorrhagic).
- Fifty per cent originate from ICA/middle cerebral artery (MCA) origin.
- Twenty-five per cent small vessel disease (intrinsic cerebral vessels).
- Fifteen per cent cardiogenic.
- Mortality: 20–30%.
- Of the survivors, 33% fully recover, 33% recover with mild deficits, 33% recover with significant deficits.

Carotid artery disease
- Twelve per cent of patients >65 years have a carotid bruit on auscultation.
- Twenty-five to fifty per cent of 'symptomatic' carotid patients will have a bruit.
- Thirty per cent of symptomatic patients with carotid stenosis 70–90% will NOT have a bruit.
- Sixty per cent of symptomatic patients with carotid stenosis 90–99% will NOT have a bruit.

- Fifteen per cent of CVAs are secondary to carotid artery stenosis.
- ≥70% stenosis (≥60% USA) should be repaired (especially if symptomatic):
  - Symptomatic: NNT = 15.
  - Asymptomatic: NNT = 50.
- A symptomatic patient is one who has had symptoms within 6 months.
- Three to five per cent operative risk of CVA, 1% risk of cranial nerve injury.
- One to two per cent operative mortality.

Lower limb ulceration
- Eighty per cent have evidence of venous disease.
- Ten to twenty-five per cent have evidence of arterial insufficiency to a variable degree.
- Twelve per cent have co-existing diabetes.
- Chronic venous insufficiency affects 2–10% of the general population.
- Fifty per cent of ulcers have been present for >1 year.
- Seventy-five per cent of ulcers are recurrent.

Peripheral vascular disease
- Asymptomatic PVD is prevalent in 7–15% of men >55 years.
- Sixty-five per cent have significant femoral artery atherosclerosis of which only 10% are symptomatic.
- PVD is an independent predictor of both stroke and MI risk.
- Intermittent claudication affects 1–2% of the general population under 60 years.
- Thirty-three per cent of patients improve, 33% remain stable and 33% will deteriorate with BMT and exercise/life-style adjustment alone (typically over a 6-month period).
- Five per cent deteriorate significantly to warrant more urgent revascularisation.
- One to two per cent will require amputation.
- Patients with PVD have a 25% higher mortality than those without.
- Absolute coronary risk of 30% over 10 years.
- There is a 3–5% CVA risk per annum with PVD.

Critical limb ischaemia
Definition
- Ankle systolic pressure <50 mmHg (toe <30 mmHg). ABPI <0.4
- Rest pain >2 weeks' duration requiring regular analgesia.
- Tissue loss/gangrene.

Outcomes
- About 70% are suitable for revascularisation with a 75% limb salvage rate.
- Amputation rate 21% (40% <6 months).
- Mortality rate of 13–15% (50% at 5 years, 80% at 10 years).

Critical arterial stenosis
- Velocity >250 cm/s (2.5 M/s) across a stenosis.
- ≥3 velocity ratio across a stenosis.
- Marked spectral broadening across a stenosis.
- >75% cross-sectional area reduction.
- Resting systolic pressure gradient difference ≥15 mmHg.

Overview

Vascular surgery arguably has some of the strongest evidence base behind it of all the surgical disciplines, particularly in carotid endarterectomy (CEA) and AAA repair. This chapter summarises some of the most well-known trials in the 'big three' vascular operations that have changed practice along with their headline contributions, or, in some cases, consensus documents that have consolidated previous research. Of course, this is the tip of the iceberg!

Carotid
North American Symptomatic Carotid Endarterectomy Trial (NASCET)[1]
• Multicentre randomised controlled trial of CEA versus BMT in symptomatic patients (1991, NEJM).
• N = 1415.
• Demonstrated a highly beneficial effect of CEA in high-grade carotid stenosis (70–99%). Modest benefit for moderate-grade stenosis (50–69%)

European Carotid Surgery Trial (ECST)[2]
• Multicentre randomised controlled trial of CEA versus BMT in symptomatic patients (1991, Lancet).
• N = 3024.
• The same principal result: demonstrated a highly beneficial effect of CEA in high-grade carotid stenosis (70–99%); modest benefit for moderate-grade stenosis (50–69%).

Carotid Endarterectomy Trialists Collaboration[3]
The above 2 studies along with a similar study, the Veteran's Affairs trials, were amalgamated into one very large dataset of over 6000 patients. This has provided the best evidence for CEA, and the group have published several papers. Essential points:
 Numbers Needed to Treat to prevent a stroke at 5 years:
• Stenosis 70–99% = 6 patients.
• Stenosis 50–69% = 13 patients.
• Stenosis <50% or completely occluded = no benefit.
• Subgroup analysis shows maximum benefit in recently symptomatic patients (best within 2 weeks).
Interpretation of symptomatic CEA trials: patients with a 70–99% stenosis should undergo CEA within 2 weeks. Occluded carotids do not benefit from surgery. Stenoses 50–69% are contentious. Stenoses <50% have no benefit.

Asymptomatic Carotid Atherosclerosis Study (ACAS)[4]
• Multicentre randomised controlled trial of CEA versus BMT in asymptomatic patients (1995, JAMA).
• N = 1662.
• In patients with a 60–99% stenosis, very modest benefit of CEA.
• Numbers Needed to Treat to prevent a stroke at 5 years = 20 patients.

Asymptomatic Carotid Surgery Trial[5]
• Multicentre randomised controlled trial of CEA versus BMT in asymptomatic patients (2004, Lancet).
• N = 3120.
• Confirmed the findings of ACAS, similar figures.

Interpretation of asymptomatic CEA trials: surgeons differ in how they interpret these trials. Some never offer CEA for asymptomatic carotids, some always do, some offer selectively. Subgroup analysis of these trials has shown, for instance, that there is no benefit of CEA in asymptomatic women aged over 75.

Abdominal aortic aneurysms
UK Small Aneurysm Trial[6]
• Multicentre randomised controlled trial of elective AAA repair or U/S surveillance in AAAs 4.0–5.5 cm diameter (1998, Lancet).
• N = 1090.
• No difference in survival between the groups at 6 years; therefore supports 5.5 cm minimum threshold for elective surgical repair.

US Aneurysm Detection and Management (ADAM)[7]
• Multicentre randomised controlled trial of elective AAA repair or U/S surveillance in AAAs 4.0–5.4 cm diameter (2002, NEJM).
• N = 569.
• No difference in survival between the groups; therefore supports 5.5 cm minimum threshold for elective surgical repair.
Interpretation of small aneurysm trials: no benefit in operating on aneurysms smaller than 5.5 cm.

Multicentre Aneurysm Screening Study (MASS)[8]
• Multicentre population-based screening study of men aged 65–75 (2002, Lancet).
• N = 67,800.
• Forty-two per cent risk reduction in aneurysm-related death in the invited group.
Interpretation of screening trials (such as MASS): screening older men brings cost-effective health benefits.

Endovascular Aneurysm Repair Study–1 (EVAR-1)[9]
• Multicentre randomised controlled trial of open or endovascular repair of AAAs in patients suitable (and fit) for either (2004, Lancet).
• N = 1082.
• Lower 30-day mortality in the EVAR group (1.7%) compared with open group (4.7%). Higher rate of graft-related complications with EVAR.
Interpretation: EVAR is at least as safe as open repair in patients fit enough for either, may have lower mortality but has drawback of long-term surveillance of stent + reinterventions.

Endovascular Aneurysm Repair Study–2 (EVAR-2)[10]
• Multicentre randomised controlled trial of open or endovascular repair of AAAs in patients unfit for open repair, randomised to EVAR or BMT (2005, Lancet).
• N = 338.
• No difference in all-cause mortality between the groups.
Interpretation: patients unfit for open repair are likely to die of other causes anyway, mitigating against any benefit in repair. There are criticisms of this study, however, such as delay in treatment in those randomised to surgery resulting in rupture before the opportunity for repair. Many surgeons will still offer EVAR to patients unfit for open repair.

Peripheral vascular disease
Chronic
Trans-Atlantic Inter-Society Consensus Working Group (TASC-II)[11]

The TASC group have consolidated evidence and expert opinion on the best management of atherosclerotic lesions. They provide guidelines regarding whether open surgery or an endovascular approach is best suited to differing kinds of lesions in the various anatomical sites.

Bypass versus Angioplasty in Severe Ischaemia of the Leg (BASIL)[12]
• Multicentre randomised controlled trial of angioplasty versus infrainguinal bypass (2005, Lancet).
• N = 452.
• Surgery had a higher morbidity (mainly MI and wound problems); however, the results were more durable than angioplasty. No difference in overall mortality, quality of life or amputation rate.

Interpretation: surgery is better for fit patients if a suitable vein is available. Despite this, endovascular approaches to PVD are still often used as first line.

Acute
Surgery versus Thrombolysis for Ischaemia of the Lower Extremity (STILE)[13]
• Multicentre randomised controlled trial of intra-arterial thrombolysis versus surgery in acute leg ischaemia (1994, Ann Surg).
• N = 393.
• No difference in amputation-free survival between the two groups. Many criticisms about the methodology of the study.

Thrombolysis or Peripheral Arterial Surgery (TOPAS)[14]
• Multicentre randomised controlled trial of thrombolysis with urokinase versus open surgery in acute (<14 days) limb ischaemia (1998, NEJM).
• N = 246.
• Amputation-free survival was similar in both groups. The thrombolysis group had a higher frequency of haemorrhagic complications and reduced need for open surgical procedures.

Interpretation of thrombolysis versus surgery in acute leg ischaemia: equivocal. No strong evidence either way; therefore dealt with on case-by-case basis depending on departmental availability.

References
1 North American Symptomatic Carotid Endarterectomy Trial Collaborators (1991) Beneficial effect of carotid endarterectomy in symptomatic patients with high-grade carotid stenosis. *New England Journal of Medicine*, 325 (7), 445–453.

2 European Carotid Surgery Trialists' Collaborative Group (1991) MRC European Carotid Surgery Trial: interim results for symptomatic patients with severe (70–99%) or with mild (0–29%) carotid stenosis. *Lancet*, 337, 1235–1243.

3 Carotid Endarterectomy Trialists Collaboration (2003) Analysis of pooled data from the randomised controlled trials of endarterectomy for symptomatic carotid stenosis. *Lancet*, 361 (9352), 107–116.

4 Executive Committee for the Asymptomatic Carotid Atherosclerosis Study (1995) Endarterectomy for asymptomatic carotid artery stenosis. *Journal of the American Medical Association*, 273 (18), 1421–1428.

5 MRC Asymptomatic Carotid Surgery Trial (ACST) Collaborative Group (2004) Prevention of disabling and fatal strokes by successful carotid endarterectomy in patients without recent neurological symptoms: randomised controlled trial. *Lancet*, 363, 1491–1502.

6 UK Small Aneurysm Trial Participants (1998) Mortality results for randomised controlled trial of early elective surgery or ultrasonographic surveillance for small abdominal aortic aneurysms. *Lancet*, 352 (9141), 1649–1655.

7 Lederle, F.A., Wilson, S.E., Johnson, G.R., Reinke, D.B., Littooy, F.N., Acher, C.W. et al. (2002) Immediate repair compared with surveillance of small abdominal aortic aneurysms. *New England Journal of Medicine*, 346, 1437–1444.

8 Multicentre Aneurysm Screening Study Group (2002) The Multicentre Aneurysm Screening Study (MASS) into the effect of abdominal aortic aneurysm screening on mortality in men: a randomised controlled trial. *Lancet*, 360 (9345), 1531–1539.

9 EVAR Trial 1: Comparison of endovascular aneurysm repair with open repair in patients with abdominal aortic aneurysm; 30-day operative mortality results: randomised controlled trial (2004) *Lancet*, 364: 843–848.

10 EVAR Trial 2: Endovascular aneurysm repair and outcome in patients unfit for open repair of abdominal aortic aneurysm; randomised controlled trial (2005) *Lancet*, 365 (9478), 2187–2192.

11 Inter-Society Consensus for the Management of Peripheral Arterial Disease (TASC II). *Journal of Vascular Surgery*, 2007, 45: Suppl S:S5–67.

12 Bypass versus angioplasty in severe ischaemia of the leg (BASIL): multicentre, randomised controlled trial (2005) *Lancet*, 366 (9501), 1925–1934.

13 STILE Trial Investigators (1994) Results of a prospective randomized trial evaluating surgery versus thrombolysis for ischemia of the lower extremity. *Annals of Surgery*, 220 (3), 251–266.

14 Thrombolysis or Peripheral Arterial Surgery (TOPAS) (1998) A comparison of recombinant urokinase with vascular surgery as initial treatment for acute arterial occlusion of the legs. *New England Journal of Medicine*, 338 (16), 1105–1111.

Appendix 1: Wires commonly used during angiography and angiointervention

Wire	Length (cm)	Diameter (inches)	Function and comments
General and access wires			
Bentson (Cook Medical)	145, 180	0.035	20 cm flexible tip with 6 cm flexible tip. Straight wire made from stainless steel. Cheap and easy to use.
Newton (Cook Medical)	145, 180	0.035	10–15 cm flexible tip with J-shaped tip. Made from stainless steel. Cheap and easy to use.
Selective catheterisation wires			
Glidewire (Terumo)	150, 180, 260	0.018, 0.025, 0.035	Most versatile and widely used wire. Straight, angled or J-tipped ends. Very flexible, hydrophilic coating. Best for crossing all manner of lesions as well as selective catheterisation. Its excellent flexibility means it offers little stability once across a lesion so that it must be exchanged for a stiffer wire before intervention carried out.
Wholey (Coviden)	145, 175, 260, 300	0.018, 0.035	Floppy and malleable tip. Useful for selective catheterisation. Steel shaft makes it more rigid. Useful for antegrade femoral puncture. Better torqueability than Glidewire.
Exchange wires			
Rosen (Cook Medical)	145, 180, 260	0.035	Least stiff of the exchange wires, but good for most general use intervention. J-tipped. Excellent for navigation and exchange around tortuous vessels.
Amplatz Extra-stiff (Cook Medical)	145, 180, 260, 300	0.035, 0.038	Excellent general use wire. Stiffer than Rosen wire. Straight with 1 cm flexible tip. Excellent for exchange of stiff angiointervention devices.
Lunderquist (Cook Medical)	260, 300	0.035	Very stiff, made from stainless steel. Best for very stiff devices in large stiff, tortuous vessels (e.g. EVAR). Floppy tip to minimise vessel injury during navigation.

Note: Selection of wires commonly used during angiography and angiointervention. There are many other products on the market and the specifications and manufacturing companies are prone to change and re-invention. Other 'specialty' wires are not mentioned here.

Vascular and Endovascular Surgery at a Glance, First Edition. Morgan McMonagle and Matthew Stephenson.

Appendix 2: Catheters commonly used during angiography and angiointervention

Catheter	Length (cm)	Calibre (Fr)	Function and comments
Flush catheters			
Pigtail	65, 90, 100	4, 5	Curled tip when wire removed. Good general flush catheter. Multiple holes for high-volume, high-pressure contrast administration.
Omni-flush (angiodynamics)	65	4, 5	Tip shaped like a shepherd's hook. Good general flush catheter especially in aorta. Occasionally used for selective catheterisation (e.g. crossing aortic bifurcation). Multiple holes for high-volume, high-pressure contrast administration.
Exchange catheters			
Straight	70, 90, 100	4, 5	Designed for ease of inserting (exchanging) a stiffer wire. May also be used as a flush catheter.
Simple selective catheters (single [primary] curve)			
Teg-T	70, 100	4, 5	Short angled tip 30°.
Kumpe (KMP)	40, 65	4, 5	Short angled tip 45°.
DAV	100	4, 5	Short angled tip (shorter than KMP).
Vert	100	4, 5	Similar angle to DAV, but longer tip.
RIM	65	4, 5	More acute angled tip. Excellent for tight curves (e.g. tight aortic bifurcation).
MPA and MPB	65, 100	4, 5	Longer angled tip 45° (A) or 70° (B).
Berenstein	65, 100, 130	4, 5	Short angled tip similar to KMP.
Hook/Shepherd's hook	65	4, 5	Shaped like a hook for difficult curves and angles.
Complex selective catheters (Usually two curves [primary and secondary])			
Cobra	65, 80	4, 5	C2 most commonly used for difficult angled cannulation for any vessel or contralateral EVAR limb cannulation.
Vitek (VTK)	100, 125	5	Acute primary and secondary curves. Excellent for aortic branches and cerebral access.
Simmons	100	5	Complex dual curve. Excellent for aortic arch branches and visceral branch cannulation.

Note: Selection of catheters commonly used during angiography and angiointervention for travel, exchange and selective access to a lesion or vessel (or branch). There are many other products on the market and the specifications and manufacturing companies are prone to change and re-invention. Other 'specialty' catheters (e.g. complex cerebral intervention) are not mentioned here. RIM = right internal mammary. MPA/B = multipurpose A/B. Vert = vertebral.

Vascular and Endovascular Surgery at a Glance, First Edition. Morgan McMonagle and Matthew Stephenson.
© 2014 John Wiley & Sons, Ltd. Published 2014 by John Wiley & Sons, Ltd. Companion website: www.ataglanceseries.com/vascular

Index

Page numbers in *italics* denote figures, those in **bold** denote tables.

Vascular and Endovascular Surgery at a Glance, First Edition. Morgan McMonagle and Matthew Stephenson.

154 © 2014 John Wiley & Sons, Ltd. Published 2014 by John Wiley & Sons, Ltd. Companion website: www.ataglanceseries.com/vascular

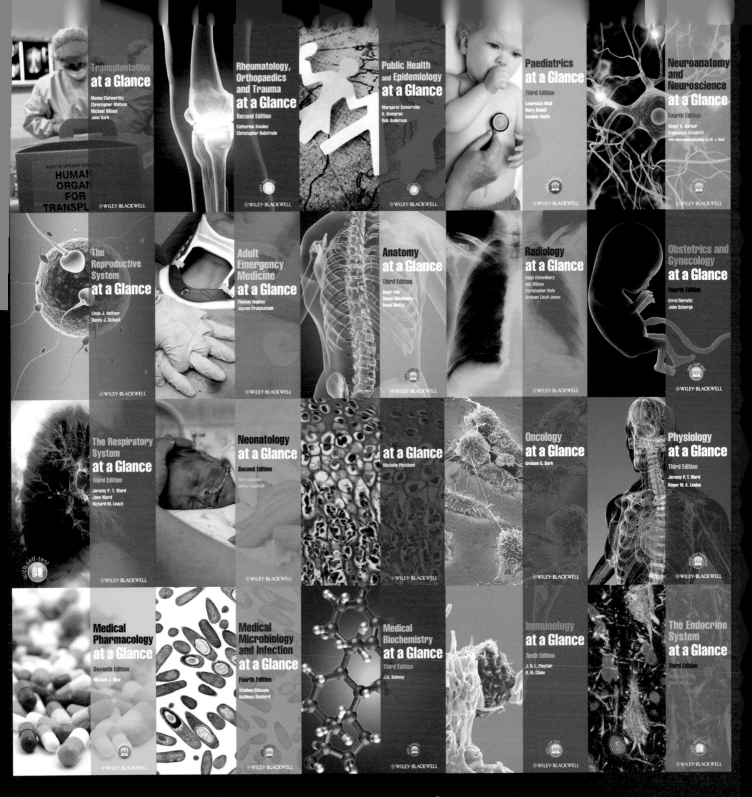

The at a Glance series

The market-leading *at a Glance* series is used world-wide by medical students, residents, junior doctors and health professionals for its concise and clear approach and superb illustrations. Each topic is presented in a double-page spread with clear, easy-to-follow diagrams, supported by succinct explanatory text. Covering the whole medical curriculum, these introductory texts are ideal for teaching, learning and exam preparation, and are useful throughout medical school and beyond.